D0710505

The Man Who Crucified Himself

Clio Medica

STUDIES IN THE HISTORY OF MEDICINE AND HEALTH

VOLUME 97

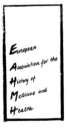

The titles published in this series are listed at *brill.com/clio*

The Man Who Crucified Himself

Readings of a Medical Case in
Nineteenth-Century Europe

By

Maria Böhmer

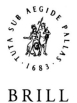

BRILL

RODOPI

LEIDEN · BOSTON

Cover illustration: This is one of the two copperplate engravings included in the first publication on Lovat's case (1806) by the physician Cesare Ruggieri. The figure appears in the book as illustration 1A.

Library of Congress Cataloging-in-Publication Data

Names: Böhmer, Maria, 1950- author.
Title: The man who crucified himself : readings of a medical case in
    nineteenth-century Europe / by Maria Bohmer.
Description: Leiden ; Boston : Brill/Rodopi, [2019] | Includes
    bibliographical references.
Identifiers: LCCN 2018047056 (print) | LCCN 2018048547 (ebook) | ISBN
    9789004353602 (E-book) | ISBN 9789004353596 (hardback : alk. paper)
Subjects: LCSH: Medicine--Europe--History--19th century--Case studies.
Classification: LCC R484 (ebook) | LCC R484 .B64 2019 (print) | DDC
    610.94--dc 3
LC record available at https://lccn.loc.gov/2018047056

Typeface for the Latin, Greek, and Cyrillic scripts: "Brill". See and download: brill.com/brill-typeface.

ISSN 0045-7183
ISBN 978-90-04-35359-6 (hardback)
ISBN 978-90-04-35360-2 (e-book)

Contents

Acknowledgements

I am indebted to many friends, colleagues and institutions for their support in carrying out the research for this study and in writing up this book.

I greatly appreciate the financial, logistic and scientific support provided by different institutions. The research upon which this book is based was funded by a three-year grant from the *Deutscher Akademischer Austauschdienst* (DAAD) for the doctoral programme of the Department of History and Civilization at the *European University Institute* (EUI) in Florence, Italy, and by a one-year completion grant from the EUI. Research missions to various places were supported by generous travel and accommodation funding from the EUI as well as by grants of the *Deutsches Studienzentrum in Venedig* and by the *Deutsches Historisches Institut Paris*. I wish to acknowledge the help of the administrative and scientific staff of these institutions who ensured the success of my research missions. My special thanks are extended to the staff of the various libraries and archives I used during my research, in particular Luigi Armiato and Fiora Gaspari from the archive of San Servolo in Venice.

I am particularly grateful to Antonella Romano, who as my mentor during the four years of the doctoral programme at the EUI has accompanied the development of my research project from the very beginning. My research on Lovat's case has also benefitted enormously from the advice given by the second readers of my thesis, Giulia Calvi and Lucy Riall, as well as by the external members of my dissertation committee, Flurin Condrau and Gianna Pomata. The latter has introduced me to the world of 'thinking in cases' – I owe her my greatest thanks. Over the years, many other persons at different places have kindly helped me with their advice on different questions, notably Klaus Bergdolt, Jacqueline Carroy, John Davis, David Gentilcore, Philip Rieder, Elena Vanzan Marchini, and Sebastiano Vassalli.

Turning the thesis into this book has been a long process, which has only been possible thanks to the time I was able to dedicate to it in the context of my postdoc position at the *Institute of Biomedical Ethics and History of Medicine* at the *University of Zurich*, Switzerland, from 2014 onwards. I greatly appreciate the support and encouragement given by Flurin Condrau during this process. James Kennaway has been a fantastic proofreader and Jermain Heidelberg has helped me with various technical details – many thanks for their precious work. Last but not least, I would like to thank the editors of the Clio Medica Series for including my book into this series.

Without the enduring encouragement and help of many friends, the writing up of this book would not have been possible. My warmest thanks go to

Katharina Böhmer, Laura Binz, Janina Kehr, Matthias Pohlig, Franziska Solte, Frédéric Vagneron, Martina Wernli and Anita Winkler. My very special thanks are owed to my family: to my mother and father, whose professional backgrounds have aroused my curiosity in both medical and religious topics, and to my husband Caspar Bresch for his never-ending encouragement and support. I dedicate this book to our two children: Helen, who arrived right after the defence of my thesis, and Simon, who joined us shortly before the publication of this book.

Illustrations

Introduction

Die Geschichte des Kasus und der Wanderungen und Wandlungen
einzelner Kasus [...] wäre eine schöne Aufgabe.
ANDRÉ JOLLES

In 1805 a shoemaker in Venice called Mattio Lovat (or Casale) attempted to
crucify himself in a public street. He constructed a wooden cross, inflicted a
wound on his own side, and put a crown of thorns on his head. In order to re-
enact the Passion of Jesus Christ, he then fixed himself to the cross with nails.
Using a net that tied his body to the wooden beam, he finally hung himself and
the cross out of the window of his room. With his left arm nailed to the cross,
and his right hanging down, Lovat was found alive in the early morning by
some passers-by who took him down from the cross and put him to bed. The
Venetian physician Cesare Ruggieri, who had come to the spot out of curiosity, made sure that Lovat was immediately admitted to the Clinical School of
Venice at which he himself was Professor of Surgery. For several weeks Ruggieri
treated and observed Lovat at his bedside until he had physically recovered.
Due to Ruggieri's diagnosis of a persistent mental disorder, Lovat was then
transferred to the hospital of San Servolo, an early mental asylum situated on
an island with the same name in the Venetian lagoon, where Lovat died in
April 1806 from some unspecified disease of the chest.

As far as Venetian institutions were concerned, the case was closed. Soon,
however, Ruggieri wrote down the medical case history of his patient:[1] He felt
entitled to do this in his capacity as Lovat's first physician. In his case narrative, entitled in Italian *Storia della crocifissione di Mattio Lovat da se stesso
eseguita*, Ruggieri put forward a tentative diagnosis to explain Lovat's physical
and mental condition. He suggested that Lovat had suffered from a particular
kind of mental disorder that was somehow connected with his religious convictions, and he also observed several physical symptoms in his patient that
he believed to result from a certain local disease called pellagra. To visualise
Lovat's self-crucifixion, Ruggieri commissioned a Venetian painter to produce

---

1 Throughout this book, I use the terms medical case history and medical case narrative alternatively, indicating the narrative account of the course of a disease in an individual patient.
All translations in this book from German, Italian and French into English are mine unless
otherwise indicated. All quotations from manuscript and printed sources are kept in their
original spelling and punctuation.

© KONINKLIJKE BRILL NV, LEIDEN, 2019 | DOI:10.1163/9789004353602_002

two illustrations of the incident, which he included in his publication, one showing Lovat hanging on the cross, the other displaying the instruments that Lovat had used for his crucifixion – the wooden cross, the nails and the crown of thorns (see illustrations 1A and 1B).

Ruggieri was eager to make Lovat's case known to a broader public. Between 1806 and 1814, he published his illustrated case history in two Italian versions and one in French, thereby providing slightly different editions of his text and opening up different paths for its dissemination.[2] Subsequently the narrative of Lovat's self-crucifixion was read, commented on, rewritten and reproduced by editors and authors in Italy, France, Germany and Britain throughout the nineteenth century. It circulated not only between medical writers and in between different scientific disciplines, but also entered popular debates about medicine, madness, suicide and religion. In the process of its Europe-wide dissemination, various authors and editors interpreted Ruggieri's original case narrative in different ways, charged it with different meanings and used it for different epistemic and literary purposes. This resulted in multiple transformations of both the narrative's form and content, which were realised in numerous reproductions of Lovat's case in diverse media.

This book tells the story of Lovat's case as a 'travelling case' in nineteenth-century Europe. It is not a biography of Mattio Lovat as a person, or of his physician Cesare Ruggieri, although both play an important part in the story. There would not be a case without Lovat and his public self-crucifixion, and we would know very little if anything about his case if Ruggieri had not written down and published his treatise. Yet while travelling through various times and locations of the nineteenth century, the case narrative about the man who crucified himself developed a life of its own – and it is this life that fascinates me. One could thus say that this book presents the history of a medical case that outlived both its author and protagonist.

---

2   C. Ruggieri, 'Storia della crocifissione di Matteo Lovat da se stesso eseguita. Comunicata in lettera da Cesare Ruggieri. Medico fisico, e di clinica chirurgica a Venezia. Ad un medico suo amico', in C. Amoretti (ed.), *Nuova scelta di opuscoli interessanti sulle scienze e sulle arti tratti dagli atti delle accademie, e dalle altre collezioni filosofiche e letterarie, dalle opere più recenti inglesi, tedesche, francesi, latine, e italiane, e da' manoscritti originali, e inediti*, vol. 1, no. 6, Milan, Presso Giacomo Agnelli successore Marelli Librajo-Stampatore in S. Margherita, 1804–1807, 403–412; C. Ruggieri, *Histoire du crucifiement éxécuté sur sa propre personne par Mathieu Lovat, communiqué au public dans une lettre de César Ruggieri docteur en medecine et professeur de chirurgie clynique à Venise. A un medecin son ami*, s.l., s.n., s.d.; C. Ruggieri, *Storia della crocifissione di Mattio Lovat da se stesso eseguita. Comunicata in lettera da Cesare Ruggieri medico fisico, e di clinica chirurgica in Venezia elettore nel collegio dei dotti, socio corrispondente delle accademie i.r. giuseppina medico-chirurgica di Vienna, reale di Madrid, della facoltà e società medica d'emulazione di Parigi ec.ec. Ad un medico suo amico*, Venice, Nella Stamperia Fracasso, 1814.

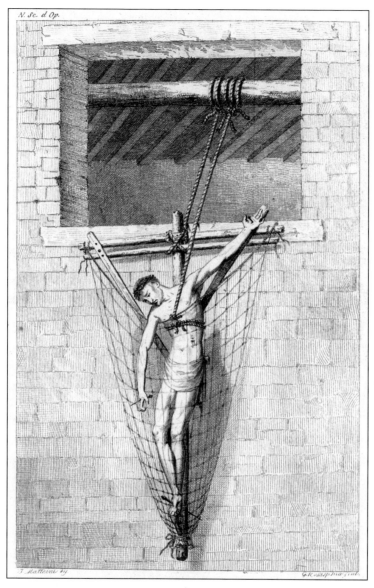

ILLUSTRATION 1A Ruggieri, *Storia della crocifissione di Matteo Lovat*, ed.
Amoretti, 1806, tav. XII.

1 A Popular Case

As a Venetian anecdote, the story of a remarkable and singular event, Lovat's
self-crucifixion is well known to this day, especially in Italy. I learned about
the case for the first time in 2009 while doing research in the archive of the

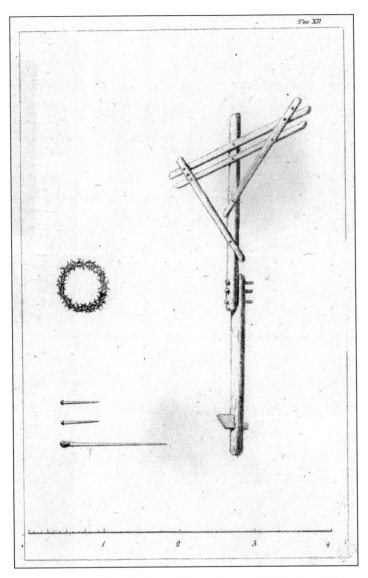

ILLUSTRATION 1B   Ruggieri, *Storia della crocifissione di Matteo Lovat,* ed.
                  Amoretti, 1806, tav. XII.

Venetian mental asylum of San Servolo, the very place where Lovat had
died in 1806. San Servolo was one of the first Italian asylums to be shut down
as a consequence of the Italian anti-psychiatric movement and the Italian
law of 1978, which demanded the closing-down of all mental asylums in

Italy.[3] After the closure of the hospital, a foundation was installed which grants access to the hospital's archive and, in 2006, also established a museum.[4] It was in this local museum that my attention was first drawn to Lovat's case. Visitors to the museum learn that Lovat was one of the first and the most famous patients in the early history of San Servolo as a mental asylum. His case is revealed to the public with a reproduction of the compelling picture illustrating Lovat's self-crucifixion taken from Ruggieri's case history.[5]

Lovat's case is thus not 'my' case in the sense that I discovered it in the archive and preserved it from oblivion. Thanks to Ruggieri's case history and its wide reception during the nineteenth century, the incident of Lovat's self-crucifixion has never been completely forgotten. In the 1980s the Venetian historian Mario Galzigna re-introduced the case into modern academic debates. In two books, his co-edited book on the history of the asylum San Servolo and his monograph on the origins of modern psychiatry, Galzigna edited and commented the few existing documents related with Lovat's case.[6] He also pointed to the remarkable international dissemination of Ruggieri's case history in the nineteenth century, by discussing how two French physicians adopted Lovat's case in their works.[7] Galzigna's interest in Lovat's case primarily lay in his depiction of the case as the object of an evolving psychiatric gaze, which was more pronounced in France than elsewhere in Europe. Although he mentioned the existence of Ruggieri's original treatise, the *Storia della crocifissione*, Galzigna did not examine and contextualise this publication in any great detail, because from his point of view, it contained no specifically psychiatric argument.[8]

---

3 This was the so-called Legge no. 180/1978. *Accertamenti e trattamenti sanitari volontari e obbligatori*. See for an online edition http://www.salute.gov.it/imgs/C_17_normativa_888_allegato .pdf, (accessed 15 March 2016). The most famous figure in this movement was the Italian psychiatrist Francesco Basaglia who published several pivotal books that criticised the conditions in Italian mental asylums.

4 Fondazione San Servolo I.R.S.E.S.C. (Istituto per le Ricerche e per gli Studi sull'Emarginazione Sociale e Culturale), [website], http://www.fondazionesanservolo.it/html/fondazione.asp, (accessed 15 March 2016).

5 The case is however not described in the exhibiton catalogue, see M. Galzigna (ed.), *Museo del manicomio di San Servolo. La follia reclusa*, Verona, Arsenale Editrice, 2007.

6 M. Galzigna and H. Terzian (eds.), *L'archivio della follia. Il manicomio di San Servolo e la nascita di una fondazione. Antologia di testi e documenti*, Venice, Marsilio, 1980, 75–83; M. Galzigna, *La malattia morale. Alle origini della psichiatria moderna*, Venice, Marsilio, 1988, 41–74.

7 Ibid., 53.

8 Ibid., 48.

Galzigna's contributions generated a wider academic interest in Lovat's case, and subsequently Ruggieri's original case history received renewed attention. Over the past three decades, various scholars and publishers have re-edited different versions of the *Storia della crocifissione*.[9] However, the particular way that Galzigna presented Lovat's case in his works on the history of psychiatry also implied that Lovat's case is primarily known as a noteworthy case from the early history of Italian psychiatry. This book shows that this is a partial view on Lovat's case. It is true that in the course of the nineteenth century, many of the new specialists on mental diseases came to be interested in Lovat's case, especially in France and Germany. They used it in their works for various purposes, but most importantly to develop the clinical picture of 'religious madness', a special kind of insanity that they believed was the result of exaggerated or erroneous religiosity. How and why Lovat's case was gradually transformed into a 'psychiatric case' is therefore an important part of the story I am going to tell. But this is only one part of a broader picture that develops if we follow Lovat's case through from its Venetian context of origin to the various new contexts in Europe where it became important. There were many more people interested in the case who attached various diagnoses and meanings to it, and some of them had little or nothing to do with the case's original context and the rise of the psychiatric profession.

In the wake of increasing academic attention to Lovat's case since the 1980s, the novel *Marco e Mattio* by the Italian writer Sebastiano Vassalli spurred public interest in the story.[10] In this half-historical, half-fictional book Vassalli narrates the story of Mattio's life, and that of his dubious companion Marco. By describing how Mattio's destiny was determined by the local political, economic and social upheavals in Northern Italy around 1800, Vassalli sets out a history of Lovat's life *before* his self-crucifixion in Venice in 1805, using the historical Lovat as a model for one of the protagonists of his story. While his main source regarding Mattio's biography is Ruggieri's case history, the broader historical context is that of the political and social disruption caused by the occupation of Venetian territory by Austrian and Napoleonic troops, the fall of the Venetian Republic in 1797, and the subsequent alternating French and

---

9   For an Italian reprint of the original text see C. Ruggieri, *Storia della crocifissione di Mattio Lovat da se stesso eseguita*, Crema, Amici del Museo, Arti grafiche, 1996. A German facsimile of the German translation from 1807 was published in 1984, see C. Ruggieri, *Selbstkreuzigung: Der Fall Matteo Lovat*, Munich, Belleville, 1984.

10   S. Vassalli, *Marco e Mattio*, Turin, Einaudi, 1992.

Austrian dominion in Venetia. By telling Mattio's story, Vassalli focuses on the effects these historical events had on the specific region where Mattio grew up, the Zoldo valley, and describes how the local population experienced these events primarily from a religious perspective, interpreting them as the arrival of the Antichrist and the end of the world. Vassalli characterises Mattio's valley as one where superstition and famine reigned, and speculates about how both circumstances severely affected people's lives, and in particular Mattio's character and health. Like many others, Mattio became afflicted by pellagra, a disease of famine that induced mental disorder. The apocalyptic belief of clerks also had an effect on him. The narrative further suggests that Lovat had homosexual tendencies, which he himself considered a sin for which he had to do penance by emasculating himself. On the whole, *Marco e Mattio* thus explains Mattio's self-crucifixion as the logical act of a man who, against the background of the upheavals of his time, desired to atone and to release mankind from its sinfulness.[11]

In his novel, Vassalli explicitly refers to Ruggieri's *Storia della crocifissione* as his source of inspiration and draws on additional historical documents related with Lovat's case and with local history. Yet he was not interested in the nature of Ruggieri's publication as a medical case history, nor in Ruggieri as its author. What happened with the case narrative of Lovat's self-crucifixion after its publication – the question of this book – is not the topic of *Marco e Mattio*. Vassalli, who died in the summer of 2015, was a famous Italian writer, and his novel is still widely read. As a result, Lovat is known to many readers of Italian literature as the man who crucified himself in Venice in the early nineteenth century.[12] Lately, Lara Pavanetto, a Venetian writer of historical novels and crime stories, has published another literary adaptation of Lovat's case.[13]

Hence, more than two hundred years after the first publication of the *Storia della crocifissione*, the case continues to fascinate people in both academic and

---

11 For a literary critique of this novel see the unpublished German dissertation by T. Hardtke, *Wahn-Glaube-Fiktion. Die Pathologie devianter Religiosität im medizinischen, religiösen und literarischen Diskurs seit 1800*, Freie Universität Berlin, 2016, 189–194 and P. Muri, 'E Mattio sclese di salire sulla croce', *La Repubblica*, 9 June 1992, http://ricerca.repubblica.it/ repubblica/archivio/repubblica/1992/06/09/mattio-scelse-di-salire-sulla-croce.html, (accessed 1 August 2017).

12 Lovat's case appears in popular books collecting Venetian tales such as G. Nosenghi, *Il grande libro dei misteri di Venezia risolti ed irrisolti*, Rome, Newton Compton Editori, 2010.

13 L. Pavanetto, *Crocifissione di Matteo Lovat*, Catania, Villagio Maori, 2017.

popular contexts. The starting point for this study was my curiosity about the remarkable longevity and impact of Lovat's case. In this regard, this book is the opposite of previous books on individual case histories from the nineteenth century, for instance Michel Foucault's famous study of the parricide case of Pierre Rivière, or, more recently, Jan Goldstein's fine edition of the medical case of the 'hysteric' Nanette Leroux.[14] While these studies both examine case records that have remained hidden in the archives as manuscripts until their discovery by modern scholarship, this book explores the history of a medical case narrative that has not only survived in printed and published versions but that became an object of public debate soon after the incidents it concerns.

The many-voiced response to Lovat's case is even more surprising if one considers that neither the author, Ruggieri, nor the patient, Lovat, were famous people in their lifetime. Ruggieri was a physician from Northern Italy who had come to Venice after having obtained a double degree in medicine and surgery. His academic career, which eventually led him to a professorship at the famous university in Padua, is representative for the time in so far as it mirrors the advancement of surgery as a science. But Ruggieri did not leave behind an oeuvre that made him famous; nineteenth-century physicians knew him only as the author of the *Storia della crocifissione*, if at all. As regards Mattio Lovat, his social background suggests that he was one of those obscure individuals who usually do not leave much of a trace in historical records, and therefore tend to be marginalised in historical scholarship. His life thus resembles those 'lives of infamous men' that Michel Foucault characterised as 'Lives of a few lines or a few pages, countless misfortunes and adventures, gathered together in a handful of words'.[15] As in the case of Foucault's obscure men, it is only thanks to Lovat's encounter with institutions that a few traces from his life have survived at all. Hence the fact that both Ruggieri and Lovat were

---

14   M. Foucault, *Moi, Pierre Rivière, ayant égorgé ma mère, ma soeur et mon frère...Un cas de parricide au XIXe siècle*, présenté par Michel Foucault, Paris, Gallimard, 1973; J. Goldstein, *Hysteria Complicated by Ecstasy: The Case of Nanette Leroux*, Princeton, Princeton University Press, 2011. See in particular Goldstein's sharp reflections of the problem of contextualisation when examining individual medical cases from a micro-historical perspective: Ibid., 18–20.

15   M. Foucault, *Power, Truth, Strategy*, Sydney, Feral Publications, 2006, 76. For another historiographical reflexion on how to deal with unknown individuals in nineteenth-century history, see A. Corbin, *Le monde retrouvée sur les traces d'un inconnu, 1798–1876*, Paris, Flammarion, 1998.

relatively unknown makes the case distinct from many other contemporary medical cases that became public not only thanks to their repeated publication by physicians, but probably also thanks to the social rank and celebrity of the patients involved.[16] Although Lovat's case was discussed intensively in nineteenth-century media, it is in many ways different from the phenomenon of 'celebrity patients' that emerged only during the twentieth century, as described by Barron H. Lerner.[17]

Lovat's self-crucifixion was an exceptional and solitary action that initially did not have much of an impact in the local context – only Ruggieri's publications and the different translations attracted the attention of a broader medical and non-medical European public. The great publicity and popularity of Lovat's case in nineteenth-century debates therefore raises a number of basic questions: How could a medical case narrative be so powerful and productive as to provoke discussions over such a long period of time? What was the particular allure of Lovat's case for the contemporaries of the nineteenth century? And how, in fact, did Lovat's case become a famous case?

2   A Travelling Case

These questions lead us into the broader academic debate on the case as a style of thinking and as a particular form of writing about individuals, a lively debate that has developed in the humanities and social sciences over the past three decades – which some have described as a 'renaissance of casuistry'.[18] The medical case has attracted particular attention in this debate. John Forrester's work on cases has been particularly influential. With his 1996 seminal article 'If p – Then What? Thinking in Cases', he opened up various ways of inquiry. He described the nature of the case as a form of reasoning that oscillates between the particular and the general, between practice and theory. Also,

---

16   See for instance the case of the Swiss natural scientist Horace-Bénédict de Saussure, described in L. Odier, *Les honoraires médicaux et autres mémoires d'éthique médicale*, Paris, Classiques Garnier, 2011, 123.

17   B.H. Lerner, *When Illness Goes Public. Celebrity Patients and How We Look at Medicine*, Baltimore, Johns Hopkins University Press, 2008.

18   C. Zelle, 'Einleitung', in C. Zelle and A. Zein (eds.) *Casus. Von Hoffmanns Erzählungen zu Freuds Novellen. Eine Anthologie der Fachprosagattung 'Fallerzählung'*, Hannover, Wehrhahn Verlag, 2015, 7–28, 7. On the contemporary rise of casuistry see C. Ginzburg, 'Ein Plädoyer für den Kasus', in J. Süßmann, S. Scholz, and G. Engel (eds.), *Fallstudien. Theorie – Geschichte – Methode*, Berlin, trafo, 2007, 28–48.

Forrester pointed to the fact that medical cases have an autonomous history, and that this history still needed to be explored.[19] Parallel to the contemporary reassessment of case reports in modern medicine itself,[20] medical case narratives have since then become an object of intense study in the fields of the history of science and philosophy and literary studies. This work has not only highlighted the important epistemic role medical cases have played – and still play – in medical culture, but it has also revealed their significance in the realm of literature.[21]

A frequently cited definition of the case as a particular narrative form comes from the literary historian André Jolles. In his 1930 book *Einfache Formen*, he described the case (*Kasus*) as a 'simple form'.[22] Jolles claimed that the case is different from an example because it does not simply illustrate a general concept or practical rule; rather, a case indicates conflicting norms and points to an unsolved problem. According to Jolles, it calls for the application of a legal or moral norm: 'At the root of the case [...] is the weighing and counterweighing of different norms in the attempt to apply them to a challenging set of

19   J. Forrester, 'If p – Then What? Thinking in Cases', *History of the Human Sciences*, vol. 9, no. 3, 1996, 1–25. See also his recent collection of articles related to the topic: J. Forrester, *Thinking in Cases*, Cambridge and Malden, Polity Press, 2017. In the following years, scholars from different disciplines have taken up Forrester's call, see J.-C. Passeron and J. Revel, 'Penser par cas. Raisonner à partir des singularités', in J.-C. Passeron and J. Revel (eds.), *Penser par cas*, Paris, EHESS, 2005, 9–44. For a recent overview of the developments in the field see the special issue 'Medical Case Histories as Genre: New Approaches', *Literature and Medicine*, vol. 32, no. 1, 2014. For the German-speaking context see for instance R. Hackler and K. Kinzel (eds.), *Paradigmatische Fälle. Konstruktion, Narration und Verallgemeinerung von Fall-Wissen in den Geistes- und Sozialwissenschaften*, Basel, Schwabe, 2016.

20   On the epistemic role of cases in modern medicine see R.A. Ankeny, 'The Case Study in Medicine', in M. Solomon, J.R. Simon, and H. Kincaid (eds.), *The Routledge Companion to Philosophy of Medicine*, New York and London, Routledge, 2017, 310–318; R.A. Ankeny, 'The Overlooked Role of Cases in Casual Attribution in Medicine', *Philosophy of Science*, vol. 81, no. 5, 2014, 999–1011. With a focus on narrativity see B. Hurwitz, 'Narrative Constructs in Modern Clinical Case Reporting', *Studies in History and Philosophy of Science*, vol. 62, 2017, 65–73.

21   See the literature cited in the following and in the different chapters. For a review of the debate see R. Leventhal, 'Der Fall des Falls: Neuere Forschung zur Geschichte und Poetik der Fallerzählung im 18. Jahrhundert', *Das Achtzehnte Jahrhundert*, vol. 41, no. 1, 2017, 93–102 and M. Wernli, 'Sammelrezension Fallgeschichten' H-Soz-Kult, 16 February 2017, www.hsozkult.de/publicationreview/id/rezbuecher-26171, (accessed 6 October 2017).

22   A. Jolles, *Einfache Formen: Legende, Sage, Mythe, Rätsel, Spruch, Kasus, Memorabile, Märchen, Witz*, Tübingen, Max Niemeyer Verlag, 1968 (first edition 1930), 171–199. It should be mentioned that the art and literary historian André Jolles (1874–1946) was a member of the German NSDAP since 1933, on Jolles see H. Rosenfeld, 'Jolles, André' in *Neue Deutsche Biographie*, vol. 10, 1974, 586 f., https://www.deutsche-biographie.de/pnd122521102.html#ndbcontent, (accessed 4 June 2018).

circumstances'.[23] A case narrative therefore typically raises a question that it-self does not give an answer to; once the answer is given, the case ceases to be a case.[24] The history of Lovat's case as explored in this book fits well with Jolles' description of the case. It is a narrative description of an incident which raises various questions, challenges moral norms and for this reason provokes a ma-ny-voiced discourse which, in the search for answers, attributes meaning to it.

Following the definition proposed by the historian Gianna Pomata, it is helpful to understand the medical case narrative not only as a literary but as an 'epistemic genre'. As the written report of a medical observation of an in-dividual patient, it is the immediate product of medical practice and pursues cognitive rather than aesthetic or expressive goals.[25] Pomata has demonstrated that for learned physicians in the early modern period, the writing of medical case histories was not only important to document the treatment of a single case, but it was also a means to share practical knowledge with colleagues. Physicians communicated their first-hand observations of individual cases to other physicians in letters, or published them in print as case collections, as so-called *observationes*.[26] For this reason, Pomata argues that the *observatio-nes* provided 'knowledge that can travel' and essentially meant 'sharing cases'. Within the broader Republic of Letters, the rise of the genre contributed to the construction of a *res publica medica*, and helped to constitute 'communities of learned experience'.[27] Ruggieri's *Storia della crocifissione* clearly tied in with this early modern tradition of the *observationes*. It was an empirical medical observation that was communicated in the conventional form of this genre to be shared with other physicians. By following the trajectories of Lovat's case, this book thus transfers the question of the shared cases into the nineteenth

---

23   Pomata on Jolles in G. Pomata, 'The Medical Case Narrative: Distant Reading of an Epis-temic Genre', *Literature and Medicine*, vol. 32, no. 1, 2014, 1–23, 1.

24   See Jolles, *Einfache Formen*, 190f.

25   See Pomata, *The Medical Case Narrative*. Gianna Pomata's important contributions spot-light the history of the case history as an epistemic genre in a longue durée perspective, evidencing the long tradition of medical cases in European culture and sciences since antiquity. Pomata is currently preparing a monograph on the early modern history of the case history from a cross-cultural perspective (Europe and China).

26   G. Pomata, 'Sharing Cases: The Observationes in Early Modern Medicine', *Early Science and Medicine*, vol. 15, no. 3, 2010, 193–236. On the form of the *observatio* see also V. Hess, 'Observatio und Casus: Status und Funktion der medizinischen Fallgeschichte', in S. Düwell and N. Pethes (eds.), *Fall – Fallgeschichte – Fallstudie. Theorie und Geschichte einer Wissensform*, Frankfurt, campus, 2014, 34–59 and M. Stolberg, 'Formen und Funktionen medizinischer Fallberichte in der Frühen Neuzeit (1500–1800)', in J. Süßmann, S. Scholz, and G. Engel (eds.), *Fallstudien. Theorie – Geschichte – Methode*, Berlin, trafo, 2007, 81–95.

27   Pomata, *Sharing Cases*, 199. On the travelling of cases in letters and 'communities of learned experience' see N.G. Siraisi, *Communities of Learned Experience. Epistolary Medi-cine in the Renaissance*, Baltimore, Johns Hopkins University Press, 2012.

century, the period which historians of medicine generally refer to as a turning point in medicine, brought about by medical professionalism, the rise of specialised hospitals, and new state health policies. In which ways were medical cases disseminated in this period, and how did they circulate across territorial and language borders, between different people, and within different media?

In dealing with these questions, the notion that medical cases have the ability to 'travel' is particularly revealing. Rachel Ankeny has argued that in modern medicine, medical cases circulate effectively between different actors because they contain scientific facts observed in individual patients, and therefore transmit new empirical knowledge. Case narratives play a crucial role in establishing novel diagnoses in that they help physicians to create 'generic facts by making particular facts travel together'.[28] She suggests that a medical case itself functions as a 'vehicle' of knowledge: it consists in a set of facts that travel together like in a coach of a train while their concrete relation is not yet established. Working on a specific case, physicians identify and determine how the facts are actually related to each other:

> By organizing (and re-organizing) the various facts, medical practitioners can propose a diagnostic category that establishes which facts are relevant and how they are interrelated. Those facts that are most essential will be upgraded to travel together in a first class cabin and given a place of prominence within the case as the main symptoms associated with the diagnostic category; other facts that are relevant but less central will stay in the carriage, that is, remain part of the diagnostic category captured by the case, but de-prioritised and hence relegated to second class. Some will join the existing cluster of facts as late arrivals, and some will be pushed off the train (out of the case) altogether.[29]

Ankeny's metaphor of the case as a train carrying different facts is helpful to understand why and how Lovat's case could take on different meanings along its journey in nineteenth-century Europe. Because Lovat's self-crucifixion in its original form of the *Storia della crocifissione* was presented as a medical case history, it is not surprising that many physicians felt a need to deal with it. They applied various medical terms and diagnoses to it in order to explain

---

28   R.A. Ankeny, 'Using Cases to Establish Novel Diagnoses: Creating Generic Facts by Making Particular Facts Travel Together', in P. Howlett and M.S. Morgan (eds.), *How Well Do Facts Travel? The Dissemination of Reliable Knowledge*, Cambridge, UK, Cambridge University Press, 2011, 252–273.

29   Ibid., 255.

what, in their view, Lovat had suffered from. In the *Storia della crocifissione*, the essential facts travelling together (i.e. those that were given importance) were on the one hand related to the diagnosis of pellagra, on the other hand to the diagnosis of a specific mental disorder. The specific relation between these facts, however, remained unclear in Ruggieri's account, and so did the relationship between Lovat's presumed mental disorder and his religious convictions. It turns out that it was exactly this vagueness in the first description of Lovat's case that allowed foreign editors and authors to continuously reorganise the facts in Lovat's case according to their interests. They picked up particular aspects of it, ignored others, or added additional facts that helped them to establish their own readings of the case. Therefore, what might at first sight appear as a weakness of Ruggieri's original case description ultimately turns out to be an epistemic strength that is vital for the case's career. As Ankeny puts it, the 'qualities of openness to the entrance of new facts, as well as the reorganisation and re-prioritisation of the existing facts, are precisely what gives cases epistemic strength'.[30]

Because none of the medical commentators had themselves observed Lovat, they all relied on different sources of information, that is, narratives about the case that they had found in different publications and which, in most cases, had already been transformed from Ruggieri's original account. This means that what many of them did is *retrospectively* diagnose Lovat by applying the knowledge, terms and diagnoses available to them in their respective cultural contexts and time. In studying the medical readings of Lovat's case, my intention is not to judge whether the disease categories that the contemporaries of the nineteenth century applied to Lovat's case are right or wrong according to our modern knowledge, but to historicise them and to explain how they tried to frame and capture the individual case.[31] In so doing, this book is also an attempt to shed light on the role of cases in the invention and transformation of disease categories in nineteenth-century medicine and psychiatry.

The potential of medical case narratives to travel also means that their dissemination often remains not necessarily restricted to the medical context – they also enter popular debates and genres.[32] In this regard, the nineteenth century is a particularly interesting period to study as it saw not only the

---

30   Ibid., 267.

31   On the problem of retrospective diagnosis in the history of medicine see A. Cunningham, 'Identifying Disease in the Past: Cutting the Gordian Knot', *Asclepio*, vol. 54, 2002, 13–34.

32   André Jolles has mentioned the kinship between the case and the literary genre of the *novella*, see Jolles, *Einfache Formen*, 182. For narrative similarities between the novella and the case history in medicine see also S. Goldmann, 'Kasus-Krankengeschichte-Novelle', in S. Dickson, S. Goldman and C. Wingertszahn (eds.), *'Fakta, und kein moralisches*

expansion of medical journalism, but also that of national bookmarkets as well as the emergence of a wider literate reading public.[33] In fact, literary scholars have observed that in this period, many medical cases migrated into literature and delivered documentary material for the literary works of writers.[34] The main reason for this seems to be that medical cases not only transmit medical knowledge, but also tell stories about individuals and their physical and mental conditions. This focus on the individual corresponds well with various literary genres that flourished in the eighteenth and nineteenth centuries which explored the psychological development of characters. To be sure, Lovat's case did not become a famous piece of literature and did not enter the literary canon: at least in the nineteenth century, no famous writer made a novel or novella out of it. But the literary adaptations of Lovat's case examined in this book take place in the context of nineteenth-century popular journalism where case narratives were not used to produce scientific knowledge, but primarily served to morally instruct and entertain a broader literate readership. While it travelled between various actors and publications, not only medical diagnoses but also popular notions concerning madness, suicide and religion got on and off the train of Lovat's case.

Drawing on sources that were produced in scientific contexts as well as on sources that were produced in literary and journalistic contexts, this book raises the question of how to understand the relation between epistemic genres, as conceptualized by Pomata,[35] and literary genres. In the past two decades, scholars of literature, in particular of German literature, have intensively debated the question of how to define the 'literary case narrative' (*literarische Fallgeschichte*), as they call literary presentations of cases, in terms of genre. Extending their focus to smaller forms of literature beyond the classical canon and genres, their special interest in case narratives arises from the observation that many literary texts rely on authentic documents from different professional fields, particularly

Geschwätz'. Zu den Fallgeschichten im 'Magazin für die Erfahrungsseelenkunde' (1783–1793), Göttingen, Wallstein, 2011, 33–64.

33   See for instance the contributions in W.F. Bynum, S. Lock, and R. Porter (eds.), *Medical Journals and Medical Knowledge. Historical Essays*, London and New York, Routledge, 1992. For further literature on this topic see Chapter 3.

34   See for instance A. Košenina, 'Fallgeschichten. Von der Dokumentation zur Fiktion', *Zeitschrift für Germanistik. Neue Folge*, vol. 19, no. 2, 2009, 283–287. For further literature see below.

35   Pomata, *The Medical Case Narrative* and Idem, 'The Recipe and the Case: Epistemic Genres and the Dynamics of Cognitive Practices', in K. von Greyerz, S. Flurbacher, and P. Senn (eds.), *Wissenschaftsgeschichte und Geschichte des Wissens im Dialog – Connecting Science and Knowledge*, Göttingen, V&R unipress, 2013, 131–154.

on individual cases registered in law or medicine.[36] Well-known examples from German literature are Karl Philipp Moritz's novel *Anton Reiser* (1785–90) and Georg Büchner's novella *Lenz* (1836), to name only the most famous ones.[37] Recent work demonstrates that the exchange between medical cases and literature was particularly fertile during the late eighteenth and early nineteenth centuries, and that the influence was reciprocal.[38]

This focus on the role of authentic cases in literature and their narrative structures contributes to the broader debate on how literary production and the production of scientific knowledge are interrelated more generally,[39] and in particular in the case of medical case narratives.[40] Scholar of literature Nicolas

---

36   Košenina, *Fallgeschichten*.

37   For further examples from German literature see N. Pethes, *Literarische Fallgeschichten. Zur Poetik einer epistemischen Schreibweise,* Konstanz, Konstanz University Press, 2016. On Büchner's *Lenz* see recently Y. Wübben, *Büchners 'Lenz'. Geschichte eines Falls*, Konstanz, Konstanz University Press, 2016.

38   Scholarship on the topic is abundant, in particular German publications. The most recent contributions include S. Retzlaff, *Observieren und Aufschreiben: Zur Poetologie medizinischer Fallgeschichten (1700–1765)*, Munich, Wilhelm Fink, 2018; M. Krause, *Infame Menschen: Zur Epistemologie literarischer Fallgeschichten 1774–1816*, Berlin, Kadmos Kulturverlag, 2017; S. Vasset, *Medicine and Narration in the Eighteenth Century*, Oxford, Oxford University Press, 2013. For further contributions see the most recent collective and interdisciplinary volumes: Behrens, Bischoff, and Zelle (eds.), *Der ärztliche Fallbericht*; Y. Wübben and C. Zelle (eds.), *Krankheit schreiben. Aufzeichnungsverfahren in Medizin und Literatur*, Göttingen, Wallstein, 2013.; S. Düwell and N. Pethes (eds.), *Fall – Fallgeschichte – Fallstudie. Theorie und Geschichte einer Wissensform*, Frankfurt, campus, 2014; L. Aschauer, H. Grunder, and T. Gutmann (eds.), *Fallgeschichten. Text- und Wissensformen exemplarischer Narrative in der Kultur der Moderne*, Würzburg, Königshausen&Neumann, 2015; Hackler and Kinzel, *Paradigmatische Fälle*. On the exchange between psychiatry and literature see Y. Wübben, *Verrückte Sprache: Psychiater und Dichter in der Anstalt des 19. Jahrhunderts*, Konstanz, Konstanz University Press, 2012 and M. Wernli, *Schreiben am Rand: Die 'Bernische Kantonale Irrenanstalt Waldau' und ihre Narrative (1895–1936)*, Bielefeld, transcript, 2014.

39   On the narrative conditions of knowledge see J. Vogl, 'Einleitung', in J. Vogl (ed.), *Poetologien des Wissens um 1800*, Munich, Wilhelm Fink, 1999, 7–16. The literature is abundant, see for instance A. Höcker, J. Moser, and P. Weber (eds.), *Wissen. Erzählen. Narrative der Humanwissenschaften*, Bielefeld, transcript, 2006. On the interrelations between medicine and literature in France see M. Föcking, *Pathologia litteralis. Erzählte Wissenschaft und wissenschaftliches Erzählen im französischen 19. Jahrhundert*, Tübingen, Gunter Narr, 2002, 170–209; A. Carlino and A. Wenger (eds.), *Littérature et médecine. Approches et perspectives (XVIe –XVIe siècle)*, Geneva, Droz, 2007; S. Vasset and A. Wenger (eds.), *Raconter la maladie. Dix-huitième siècle n°47*, Paris, La Découverte, 2015; A. Wenger, 'From Medical Case to Narrative Fiction: Diderot's *La Religieuse*', *SVEC*, vol. 4, 2013, 17–30.

40   S. Willer, 'Fallgeschichte', in B. von Jagow and F. Steger (eds.), *Literatur und Medizin. Ein Lexikon*, Göttingen, Vandenhoeck & Ruprecht, 2005, 231–235; C. Frey, 'Fallgeschichte', in R. Borgards et al. (eds.), *Literatur und Wissen. Ein interdisziplinäres Handbuch*, Stuttgart and

Pethes, for instance, has suggested a functional perspective on case narratives that downplays the boundaries between scientific and literary writing, arguing that various scientific disciplines and literature shared an 'epistemic mode of writing' that built its own 'poetics'.[41] He demonstrates that the form of the case narrative had the potential to communicate between the professional fields of law, medicine and literature and to thereby popularise scientific knowledge.[42] It helped authors to contribute to knowledge-in-the-making in various emerging professional debates.[43] For Pethes, case narratives therefore do not constitute a genre per se with distinct formal characteristics. Rather, their great heterogeneity reflects a certain 'writing against genre' that allowed for an exchange between different disciplines, and especially between the fields of literature and medicine.[44]

Considering how Lovat's case criss-crossed various professional and popular debates and thereby permanently changed its narrative form, Lovat's case seems to confirm Pethes' observations and one could therefore argue that the question of genre is somewhat obsolete. Literary conventions and narrative structures are fundamental to both literature and science, and any rigid distinction between epistemic and literary genres is therefore artificial. However, for my study of Lovat's case, the analytical distinction between epistemic and literary genres has proven to be very useful: it allows us to distinguish the

---

Weimar, Metzler, 2013, 282–287; C. Zelle, "'Die Geschichte bestehet in einer Erzählung". Poetik der medizinischen Fallerzählung bei Andreas Elias Büchner (1701–1769)', in R. Behrens, N. Bischoff, and C. Zelle (eds.), *Der ärztliche Fallbericht. Epistemische Grundlagen und textuelle Strukturen dargestellter Beobachtung*, Wiesbaden, Harrassowitz, 2012, 301–316.

41 Pethes, *Literarische Fallgeschichten*, 15. To denote the interdependencies between medical and literary narratives, he has also coined the term 'Medizinische Schreibweisen' (medical modes of writing) in an earlier co-edited volume, see N. Pethes and S. Richter (eds.), *Medizinische Schreibweisen. Ausdifferenzierung und Transfer zwischen Medizin und Literatur (1600–1900)*, Tübingen, Max Niemeyer Verlag, 2008.

42 N. Pethes, 'Vom Einzelfall zur Menschheit. Die Fallgeschichte als Medium der Wissenspopularisierung in Recht, Medizin und Literatur', in G. Blaseio, H. Pompe, and J. Ruchatz (eds.), *Popularisierung und Popularität*, Cologne, Dumont, 2005, 63–92, 76. See also S. Düwell, 'Populäre Falldarstellungen in Zeitschriften der Spätaufklärung: Der spektakuläre Fall des "Menschenfressers" Goldschmidt', in S. Düwell and N. Pethes (eds.), *Fall – Fallgeschichte – Fallstudie. Theorie und Geschichte einer Wissensform*, Frankfurt, campus, 2014, 293–314.

43 S. Düwell and N. Pethes, 'Noch nicht Wissen. Die Fallsammlung als Prototheorie in Zeitschriften der Spätaufklärung', in M. Bies and M. Gamper (eds.), *Literatur und Nicht-Wissen. Historische Konstellationen 1730–1930*, Zurich, Diaphanes, 2012, 131–148.

44 N. Pethes, 'Telling Cases: Writing against Genre in Medicine and Literature', *Literature and Medicine*, vol. 32, no. 1, 2014, 24–45. For other reasons, medical historian Volker Hess has also criticised the notion of the medical case as a genre, see Hess, *Observatio und Casus*.

individual framings, appropriations and transformations to which Lovat's case was subjected, and to identify where and why the case lost its epistemic functions to assume a more literary guise. Following Pomata, I use the distinction between epistemic and literary genres not as clear-cut categories but rather as a heuristic tool that allows me to identify their particularities and to investigate the fluent boundaries between them.[45] Indeed, as Pomata argues, depending on the context in which they appear, certain forms of texts can have both a history as an epistemic genre and another history as a literary genre.[46] As Lovat's case shows, some medical cases require to acknowledge both histories, as they travel within and between different publication formats and, due to their narrative form, frequently oscillate between cognitive and aesthetic goals.

Much of the existing scholarly work on the history of medical case narratives has concentrated on the eighteenth and nineteenth centuries, suggesting a direct link between the rise of empirical psychology, psychiatry and psychoanalysis, and the predominance of the case genre.[47] In contrast to this modernist focus, Gianna Pomata's recent works propose a 'distant reading' of the genre of the medical case history over the centuries.[48] Against this background, my book proposes another approach: no work has so far zoomed in on the travelling of individual medical cases between scientific and popular cultures and across different national contexts in nineteenth-century Europe.[49] As Jolles suggested long ago, 'the history of the case (*Kasus*) and of the journey and transformations of individual cases [...] would be a nice challenge'.[50] Because of its Europe-wide reception, Lovat's case is particularly revealing for such an endeavour. By offering a thick description of the *Storia della crocifissione* as a travelling case narrative, this book thus proposes that we can learn a lot about

---

45 Pomata, *The Medical Case Narrative*, 3.

46 Ibid.

47 This focus has, at least in part, been inspired by Michel Foucault's works on 'the birth of the clinic' and other institutions of power, which allegedly turned individuals into administrated, normalised cases, see M. Foucault, *The Birth of the Clinic: An Archaeology of Medical Perception*, London, Routledge, 1997. For Foucault's description of the case as the product of techniques of writing see M. Foucault, *Discipline and Punish: The Birth of the Prison*, London, Allen Lane, 1979, 185–191.

48 Pomata, *The Medical Case Narrative*. For a critique of Foucault's partial view see also Forrester, *Thinking in Cases*, 12–16.

49 A brilliant study of a famous individual criminal case that became a media event in early twentieth-century Germany is M. Hagner, *Der Hauslehrer – Die Geschichte eines Kriminalfalls. Erziehung, Sexualität und Medien um 1900*, Frankfurt, Suhrkamp, 2010. For a history of an individual literary case narrative see Wübben, *Büchners 'Lenz'*.

50 Jolles, *Einfache Formen*, 194: 'Die Geschichte des Kasus und der Wanderungen und Wandlungen einzelner Kasus, auf die ich hier verzichte, wäre eine schöne Aufgabe'.

the medical case and its epistemic and literary significance in nineteenth-century Europe if we take a close look at the trajectories of one particular case. What exactly made Ruggieri's case narrative (including the pictures) travel? Who were the readers and authors who triggered the interest in Lovat's case? And what happened to the case's format while travelling?

3   Interpretive Communities

To answer these questions, this book analyses the different readings and re-writings of Lovat's case by a large number of nineteenth-century authors and editors, from Italy, Germany, France and Britain. While some of these authors are well-known figures in the history of nineteenth-century medicine and psychiatry, such as the French alienist Étienne Esquirol or the German psychiatrist Emil Kraepelin, many others are less prominent or even unknown. According to their professional interests and needs, authors and editors engaged with different aspects of Lovat's case, and in so doing, shaped and perpetuated distinct readings of the case in specific scientific and popular contexts. As a result, the narrative of Lovat's self-crucifixion had undergone significant transformations in its form and content by the end of the nineteenth century. Originally a medical case history that was communicated by an Italian Professor of Surgery in the epistemic genre of the *observationes*, Lovat's case had assumed two principal guises. While in the literary field it circulated as a popular anecdote about an eccentric character, it was handed on in scientific publications as a paradigm case for the psychiatric disease classification of 'religious madness'. The travelling of Lovat's case was provoked by 'interpretive communities', that is, multiple readerships that built communities of interest around the case and produced different interpretations of the narrative's content.[51] The interpretive communities appropriated Lovat's case in different ways and thereby defined which elements and meanings of Lovat's case became important, and which narrative form it assumed. My book is concerned with these various appropriations of Lovat's case.

---

51   R. Chartier, 'Texts, Printings, Readings', in L. Hunt (ed.), *The New Cultural History*, Berkeley, University of California Press, 1989, 154–175, 158. The term 'interpretive community' was first used by S. Fish, *Is There a Text in This Class? The Authority of Interpretive Communities*, Cambridge, MA, Harvard University Press, 1982, 167–173. W.F. Bynum and M. Neve have proposed a similar focus on changing interpretations of a literary character, see W.F. Bynum and M. Neve, 'Hamlet on the Couch: Hamlet Is a Kind of Touchstone by Which to Measure Changing Opinion – Psychiatric and Otherwise – about Madness', *American Scientist*, vol. 74, no. 4, 1986, 390–396.

Examining in this way the history of a case narrative and its transformations implies taking for granted that material scientific objects – in our case a particular text – are relevant to the history of science and can be seen as having proper 'biographies', as Lorraine Daston and others have suggested.[52] In *How Well Do Facts Travel?* Peter Howlett and Mary S. Morgan have taken up the idea that objects can have proper lives and have suggested that facts, understood as 'pieces of knowledge', can have lives of their own, and that the 'life stories of certain facts' can be investigated by following the ways in which they travel.[53] Although my book has been inspired by these approaches, it shows that the history of a medical case cannot be fruitfully described as a biography with a clear beginning and ending – rather, it requires tracing its various journeys in different contexts.

Following the trajectories of Lovat's case, national contexts matter. Most obviously, they determine the language in which the narrative is translated and conveyed, but they also provide the broader cultural and political framework for the readings of Lovat's case in the different languages. However, this book is not structured according to the four national contexts of Germany, Italy, France and Great Britain and does not offer a symmetrical story of its reception in the four countries. Using national contexts as an analytical category seems problematic when considering the political situation of the German and the Italian States as well as that of Great Britain and France in the nineteenth century. It suggests that we speak of stable nation states in our modern sense whilst the rise of these nations with distinct national cultures was only a product of the nineteenth century and of nineteenth-century nationalism.[54] The comparative approach of this book thus comes closer to that of a *histoire croisée* which seeks to transcend the nation as a preconceived unit of analysis by offering multiple perspectives, than to classic ideas of historical comparison.[55] I include the comparative perspective within the broader themes characterizing the reception of Lovat's case – religion, madness and suicide – by paying attention to national specificities and differences. By focusing on interpretive communities, my analysis of the readings of Lovat's case seeks to pay tribute

---

52   L. Daston (ed.), *Biographies of Scientific Objects*, Chicago, University of Chicago Press, 1999. On 'biographies' of scientific artefacts in the museum see S.J.M.M. Alberti , 'Objects and the Museum', *Isis*, vol. 96, no. 4, 2005, 559–571.

53   Howlett and Morgan, *How Well Do Facts Travel?*, xv and 5.

54   D. Langewiesche, 'Nation', 'Nationalismus', 'Nationalstaat' in der europäischen Geschichte seit dem Mittelalter – Versuch einer Bilanz, http://www.db-thueringen.de/servlets/DerivateServlet/Derivate-1344/langewiesche.pdf, 68 (accessed 4 June 2018).

55   M. Werner and B. Zimmermann, 'Penser l'histoire croisée: entre empirie et réflexivité', *Annales*, vol. 58, 2003, 7–36 and Idem, 'Beyond Comparison. Histoire Croisée and the Challenge of Reflexivity', *History and Theory*, vol. 45, 2006, 30–50.

to the fact that the contexts of its reception are neither confined to territorial nor language boundaries but that the trajectories of the case are transnational. Focusing on the multiple readerships of Lovat's case allows me to highlight the transnational contacts and exchanges that enabled it to permanently cross territorial, cultural and linguistic boundaries. In fact, my study of Italian, German, French and English sources reveals that the various readings of Lovat's case that we find in the media of the different countries are not self-contained but are interdependent and communicate with each other.

Lovat's case travelled in several senses. It travelled within and between scientific disciplines, within different publication formats and between different readerships, across geographical and territorial space, and across time. These different journeys did not take place independently from each other; rather, they happened simultaneously. However, for the sake of presentation and readability, my book deals with the implications of these different ways of travelling by focusing on different aspects in seven chapters:

The first chapter, *The Man Who Crucified Himself*, introduces Lovat's case in greater detail. It discusses several basic questions that immediately come up when talking about it and that concern the historical circumstances of Lovat's case: Who was Mattio Lovat? Why did he try to crucify himself? Was he ill, and what did he suffer from? How did he manage to put himself on the cross? And was his self-crucifixion a unique case in nineteenth-century Europe? Although these questions do not directly concern the case's travels, they reveal its blank spaces and open questions, and these gaps are important for understanding why it piqued the interest of readers throughout the nineteenth century. By discussing the questions raised above, the chapter explores Lovat's case as a discursive event within the local urban context of Venice. Drawing on both information taken from Ruggieri's case history and from additional sources gathered in the Venetian archives, it describes the incidents surrounding Lovat's attempted self-crucifixion, and shows how the local authorities negotiated the case.

The second chapter *The* Storia della crocifissione *as an Epistemic Genre* takes a close look at Ruggieri's original case history and explores its nature as an epistemic genre, one that is rooted in the medical practice of observing individual cases. For this purpose, I focus on the author of the *Storia della crocifissione*, Cesare Ruggieri, and his individual interest in publishing Lovat's case. Why did a Professor of Surgery consider it important to communicate such an extraordinary case to an international audience? On which documentary basis did he produce his narrative? And why did he publish three versions of his case narrative? I examine the Venetian Clinical School of Surgery, where Ruggieri observed Lovat at his bedside, as well as the Venetian medical society of which Ruggieri was a member, as important social places that shaped his conception of case histories. The chapter thus situates Ruggieri's publishing strategy within the broader context of medical case writing at the beginning of the nineteenth century.

The third chapter *Making the Case Travel: Translation, Media, Reading* describes the various translations of the case narrative, arguing that they have to be seen in relation to a rapidly changing media landscape. Both the existence of vernacular translations and an ever-growing market for publication formats which favoured short narrative forms were fundamental preconditions that allowed Lovat's case to reach different readerships and attract the interest of various interpretive communities. The chapter serves as introduction to the Chapters 4 to 7, in which I distinguish and describe the different professional and popular readings of Lovat's case alongside the three major topics religion, madness and suicide.

The Chapters 4, 5 and 6 focus on three main themes that scholars from different disciplines associated with Lovat's case in their professional readings of it: religion, madness and suicide. In nineteenth-century Europe, these themes were scrutinised in various scientific debates. By 'professional readings' I mean those readings and appropriations of Lovat's case which were conditioned by the scientific (not only medical) interests of authors and editors, and that served specific cognitive and epistemic goals within specialist debates. I examine a broad spectrum of epistemic genres ranging from journals, monographs, encyclopaedias and textbooks where Lovat's case appeared. Through the lens of Lovat's case, I describe the role and function of case histories in the debates on religion, madness and suicide, and explain why the narrative of Lovat's self-crucifixion became a kind of touchstone for authors and editors.

In contrast, the last chapter *Popular Readings: Moral Education through Literary Entertainment* traces how authors and editors appropriated Lovat's case in the context of journalism and popular publication formats. The case narrative was included in a great variety of popular publications, such as magazines, newspapers and anthologies of criminal cases and popular anecdotes. 'Popular readings' of Lovat's case were characterised by a more general and market-orientated interest of editors in Lovat's case as an entertaining story, and in Lovat as an 'eccentric' character. Through this framing, the narrative itself lost its epistemic functions, and served primarily literary aims. Focusing in this way on the gradual transformation of a medical case history into a popular anecdote, the chapter not only explores the close relationship between medical and literary narratives, but also highlights the permeable boundaries between 'scientific' and 'popular' cultures of knowledge in nineteenth-century Europe.

Researching Lovat's case means oscillating between two impressions – that it is everywhere and at the same time nowhere. As a historiographical case, it is of continuing interest to scholars, and as a compelling anecdote it circulates beyond academia. It is a popular case, because it travels between different readerships to this day, adapting to the changing media formats of each time period. And yet, after twohundred years of discussion, it remains a case that raises many unsolved questions and is therefore a challenge for the historian. As we will see, the local archival evidence for the case itself is scarce, and Ruggieri's *Storia della crocifissione* triggers as many questions as it answers. Given this ambivalence, this book comes not with the promise of filling the gaps of Lovat's case and disclosing the mysteries surrounding Lovat himself. Instead, it seeks to explain why nineteenth-century contemporaries were puzzled by the case, and shows how *they* tried to fill its blank spaces in order to make it fit with their interests. In this way, of course, this book itself contributes to the ongoing re-reading and re-writing of Lovat's case – a case that continues to travel even in the twenty-first century.

CHAPTER 1

The Man Who Crucified Himself

1   Registering the Case

In Venice, the news about Lovat's public self-crucifixion began to spread immediately after the incident on the morning of 19 July 1805. Ruggieri writes in his published case narrative that 'in the moment when I heard the news, I was in the same neighbourhood to do my duty as a physician, and I wanted to go to the spot to see it with my own eyes, because I could not believe what people had told me'.[1] We don't know to what extent the news spread in Venice by word of mouth, and what the ordinary people thought and said about Lovat's self-crucifixion. But we know that on the very day of that incident, various Venetian institutions began to register and to deal with it in administrative terms.

The records of the Venetian police (*Direzione generale di polizia*) kept in the Venetian State Archive reveal that there was an extensive exchange of letters concerning the event.[2] The original letters are not preserved, but some records of the police have survived that briefly summarise their content. These excerpts from the letters (*Protocolli degli esibiti*) confirm that several Venetian institutions were involved in Lovat's case and commented on his self-crucifixion in the weeks after the incident. Besides the police, the Venetian tribunal of justice (*Regio tribunale criminale*), the physician Cesare Ruggieri as well as the administrative body of the Venetian hospitals (*Imperial regio capitanato provinciale di Venezia*) had noted the incident.[3]

---

1   Ruggieri, *Storia della crocifissione*, 10f.: 'Trovatomi in quel momento per oggetti di mia professione in quelle vicinanze, ed intesa tal cosa volli andar a vedere, perchè non sapeva persuadermi di quanto veniva raccontato'.

2   The Direzione Generale Polizia was established after the Austrian takeover of Venice in 1798. It formed part of the General Government and consisted in six commissioners for the different districts, who cooperated with the chief responsible of the area, see M. Gottardi, *L'Austria a Venezia. Società ed istituzioni nella prima dominazione austriaca, 1798–1806*, Milan, F. Angeli, 1993, 163–213. On the following French occupation of Venice, see A. Zorzi, *Napoleone a Venezia*, Milan, Mondadori, 2010.

3   ASV, Direzione Generale Polizia, protocolli degli esibiti, b. 18 (=anno 1805; 7.V–5.VIII, Protocollo 2761–5207). The *Protocolli degli esibiti dell'imperial regia direzione generale di polizia* list the incoming and outgoing letters in chronological order and with reference to the numbers of the registers. In order to consult the protocols, one has to use the so-called *registri*, which are classified per year, each listing the names of the cases treated by the police in alphabetical order: ASV, Direzione Generale di Polizia, indice del protocollo 1805, reg. 15 (=dal 19

On the day of the incident, a police officer in Venice delivered a report concerning 'a certain Mattio Casal who had been found in the neighbourhood of S. Alvise, on a cross in the same place where he lived in No. 2888'.[4] Similarly, the commissioner of the Venetian quarter Canal Regio (today *Cannaregio*) reported from his office on the 'surprising suicide attempted by a certain Matteo Casal from Soldo'.[5] One week after, on 25 July, the Venetian tribunal of justice announced that it 'has found out that Mattio Casal's self-crucifixion was purely an effect of mania, and that no other person was involved in the operation. However, it believes it necessary to attach the authentic denunciations as well as its protocol, so that in the event of his recovery, the police might adjust his provision and the appropriate accommodation'.[6] The following day the Venetian police registered an incoming letter from Ruggieri, which confirmed that Mattio Lovat, after he had been taken down from the cross, had been brought to the Clinical School, situated in the Venetian hospital *SS. Giovanni e Paolo*, and that it was Ruggieri himself who treated him at this hospital, in his function as Professor of Surgery: 'The venerable Professor Doctor Cesare Ruggieri describes in detail the condition and the quality of the wounds of Mattio Casal from Belluno, who stays in the venerable Clinical School of SS. Giovanni e Paolo. In the state of a melancholic delirium, he intended to crucify himself in the night of the 18th'.[7]

---

gennaio al 31 Agosto). As far as the files of the police, the so-called *atti*, are concerned, only a few are conserved for the year 1805, and they do not contain any documents regarding the self-crucifixion of Mattio Lovat: ASV, Direzione Generale di Polizia, atti, bb. 54–58 (= anno 1805).

4   ASV, Direzione Generale Polizia, protocolli degli esibiti, b. 18, numero dell'esibito 4681, 19 luglio 1805: 'Il Reverendo Comando della Guardia Militare di Polizia accompagna una referenza del Capitano [illegible; probably Katich, M.B.], relativa al rinvenimento questa mane [mattina, M.B.] di certo Mattio Casal, ritrovato nei contorni di S. Alvise trovato in una croce nella stessa casa di suo alloggio al No. 2888'.

5   ASV, Direzione Generale Polizia, protocolli degli esibiti, b. 18, numero dell'esibito 4684, 19 luglio 1805: 'Il Reverendo Comando di Polizia di Canal Regio subbordina il proprio Rapporto col sopraluoco praticato in questa mattina dal suo officio in punto di sorprendente suicidio da se tentato di certo Matteo Casal di Soldo'.

6   ASV, Direzione Generale Polizia, protocolli degli esibiti, b. 18, numero dell'esibito 4890, 25 luglio 1805: 'L'Imperiale Regio Tribunale Criminale Riscontrato che l'essersi crocefisso Mattio Casarzi [sic!] sia stato puro effetto di mania, nè siavi entrata menoma operazione di altre persone; trova perciò di dover sotto accompagnare le autentiche denunzie, e suo protocollo, acciò nel caso di suo ricupero voglia la Reverenda Direzione Generale addattarvi le providenze di sua carità, e proprie di suo instituto'.

7   ASV, Direzione Generale Polizia, protocolli degli esibiti, b. 18, numero dell'esibito 4900, 26 luglio 1805: 'Il Reverendo Professore Cesare Dottor Ruggieri (M) descrive in dettaglio lo stato particolare, e qualità, delle Ferite in Mattio Casal di Belluno, esistente nella Reverenda Scuola Clinica nello ospitale de' Santissimi Giovanni e Paolo, che dietro nello melanconico delirio,

By mid August, the police received another letter from Ruggieri. He informed the police that the five wounds that remained in Lovat's body from his self-crucifixion were by then 'perfectly healed'. Ruggieri remarked, however, that his patient still suffered from 'signs of a melancholic delirium'. Therefore, he did not want to discharge him from the hospital without receiving a relevant order from the police.[8] The cited correspondence reveals that two concerns determined the first documentation of Lovat's case in Venice: the police's concern to secure public order, and the tribunal of justice's duty to investigate a possible crime. However, as soon as it had become clear to the authorities that no other person had helped Lovat in carrying out his crucifixion, the tribunal regarded the incident as a straightforward medical matter. Subsequently, the correspondence on Lovat's case became more influenced by a medical perspective on the incident.

Reading the excerpts of the letters carefully, it indeed appears that the medical reports by Ruggieri had the strongest influence on the way that the Venetian authorities understood and dealt with Lovat's case. In the first letter the police referred to the incident simply as an extraordinary attempt at suicide ('surprising suicide').[9] Adopting Ruggieri's medical terms ('melancholic delirium'), the tribunal later declared that the incident was an 'effect of mania', and that this was a question of a mental disorder. The declaration of insanity was very important, because in the eyes of the tribunal, insanity meant an excuse for criminal actions – and according to the traditional understanding, suicide was a crime. Ruggieri's medical diagnosis therefore implied that the Venetian authorities would not consider Lovat as a criminal to be punished, but agreed

---

pensò di crocefiggersi da se stesso, la notte 18. [illegible; probably Const., M.B.]' In the files of the General Government, there is an entry of the same day stating that the Capitanato reported on the incident, see ASV, Prima Dominazione Austriaca, Governo generale, protocollo degli esibiti del governo, No. 74 (=anno 1805, dal 1. al 31. lulio), numero dell'esibito 5630626: 'Il Capitanato di Venezia comunica lo strano [sic!] emergenze per parte di Matteo Casal da Zoldo che pensò da crocifigersi da se stesso'. In his published case history, Ruggieri also refers to this letter written by him to the Venetian tribunal, see Ruggieri, *Storia della crocifissione*, 11: '[...] e di tal tenore furono le denunzie da me rassegnate su tal proposito ai competenti Tribunali'.

8   ASV, Direzione Generale Polizia, protocolli degli esibiti, b. 19 (=anno 1805; 5.VIII–31.XII, protocollo 5208–8659), numero dell'esibito 5450, 13 agosto 1805: 'Il Reverendo Professore Ruggieri Rassegnando trovarsi perfettamente guarito dalle cinque ferite Mattio Casal fattesi per la Crocifissione, rimarca, che sussistendo ancor in questo dei segni di melanconico delirio, non crede lasciarlo sortire dall'Ospitale se non dietro ordine espresso della Direzione Generale'.

9   ASV, Direzione Generale Polizia, protocolli degli esibiti, b. 18 (=anno 1805; 7.V–5.VIII, protocollo 2761–5207), numero dell'esibito 4684, 19 luglio 1805: 'Il Reverendo Comando di Polizia di Canal Regio subordina il proprio Rapporto col sopraluoco praticato in questa mattina dal suo officio in punto di sorprendente suicidio da se tentato di certo Matteo Casal di Soldo'.

that he fell under the responsibility of physicians.[10] This view of the Venetian authorities corresponds to a more general historical change in the societal attitude toward suicide in Western European societies. Christian theology had moralised and criminalised suicide as 'self-murder' for centuries. In the course of the eighteenth century, this traditional view had given way to a more secular understanding, which went hand-in-hand with a gradual medicalisation of suicide as an act of insanity. By the nineteenth century, suicide had become an object of study, a human act that could be explored and measured by all sciences concerned with human nature.[11] Like the Venetian tribunal, the police took Ruggieri's diagnosis of a mental disorder in Lovat for granted, and acted accordingly. After having received Ruggieri's second report from 13 August, which stated that Lovat's physical wounds had healed but that he still exhibited 'signs of a melancholic delirium', the police decided on the same day that the patient should be transferred to the hospital of San Servolo, situated on the island of the same name in the Venetian lagoon.

San Servolo had originally been a military hospital that since the early eighteenth century had been run by an Italian nursing order, the friars of Saint John, *fatebenefratelli* in Italian. After the fall of the Venetian Republic in 1797, the interim democratic government (*Municipalità provvisoria*) and the following first period of Austrian rule in Venice (1798–1806) instituted new health policies, which also affected the organisation of San Servolo. During the first decades of the nineteenth century, the hospital was transformed into an early mental asylum for male and female patients. Officially serving as *manicomio centrale dei due sessi* from 1804 onwards, the asylum ended the previous forms of custody of the poor insane in provisional institutions, general hospitals or prisons in Venice, and was one of the first specialised hospitals for the insane in the Italian States. In the medically informed view of the Venetian authorities,

---

10   Insanity could be considered an excuse for murder already in Early Renaissance Venice, see G. Ruggiero, 'Excusable Murder: Insanity and Reason in Early Renaissance Venice', *Journal of Social History*, vol. 16, no. 1, 1982, 109–119 and N. Vanzan Marchini, 'Diritto e follia a Venezia nel XVI secolo', *Sanità, scienza e storia*, vol. 1, 1984, 49–76. On the juridical problem of mental capacity or diminished responsibility in the eighteenth century see M. Lorenz, '"Er ließe doch nicht eher nach biß er was angefangen". Zu den Anfängen gerichtspsychiatrischer Gutachtung im 18. Jahrhundert', in R. van Dülmen, E. Chvojka, and V. Jung (eds.), *Neue Blicke. Historische Anthropologie in der Praxis*, Cologne, Böhlau, 1997, 200–222 and J. Martschukat, 'Von Seelenkrankheiten und Gewaltverbrechen im frühen 19. Jahrhundert', in R. van Dülmen, E. Chvojka, and V. Jung (eds.), *Neue Blicke. Historische Anthropologie in der Praxis*, Cologne, Böhlau, 1997, 223–247.
11   On this development see G. Minois, *History of Suicide: Voluntary Death in Western Culture*, trans. L.G. Cochrane, Baltimore, Johns Hopkins University Press, 2001. For further literature on the topic see below and Chapter 6.

San Servolo was the right institution to hospitalise Lovat because he seemed to be a madman, a so-called *pazzo* – the Italian umbrella term for mentally disturbed persons whose behaviour was considered either a threat to their own body or to social order.[12]

Lovat has left behind a few traces in the archive of San Servolo.[13] Among the documents concerning his admission, we do find the mentioned request by the police to accommodate him in San Servolo. The letter, signed by the police officer Avigni, explained that,

> Mattio Casal, a poor shoemaker, has crucified himself with the purpose of ending his life. He was rescued in time and by now his wounds are healed. This is, however, not the case for the intellectual capacities of this unhappy man, which are completely in disorder. I recommend him to the particular attention of the Supreme Father (*Padre Superiore*) in the pious place of San Servolo, and to the whole exemplary and well-deserved family of pious religious brothers.[14]

The letter commissioned the friars of San Servolo not only to care for Lovat's physical recovery, but also asked them to help him to see reason and to critically reflect upon his self-crucifixion. The act was clearly considered the result of Lovat's erroneous individual beliefs: 'They might care for the needs of Casal by applying a physical and moral cure that will, if possible, re-stabilise him, and that will enable him to recognise to what extent his attempts are contrary to the duties of a Christian, of a subject, and of man.'[15]

Lovat arrived at San Servolo a few days after that request, on 20 August in 1805. He stayed in the hospital at the expense of the government, as was the

---

12   On the hospital of San Servolo see N. Vanzan Marchini, *San Servolo e Venezia. Un' isola e la sua storia*, Venice, Caselle di Sommacampagna, 2004 and Galzigna and Terzian, *L'archivio della follia*.

13   M. Galzigna has published the few sources concerning Mattio Lovat from the archive of San Servolo: Ibid., 75–83; Galzigna, *La malattia morale*, 41–74.

14   ASS, Maniaci, Atti, b. 2, fasc. 5 (=anni 1803–1810): 'Mattio Casal calzaiolo e miserabile si era crocefisso col proponimento di perdere in tal forma la vita. Fu a tempo soccorso, ed ora le sue ferite sono sanate. Non è così per altro delle facoltà intellettuali di quest'infelice che sono tuttora in disordine. Si raccomanda alla particolar attenzione del Padre Superiore al Pio Luogo di San Servolo e di tutta quella esemplare e ospitaliera famiglia di benemeriti religiosi di applicar in bisogni del Casal quella cura tanto fisica quanto morale, che lo rimette se sia possibile in equilibrio, e lo costituisca capace di riconoscere quanto siffatti tentativi sono contrari ai doveri del Cristiano, dal suddicto, e dell'uomo. Venezia, 13. Agosto 1805 Dalla Imp. Regia Direzione Generale di Polizia. Avigni'.

15   Ibid.

case for all poor and destitute patients.[16] For this reason, it was important for the authorities to check from time to time if Lovat's hospitalisation was still necessary. This explains why in September 1805 the administrative body of the Venetian hospitals asked the police about the measures that had been undertaken after Lovat's self-crucifixion.[17] In the following months, the police in turn asked the religious director (*Padre Priore*) of the hospital to keep them informed about Lovat's state of health several times.[18] In December, Bravetti, the inspector of the hospital of San Servolo, delivered a medical-surgical report to the police, which informed them that 'the health of Mattio Casal was still not absolutely re-established'.[19] In detail, this report explained that:

> the state of health of Casal Matteo (who has crucified himself), in the course of approximately four months in which he has stayed in this pious hospital, according to the physician (*medico fisico*), has suffered and still suffers from time to time altering effects from derangements which still exist in his mind. This is why, from time to time, he experiences the most profound melancholy, refusing with all his power every

---

16   See the register of the incoming and outcoming insane (*maniaci*) of the period: ASS, Registri generali, 1 (=Elenco A dei maniaci entrati dal 25 ottobre 1725 a tutto il 24 settembre 1812): '20 Agosto 1805. Fu qui condotto per ordinanza della Regia Direzione generale di Polizia il mentecatto Mattio Casale, quale viene spesato per Reg. Conto. Morì di malattia di petto il giorno 8 aprile 1806.'

17   ASV, Direzione Generale Polizia, protocolli degli esibiti, b. 19 (=anno 1805; 5.VIII–31.XII, protocollo 5208–8659), numero dell'esibito 6721, 15 September 1805: 'Ad oggetto di prestarsi all'ordine dell' Imperiale Regia Direzione Generale, ricerca la compiacenza della Direzione Generale a volerlo poner di lumi sull'emercenza della Crocifizione di Matteo Casal e suo destino in seguito'.

18   This was the purpose of another letter from the police, addressed to the *Padre Priore* on 5 October 1805: ASS, Maniaci, Atti, b. 2, fasc. 3: 'Venezia 5 xbre 1805. Interessa la General Direzione di sapere lo stato di salute in cui si trovi Mattio Casal che attentò la propria vita crocifiggendosi. Il R.P. Priore del pio R. Ospedale di San Servolo si farà sollecita di rendernela ragguagliata. Dalla I.R. Direzione Generale di Polizia Per impedimento dell'I.R. Consigliere e Direttore Generale. Raab. Al Molto Reverendo padre Priore del Pio Ospitale di San Servolo'.

19   ASV, Direzione Generale Polizia, protocolli degli esibiti, b. 19, numero dell'esibito 8466, 11 december 1805: 'Il Reverendo Ispettore Bravetti Accompagna una Fede Medico Chirurghica di S. Servolo, dalla quale si rileva la non assoluta ripristinata salute di Mattio Casal'. Most likely, the medical-surgical report mentioned here is identical with the report sent from the *Padre Priore* to the police, dating from 10 December 1805: ASS, Rapporti sanitari, b.1, fasc. 1 (=anni 1805–1810). This document is conserved in the *rapporti sanitari* in the archive of San Servolo. The *rapporti sanitari* were reports about the health condition of patients, through which the *Padre Priore* informed the Venetian authorities about the necessity to either dismiss a patient, or to continue the treatment.

kind of food for the period of several days in a row; if we would not apply medical remedies, he would take the risk of becoming the victim of a too long an abstinence.[20]

In other words the letter claimed that because of his mental derangement, Lovat was still in need of medical assistance. The 'medical remedies' mentioned here allude to a common practice in San Servolo as well as in many other hospitals at the time – the application of force feeding using a tube in cases of refusal of food.[21] All in all the report suggested that the 'moral cure' that the police had initially requested in the admission letter had not had the effect which the Venetian authorities had hoped for Lovat.[22]

We can complement this evidence of Lovat's stay at the hospital of San Servolo with a further letter that a physician called Luigi Portalupi sent to Ruggieri after Lovat's death. In it Portalupi describes all the details he had observed in his patient until his death, including an account of the changes in Lovat's physical and mental state, of the remedies and methods used to cure him, of the ups and downs of his state of mind and his deviant behaviour. He too reported that between August 1805 and January 1806, Lovat refused to eat for several periods, and was therefore force-fed. In January, Lovat showed symptoms of typhus (*sintomi tifici*), but got better in March. Portalupi also remarked that he observed in Lovat 'a singular tendency to expose himself to the sun for continuous hours', and that the *fatebenefratelli* had to prevent him from getting burned. In April, Lovat's thorax was badly affected by a frequent cough. Portalupi concludes his observations by noting that Lovat drew his last breath on 8 April 1806.[23]

---

20 ASS, Rapporti sanitari, b. 1, fasc. 1 (=anni 1805–1810): 'Rapporti sanitari dal 1805 al 1810. 10 Dicembr. In risposta a Decreto 5 dicembre sottoscritto Raab. Lo stato di salute di Casal Matteo (che si era crocifisso), nel corso de' quattro mesi circa da che si trova in questo Pio Spedale, rapporto al fisico ha sofferto e soffre di tratto in tratto delle alternative cagionate dall'alterazione tuttavia persistente dello spirito, per cui tratto dandosi in preda alla più profonda melanconia ricusa a tutto potere per lo spazio di più giorni consecutivi qualunque sorte di refezione; per il che correrebbe rischio di restar vittima di un'astinenza troppo a lungo portratta, se non vi si ponesse riparo co'mezzi suggeriti dall'Arte medica. Ciò è quanto in esecuzione de' venerati comandi di quest' I.R. Direzione il sottoscritto ha l'onore di rassegnare'.

21 See Galzigna, *La malattia morale*, 49.

22 On the meaning of 'moral cure' in asylums led by religious orders see H. Guillemain, 'Médecine et religion au XIXe siècle. Le traitement moral de la folie dans les asiles de l'ordre de Saint-Jean de Dieu (1830–1860)', *Le mouvement social*, vol. 215, 2006, 35–49.

23 Portalupi's letter, which can be considered a small case history on Lovat on its own, is cited in Ruggieri, *Storia della crocifissione*, 18–20. Portalupi appears in the archival documentation of San Servolo already before 1797, in a list of the staff payed by the responsible congregation

Lovat thus died in the hospital of San Servolo more than nine months after his self-crucifixion. His death is also confirmed by a general chronological register conserved in the archive of San Servolo, which is the last note we have on Lovat's destiny. The patient's cause of death, written down retrospectively in the entry by the staff of San Servolo, reads 'malattia di petto', that is he died of some undesignated disease of the chest.[24] Presumingly, he was buried at the small cemetery annexed to the hospital on the same island.

Lovat's hospitalisation at San Servolo in 1805 occurred in a period in which the hospital already functioned as *ospedale dei pazzi*, the contemporary Italian term for a madhouse. The gradual transformation of the former military hospital into a proper mental asylum signaled a fundamental change in the general attitude towards the poor and sick after the end of the Venetian Republic. The new principles of health policy, as they had been expressed in several decrees by the democratic interim government, emphasised the rights of the invalid and poor to health care and their equal status as citizens (*cittadini*).[25] This change in attitude also related to the insane, who were now considered to be in need of medical assistance. Significantly, the last doge of the Venetian Republic, Ludovico Manin, left a sum of money to set up an adequate place for the so-called *pazzi* in Venice in his will. His will dating of 24 October 1802 suggests that people suffering from mental disorders were regarded as deserving

---

of the Venetian Republic, see ASS, b. 584, documenti settecenteschi 1759–1799. The respective file is entitled: *1759–1797 Deputazione delegata al pubblico spedale militare di San Servolo*. The only published work of Portalupi is a case history on a tumour operation he had carried out: G.L. Portalupi, *Storia ragionata dell'enorme tumore del nobile signore Luigi Tedeschi di Verona estirpato nel giorno 26 giugno 1823 da Fr. Gio. Luigi Portalupi*, Venice, Tipografia Armena di S. Lazzaro, 1823.

24   ASS, Registri generali, 1: '20 Agosto 1805. Fu qui condotto per ordinanza della Regia Direzione generale di Polizia il mentecatto Mattio Casale, quale viene spesato per Reg. Conto. Morì di malattia di petto il giorno 8 aprile 1806'. See also ASS, Libro dei morti dal 1 marzo 1798 a tutto il 2 febbraio 1825.

25   See the document in ASV, Miscellanea legislativa, b. 1722–1797, cited after N. Vanzan Marchini, *La follia, una nave, una citta. Storia di pazzi e di pazzie a Venezia nel '700*, Mira, Brenctani editrice, 1981, 158: 'Il governo deve garantire la vita, la proprietà, il lavoro a chi non ha proprietà, la sussistenza a chi non ha né proprietà, né è capace al lavoro. Se manca la prima garanzia il governo è tirannico, se la seconda è ingiusto, se la terza è improvvido, se la quarta è inumano [...] L'invalido deve essere assicurato della sua sussistenza dalla patria. Questa è la condizione con cui gli uomini sono uniti in società. La patria che lo soccorre paga un debito. I soli tiranni ammettevano al nome di "soccorso" il titolo di "carità" [...]'. On the similar emergence of the citizen-patient through the French Revolution, see D.B. Weiner, *The Citizen-Patient in Revolutionary and Imperial Paris*, Baltimore, Johns Hopkins University Press, 1993.

pity and as being potentially curable.[26] These broader societal changes explain why the Venetian authorities decided to hospitalise Lovat at San Servolo rather than punishing him for his self-crucifixion or abandoning him to his fate.

The cited documents are the only archival sources we have from the local context that testify to Lovat's self-crucifixion and his hospitalisation in Venice. Despite their incompleteness, they shed light on how Lovat's case was gradually established through its communication between the different Venetian authorities. However the documents also contain a serious pitfall for the historian. They suggest that we could learn from them what Lovat had actually suffered and died from. But the various symptoms and diagnoses mentioned in the cited documents are only what Lovat's attending physicians *wrote* that he suffered and died from. These sources therefore tell us something about the medical terms and diseases of the time, but they hardly tell us anything about Lovat, and nothing about his own experience of his illness.[27]

2 Mattio Lovat

So what do we know about Lovat? What did he do before coming to Venice, and why did he believe he had to die on the cross? These are questions to which the administrative sources cited before give no answer. Almost everything we know about Lovat's past and his life in Venice prior to his self-crucifixion is second- or third-hand information that we find in the *Storia della crocifissione*. Reading Ruggieri's case narrative, however, means looking at Lovat's case through Ruggieri's eyes. His perspective is that one of the physician who was directly involved in the incidents. Ruggieri had an eye for his intended readership and necessarily made choices while compiling the available information and writing down the case history of his patient. There are biographical details about Lovat he chose to tell while others he chose to hide, or simply did not know about. But a few scattered archival documents have survived which

---

26 ASV, Archivio notarile testamenti, b. 234, n. 208: '[...] Prego li soggetti che saranno in detto Dipartimento di trovar il luogo per collocare dette persone che sarebbe bene fosse uno degli ospedali [...] ordinerano sieno adatte le fabriche ad uso che dovrano servire e provederano li mobili ed utensili occorenti, per il che, destino siano loro consegnati dai miei eredi e commissari altri ducati dieci mila in moneta sonante e tutto ciò tempo un anno doppo la mia morte. Supplico essi soggetti ad impiegare la loro humanità e religione acciò li pazzi siano trattati con carità e si cerchi di risanarli [...]'.

27 On this heuristic problem see Cunningham, *Identifying Disease*, 17: Cunningham makes the point that 'you die of what your doctor says you die of'.

allow us to confirm and to complement the information on Lovat that we find in the *Storia della crocifissione*.

In summary, Ruggieri's account reads as follows: Mattio Lovat was a man of 46 years of age when he tried to crucify himself in Venice in 1805. He was the son of a certain Marco and had the nickname Casale, which referred to the place of his birth. Casale was a village in the district of Zoldo, a valley situated near the town of Belluno in the North Italian mountains. Born as the child of poor farmers, Lovat wanted to become a priest. He was taught to read and to write by the village priest. Because of the great poverty of his parents, Lovat was eventually forced to give up his studies and to become a shoemaker instead. In 1802, when still in his home village, Lovat became the subject of public attention for the first time when he carried out 'the most complete emasculation' – he amputated his genitals with his shoemaker's knife and threw them out of the window of his room.[28] Although Ruggieri mentioned this incident only briefly, this incident of Lovat's self-emasculation came to play a significant role in some later readings of the case narrative. As we shall see, some commentators of Lovat's case were even more interested in this act of self-mutilation than in his crucifixion.

As Ruggieri remarks, Lovat had already prepared herbs and bandages as remedies for his injuries, which were completely healed within a short time without any help from a surgeon.[29] The reason for this sudden action remained unknown, but the strange deed and Lovat's rapid self-healing became gossip in the village. Having become a victim of local mockery, Lovat soon withdrew from any kind of social life. On 13 November of the same year, he moved to Venice where his younger brother Angelo lived. According to Ruggieri's detailed account, Lovat changed both the places where he lived and worked in Venice several times. His brother Angelo first placed Lovat with a certain widow in the same area where he himself lived. Lovat stayed at this place for several months, working at the shop of a shoemaker close to the Venetian hospital *Ospitaletto*. On 21 September 1803, Lovat tried to crucify himself for the first time in public, but passers-by stopped him at the moment in which he tried to put a nail through his feet. In consequence of this event, Lovat's landlord sent him

---

28   Ruggieri, *Storia della crocifissione*, 5: 'A tal epoca ritirossi un giorno in una stanza di casa sua, e mediante un cattivo coltello di calzolajo eseguì su se stesso la più perfetta evirazione, gettando in seguito le recise parti dalla finestra le quali vennero raccolte da sua Madre'.

29   Ibid., 6: '[...] aveva anche pensato al modo di medicarsi; quindi aveva pronte delle erbe pestate, che diconsi da que' villici capaci a fermare il sangue, e varj pannilini per medicarsi in seguito, come realmente ha fatto, ed in breve tempo guarì senza che gli rimanesse alcune supersite incomodo in quelle parti [...]'.

away, and he went back to his home village, where he stayed for some time. Lovat later returned to Venice and worked first at the shoemaker's workshop of a certain Martin Murzani, situated close to the Church Ss. Apostoli, but then changed his workplace again in May 1805, to work at the workshop of a certain Lorenzo della Mora. At the beginning of July he finally rented a room close to the church St. Alvise at number 2888 on the street Calle delle Monache in order to live closer to where he worked. The house belonged to a certain Valentin Luccheta and the room was on the third floor. This was the very place where Lovat performed his second self-crucifixion only a few weeks later.

A birth register (*atto di battesimo*), conserved in the church archive in the village Forno di Zoldo, close to the town of Belluno, testifies Lovat's date of birth. It confirms that Lovat was born in 1761 in Casale, that his parents' names were Marco and Vittoria, and that he was baptised by a priest called Bartolo Lazaris.[30] The birth register also confirms that the full name Ruggieri reports in his case history, Mattio Lovat, was Lovat's given name – we have seen that in the administrative correspondence on Lovat's case cited at the beginning of this chapter, Lovat is not referred to as Mattio Lovat but as Mattio/Matteo Casal or Casale. It thus appears that the authorities in Venice used the designation of Lovat's home village as a nickname – either because they did not know that Mattio's actual last name was Lovat, or to indicate Lovat's status as an outsider who had come to Venice as an immigrant from the *terraferma*, the Venetian hinterland.

A second document that illuminates Ruggieri's account is a record conserved in the archives of the Venetian municipality, which lists all inhabitants of Venice in the year 1805.[31] Among the alphabetical entries, we do not find Lovat's name, but the names of two of his younger brothers, one of them Angelo, who is also mentioned in Ruggieri's case history. The record also confirms that the last place where Lovat lived in Venice in Calle delle Monache was actually inhabited by several other people coming from the region of Belluno. This

---

30   The register of birth was first discovered by the writer Sebastiano Vassalli, see Vassalli, *Marco e Mattio*, 75. It is edited in S. Bandirali (ed.), *Storia della crocifissione di Mattio Lovat da se stesso eseguita, postfazione di Sebastiano Vassalli*, Crema, Amici del Museo, Arti grafiche, 2000, 1996, 47: 'Lì 12 Settembre 1761. Matio, fig.o di Marco quondam Matio Lovat da Casal, e di Vitoria iugati fù tenuto alla porta, e al S.o Fonte da Zuane quandam Baldissare e Pia da Pra, e batezato da me P. Bartolo Lazaris cap.o [probably cappellano, M.B.]'.

31   Archivio Comunale di Venezia, Serie anagrafe, Prima Dominazione Austriaca, anagrafi generale 1805. The table indicates surname, name, father, age, religion, home city, home province, area, district, street, number of the street, civil state (married or not, widow or not, children or not), social condition (plebs or not), and profession. Lovat's brother Angelo and his brother Michiel are listed within the letters La-Le, fasc. 88. The street is Calle delle Monache No. 2888 in the area Canal Regio, contrada S. Marcola.

suggests that at Lovat's time, people from this area formed a small community
within the Canal Regio district in Venice, situated at the northern outskirts of
the city, and that Lovat lived within this community of non-Venetians.

3   The Patient's Perspective

Why did Mattio Lovat believe he had to put himself on the cross like the crucified Christ? This is the most difficult question to answer when dealing with
Lovat's case, because we simply cannot know for sure what agitated Lovat, and
what exactly persuaded him to crucify himself. Rather than searching for a
final answer to this question, this book traces the many different answers that
contemporary commentators on Lovat's case gave, to themselves and to their
readers.

The first to try to find an answer to the question was Ruggieri. Only thanks to
the *Storia della crocifissione* do we have an idea about Lovat's personal motives
at all. The answer Ruggieri gave in his case narrative was far more complex and
ambiguous than the medical explanations he had firstly put forward in his correspondence with the Venetian authorities. It appears that when investigating
Lovat's case with hindsight with the purpose of writing down his patient's case
history, Ruggieri was not only interested in finding possible medical explanations for Lovat's physical and mental condition, he was also keen to reveal
Lovat's personal reasons for his self-crucifixion as well as its obvious religious
message.

Ruggieri's account was primarily informed by the observations and inquiries he himself had made at Lovat's bedside during his recovery in the Clinical
School. Ruggieri reports how he took advantage of the rare moments in which
Lovat was lucid to inquire into the details concerning his crucifixion.[32] He reports that 'the invalid never spoke to anybody, and he was always thoughtful
while keeping his eyes closed. I interviewed him several times asking him why
he had put himself on the cross, and he always responded with the same words:
*that the pride of mankind must be chastened, and that it was therefore neces-
sary that he died on the cross*'.[33] Ruggieri also took the opportunity to interview
Lovat's brother Angelo, who accompanied Lovat when Ruggieri brought him

---

32   Ruggieri, *Storia della crocifissione*, 15f.
33   Ibid., 12f.: 'L'ammalato non parlava mai con alcuno, ed era sempre meditabondo, tenendo
       quasi sempre chiusi gli occhi. Lo interrogai varie volte sul perchè si sia posto in croce, e
       riposemi sempre le stesse parole, cioè *che la superbia degli uomini doveva esser castigata,
       ed era però necessario che ei morisse in croce*'. (Italics in the original).

by boat to the Clinical School after the incident. Again, Ruggieri renders Lovat's words in direct speech when reporting that, 'On the way, on the boat, he said to his brother Angelo, who complained about his eccentricity, only these words: *I am still unhappy!*'[34] Referring to Lovat's first attempt at public self-crucifixion in Venice, Ruggieri also notes that back then, Lovat had told his brother that this was the festive day of Saint Matthew, his titular Saint.[35]

By citing these different statements made by Lovat himself when asked for the reason for his self-crucifixion, Ruggieri already suggests to his readers that Lovat was guided by a certain Christian mission to sacrifice his body. But Ruggieri's knowledge of Lovat's personal motives did not only derive from his conversations at Lovat's bedside. He also used another important source: a short letter that Lovat had written some time before his self-crucifixion and had carried with him. Introducing Lovat's letter as one of his principal sources of information, Ruggieri explains that Lovat,

> was so convinced of his obligation to die on the cross by supreme volition that he wanted to inform the tribunal of justice in a certain way about his mission, and he did this according to his alphabetisation and the state of his imagination on a piece of paper that I still keep, written by his own hand long before his martyrdom, and with the intention that the tribunal should not believe that his deed was the act of someone else.[36]

Ruggieri reproduced a copy of Lovat's letter in a footnote to his case narrative.[37] The text is written in a north Italian dialect, and many of the phrases are fragmentary and incoherent. Although the idiosyncratic syntax of the letter makes it impossible for modern readers to grasp its full meaning, we get a vague idea about what might have occupied Lovat's mind.

The letter is addressed to the tribunal of justice in Venice. In the first part Lovat informs the reader of his intention to die on the cross, because 'this is the moment in which the prophecy comes true which has imposed me several

---

34   Ibid., 11: 'strada facendo disse a suo fratello Angelo che gli era compagno di barca, il quale lagnavasi delle sue stravaganze, queste sole parole: *sono pur infelice!*'
35   Ibid., 7.
36   Ibid., 13: '[...] ed era tanto persuaso d'esser obbligato a morir in Croce per volontà suprema, che volle in certo qual modo, e come potevano permettergli e la sua educazion letteraria, e lo stato della sua fantasia, render inteso il Tribunal di Giustizia sul destino che gli sovrastava, mediante una carta che io conservo, scritta di proprio pugno, molto tempo prima del suo martirio, affinchè non avesse a credersi questo l'opera di qualche altro'.
37   Ibid. An edition of the complete text is in Galzigna and Terzian, *L'archivio della follia*, 80f. See also Galzigna's interpretation of this text, ibid., 75–79.

times to die nailed to a cross'.[38] Lovat further explains that he was very upset that he could not become a priest 'in order to spread the Word of God'.[39] He writes in nebulous words about having lived as a good Christian, and about never having sinned against anybody, 'in particular not in terms of carnal sin'.[40] It would make no sense to involve the judiciary in his case because 'this affair is spiritual and not public.'[41] The following passage alludes to the self-mutilation Lovat had carried out in his birthplace, before his self-crucifixion in Venice. Lovat talks about his 'martyrdom' to cut away his testicles and phallus with a knife, because of a certain bewitchment (*Maggia*) he had experienced earlier from some priests (*sacerdoti*).[42] In the next passage, Lovat refers to his parents, and again several times to the priests who are mentioned in relation with some 'mistresses' and 'prostitutes' and 'scandalous dances' – apparently, these incidents gave rise in Lovat to feelings of humiliation and guilt and the wish 'to live in this world no longer'.[43] In a later passage, he writes about having been obliged by the same priests to make a sacrifice, and about forgiving them the insults he had experienced.[44] At the end of the letter, Lovat repeats his request that the 'reverend and holy government' should not intervene in his plan and should not involve the judiciary, because 'this is a spiritual affair in church'.[45]

The multiple allusions in this letter to Christian ideas of sin, repentance and sacrifice, as well as to sexual incidents obviously leave a lot of scope for interpretation. One might speculate that Lovat was a victim of sexual abuse.

---

38   Ruggieri, *Storia della crocifissione*, 13: '[...] questo è il momento che si adempisca il vaticinio che me impone più volte di far la morte inchiodato in croce [...]'.

39   Ibid.: '[...] versai abondanti lagrime di non poter arivar a la Grazia del Sacramento d'ordine sacro per predicar la parola di Dio [...]'.

40   Ibid., 14: '[...] visi da buon christiano [...] mi protesto di esser Vergine per non aver al mondo fatto sangue alle persone di nissuna condicion, specialmente in pecati di carne'.

41   Ibid.: '[...] è superfluo di tratar con la Giustizia di quest' afar perche sono cosa in spiritual e non miga di comun [...]'.

42   Ibid.: '[...] che me a do principio li sacerdoti il mio Martirio con un cortello da calegar talgido via li testicoli e membro per la Maggia [probably magia, M.B.] fatta a me da Sacerdoti'.

43   Ibid.: 'Abenche giero presente ancor io che faceva quei medesimi in compagnia dele sue Amante Done e putte insieme faceva di balli scandalosi asai e lunghe tresche d'altri giovani con tochamenti de le mani: che da per me stesso restristava l'anima mia a tali occhieti per il che non mi curavo di vivere più in Questo Mondo [...]'.

44   Ibid.

45   Ibid.: '[...] non staga a mover piedi d'Agente Soldati o qualsiasi persone a fronte degli mieii operatori [...]'; '[...] non ga da impazarsene nianche la Giustizia che è questa cosa spiritual in chiesa'. In his interpretation of Lovat's letter, Galzigna takes this phrase as a proof for a 'religious and spiritual conception of Giustizia', see Galzigna, *La malattia morale*, 43. I do not agree because it seems clear to me that 'questa' refers to the spiritual affair that is opposed to secular law.

Another hypothesis could be that some priest had told him to atone for masturbation. Historical scholarship has shown that in the discourse on *onania* that
had emerged in the Enlightenment, masturbation was moralised and patholo-
gised, and this had in turn a deep impact on the conscience of many people.
However, we do not know if any of this might have been the case with Lovat,
and due to the lack of further historical evidence, every interpretation remains
pure speculation.[46] It is clear, however, that the letter's primary motive was
Lovat's concern that the tribunal of justice should not suspect anybody else of
being involved in his self-crucifixion. Lovat was probably also afraid of being
accused of attempted self-murder. According to the legal situation of the time,
a suicide would not be granted a proper funeral and a tomb at the cemetery,
and Lovat wanted to die as a Christian, not as a self-murderer. Overall, the letter gives the impression that Lovat himself considered his two self-destructive
deeds – the self-mutilation and the self-crucifixion – as a Christian 'martyrdom' that he had to suffer in order to atone for something he had experienced
in relation with his religious educators.

   This letter is the only surviving first-person narration that we have from Lovat, and it is passed on to us only indirectly, through a reproduction in Ruggieri's case history. What is of interest here is that Ruggieri used Lovat's letter
to reconstruct Lovat's biography in his case narrative, and to shed light on the
personal motives and beliefs possibly lying behind his patient's self-crucifixion.
But even for Ruggieri, Lovat's case still raised many questions that he found difficult to answer. The most difficult question was if Lovat should be considered
a suicide or a martyr? Was his final aim to die or to suffer? We have seen before
that the Venetian tribunal did regard Lovat's self-crucifixion as a suicide attempt. In the *Storia della crocifissione*, however, Ruggieri explicitly mentions
the difficulty of considering Lovat a 'normal' suicide. While he did not find it
surprising that Lovat wanted to commit suicide, what obviously irritated Ruggieri was the particular method Lovat used. Usually, Ruggieri writes, suicides
would long for a rapid and easy death, because they were afraid of pain. And
he draws the conclusion that Lovat must either not have given any thought
to the great pain the self-crucifixion would produce, or that he must have felt
the need to make himself a proper martyr before dying.[47] This suggests quite

---

46   See A. Košenina, *Literarische Anthropologie. Die Neuentdeckung des Menschen*, Berlin,
      Walter de Gruyter, 2008, 90–93. On the discourse of onania see F.X. Eder, 'Diskurs und
      Sexualpädagogik: Der deutschsprachige Onanie-Diskurs des späten 18. Jahrhunderts',
      Paedagogica Historica, vol. 39, no. 6, 2003, 719–735; K. Braun, *Die Krankheit Onania. Kör-
      perangst und die Anfänge moderner Sexualität im 18. Jahrhundert*, Frankfurt, campus, 1995;
      J. Stengers and A. van Neck (eds.), *Storia della masturbazione*, Bologna, Odoya, 2009.
47   Ruggieri, *Storia della crocifissione*, 17f.

clearly that in Lovat's own mind, the idea of becoming a martyr by dying on
the cross predominated over the simple idea of committing suicide. While in
his letter to the Venetian tribunal, Lovat explicitly referred to his 'martyrdom'
as related to concrete personal experiences with his religious educators, he
explained his motive vis-à-vis Ruggieri in more general terms – to repent for
the pride of mankind. Indeed, the little evidence we have suggests that Lovat
actually believed that he had to imitate the sufferings of Christ by imitating the
example of his crucifixion.

4   Crucifying Onself

Ruggieri, like many other commentators on Lovat's case, was not only troubled
by the question why Lovat crucified himself, but also by the question how – in
technical terms – it was possible to crucify oneself at all. How was Lovat able to
hang himself on the cross without any help from somebody else? Here again,
we have to rely on Ruggieri's case narrative and the two illustrations as the
only surviving source describing the incident itself. We have to keep in mind,
however, that even Ruggieri's description is an account of something he had
not seen with his own eyes but that he retrospectively tried to make sense of,
because when he arrived on the spot, other people had already taken Lovat
down from the cross.

Ruggieri's meticulous description of Lovat's preparations and the technical
difficulties surrounding his self-crucifixion fills several pages of his treatise and
can be summarised as follows.[48] It was in his room in Calle delle Monache
that Lovat started thinking about how he could crucify himself once again. He
systematically prepared everything for his second self-crucifixion, including
cords, nails, a crown of thorns and a large net, with which he was going to tie
himself up to the cross.[49] First Lovat constructed a cross by using the wood
from his bed, which he then fastened with several cords to a big wooden beam
above the window. Still in the room and dressed in nothing but a small loin-
cloth, Lovat put the crown of thorns on his head. With the help of the net and
by putting nails into both of his feet, he attached himself to the cross, which
still lay on the floor. He also tried to cause himself a wound on his left side with
a shoemaker's knife – as Ruggieri assumes, Lovat probably intended to imitate
the side wound of Christ but made a mistake because, according to the Biblical

48   Ibid., 7–10.
49   Ibid., 7.

account, the wound was on the right side.[50] Lovat then sought to reveal himself to the public.[51] Because the windowsill was very low, he succeeded in moving himself, fixed with the net to the cross, out of the window. He then tried to put his hands with the nails back on the cross, but apparently did not succeed completely. When, at eight o'clock in the morning, people saw him hanging on the cross out of the window, only Lovat's left arm was fixed while his right arm was hanging down by his body.[52]

Considering the tools that Lovat used for his incident, in particular the cross, the crown of thorns, and the nails as well as the wounds he inflicted upon himself on his side and on his hands and feet, it must have been clear to the people in Venice that Lovat's self-crucifixion was in fact an attempt to imitate the Crucified according to the Biblical account of the Passion. The narrative of Christ's sufferings is at the heart of both Christian theology and iconography, deeply engrained in Catholic societies such as Venice. But, of course, Jesus of Nazareth did *not* crucify himself, he *was* crucified by his persecutors. So even from a Christian perspective, Lovat's self-crucifixion could be read in two different ways. It could be understood as a Christian martyrdom for the world's sake, as Lovat himself had probably meant it. But it could also be understood as hubris and as blasphemous provocation, because Lovat was himself in a sense claiming to be the Crucified. As the later chapters show, the second view prevailed in the various readings of Lovat's case.

Given the religious message of Lovat's self-crucifixion, it is somewhat frustrating that we do not have evidence for any involvement of the Church in Lovat's case. In Venice as elsewhere in Italy, the local parish priest traditionally acted as a mediator between parishioners and the political and religious authorities.[53] It is therefore surprising that after Lovat's self-crucifixion, the police did not interrogate the local parish priest of the area where Lovat lived in order to investigate his religious habits. It is also striking that in the files from the hospital of San Servolo, a so-called attestation of poverty (*fede di povertà*) by a priest is lacking. Along with a medical certificate, such a document was usually obligatory for admission. It might well be that these documents simply got lost. But Lovat had lived in Venice for only three years and had changed his

---

50 Ibid., 9: 'Per me credo siano queste state fatte nel cercare il sito che non opponeva esistenza alcuna al ferro che doveva in quell caso, secondo Mattio, servire di lancia'.

51 Ibid.

52 See ibid., 10.

53 D.I. Kertzer, 'Religion and Society, 1789–1892', in J.A. Davis (ed.), *Italy in the Nineteenth Century*, Oxford, Oxford University Press, 2000, 181–205, 183f.

domicile several times. Therefore, as a non-Venetian, he was maybe not properly integrated into the parish life of his neighbourhood.

Surprisingly Lovat's public self-crucifixion even went unnoticed by the contemporary Venetian newspapers, but it is extremely difficult to judge what this
means. The quarter of Venice where the self-crucifixion took place, today's
Cannaregio, is in the outermost corner in the very north of Venice. In Lovat's
time, many workers and craftsmen lived in the area. Due to the lack of sources,
it is however impossible to evaluate how many passers-by actually saw Lovat
hanging on the cross on the morning of 19 July 1805, and to what extent the
inhabitants of Venice took notice of Lovat's self-crucifixion at all. Very likely,
however, the well-to-do in Venice were not concerned with what happened in
the poorer quarters of Venice. The second point that makes it difficult to evaluate the newspaper's lacking attention to Lovat's case is the question of censorship. After the upheavals of the French occupation, the first period of Austrian
rule in Venice aimed at re-establishing public order and keeping social and
religious life under control. In order to protect the Catholic state religion, the
Austrians introduced a rigid system of censorship that sought to suppress any
sensitive discussions of controversial religious issues.[54] Publications containing ideas that were considered as heresy or superstition were forbidden. Accordingly, the situation of Venetian newspapers in 1805 was sensitive. Most of
them concentrated on news concerning politics or on events relating to people of high rank.[55] This might have been the reason for the press's silence on
Lovat's case.[56]

---

54   Gottardi, *L'Austria a Venezia*, 217. Archival documents alluding to certain measures of
     censorship in 1805 are contained in ASV, Direzione Generale di Polizia, atti, b. 52 (=anno
     1805). On censorship during the Venetian Republic see M. Infelise, 'Venezia e la circolazi-
     one delle informazioni: tra censura e controllo', *Archivio veneto*, vol. 161, 2003, 231–245
     and H. Brown, *The Venetian Printing Press, 1469–1800*, New York, G.P. Putnam's Sons, 1891.
     The Austrian system of censorship also embraced the lombardo-venetian kingdom under
     Austrian rule, see J. Marx, *Die Österreichische Zensur im Vormärz*, Vienna, Verlag für Ge-
     schichte und Politik, 1959, 19f. On Austrian policies regarding the religious life in Venice
     more in general see A. Zorzi, *Österreichs Venedig. Das letzte Kapitel der Fremdherrschaft*,
     Hamburg, Claassen, 1990, 28off.
55   Gottardi, *L'Austria a Venezia*, 244.
56   As far as I can see, the only contemporary Venetian newspapers in which Lovat's case
     could have been mentioned was *Il nuovo postiglione*, in which, however, we do not find
     any trace of the incident. This newspaper was the continuation of an older periodical
     called *Il nuovo postiglione ossia compendio de' più accreditati fogli d'Europa*. Besides that,
     in 1805 it was only *Il quotidiano veneto* that published news concerning the urban social
     life. On Venetian newspapers before the end of the Republic see M. Berengo (ed.), *Gior-
     nali Veneziani del settecento*, Milan, Feltrinelli, 1962 and R. Saccardo, *La stampa periodica
     veneziana fino alla caduta della repubblica*, Padua, Tipografia del seminario, 1942.

The Venetian authorities who dealt with Lovat's case did not comment on the religious implications of his self-crucifixion either, as they essentially understood the self-crucifixion as an attempt at suicide, resulting from mental disorder. As we have seen they nevertheless hoped that the moral treatment by the *fatebenefratelli* in San Servolo would help Lovat to recognise that, even from a Christian perspective, he was wrong. The fact that Lovat was immediately declared insane and admitted to medical institutions obviously helped to reduce public attention, and prevented the people in Venice remembering the incident as a religious martyrdom requiring devotion. Officially labelled as an act of insanity, Lovat's self-crucifixion was, in Venice, deprived of both its intrinsic religious message as well as of its provocative potential.

5   Insanity and Pellagra

But was Lovat insane? And if so, what exactly was he suffering from? As it was the case for his nineteenth-century contemporaries, probably everybody reading about Lovat's case today inevitably asks himself this question – a self-crucifixion is just too extraordinary and disturbing to be categorised as a sane and rational act. We have seen, however, that Lovat did not think about himself in terms of being ill or insane. Explicitly, he wanted his self-crucifixion to be understood as a religious matter, a 'spiritual affair', not as a juridical issue – and definitely not as a medical problem.

Ruggieri's *Storia della crocifissione* created the narrative basis for all the medical and non-medical comments later observers made on Lovat's case. As a medical case narrative written by a physician, Ruggieri's account clearly takes a medical perspective on what Lovat himself regarded as a 'spiritual matter'. Of course, as we have seen before, Ruggieri did make some effort to understand his patient's personal motives, and he also let his patient speak for himself by literally quoting Lovat's answers to his questions as well as by reproducing his letter. However, in his function as Lovat's first attending physician, Ruggieri's principal duty was to provide medical explanations. He had to explain what was wrong with Lovat and what exactly he was suffering from. And the overall answer that Ruggieri gave in his case narrative was that Lovat was mentally ill.

At the very beginning of his case narrative, Ruggieri stresses that he believes it important to say something on Lovat's 'physical and moral condition' *before* he will turn to the 'insane excess' itself.[57] This insane excess refers to

---

57   Ruggieri, *Storia della crocifissione*, 3: 'Trovo necessario, prima di entrare nella descrizione di un tal eccesso di pazzia, il premettere alcune circostanze risguardanti lo stato fisico e morale del detto Mattio'.

Lovat's self-crucifixion, and according to Ruggieri, the preconditions for this deed were to be found in several specific experiences and afflictions of Lovat's earlier life. For Ruggieri, the primary reason for the development of Lovat's insanity was that Lovat could not fulfil his wish to become a priest: 'the suppression of the will in the choice of the profession has always affected the mind even of the strongest believers', and has had terrible effects. This must have hurt strongly the sensorium of the poor Mattio. *Hinc prima mali labes* (this was the first source of misery)'.[58] Working against his true affections had thus altered Lovat's mental condition for the worse. Another factor that had affected Lovat's mental condition in a negative way was, in Ruggieri's eyes, the specific working situation of a shoemaker. Sitting all the time isolated in his shop had made Lovat turn introspective and taciturn.[59]

In Ruggieri's case narrative, the self-castration is depicted as the first outbreak of Lovat's madness. Referring to this, Ruggieri hypothesises that Lovat, because he was afraid of carnal temptation, had wished to relieve himself forever of the burden of an 'enemy'.[60] Consequently, the two attempts at public self-crucifixion in Venice in the years 1802 and 1805 are represented as the climax of a chronological development of Lovat's mental disorder. As we can see from this, Ruggieri was eager to emphasize those moments in Lovat's life that he considered to show the principal signs of the emergence of his patient's mental disorder. To this end, he employed a rhetorical device, mentioning not only the peculiarities of Lovat's behaviour, but emphasising several times the phases in which he 'did nothing extraordinary', 'never showed any sign of madness', and 'was always quiet'.[61] He underlines that Lovat did not behave in extraordinary ways until July 1802. His earlier way of life was 'good in all respects' and Lovat was even considered a very pious man because he only talked about religious issues.[62] These inconspicuous observations thus appear

---

58   Ibid., 4: 'La negazione della volontà nella elezione del proprio stato ha alterato mai sempre lo spirito anche dei creduti più forti, ed ha prodotte delle terribili conseguenze. Tal cosa deve aver molto ferito il sensorio del povero Mattio. *Hinc prima mali labes*'.

59   Ibid.

60   Ibid., 5. The italics indicate the adjuncts in the second edition. '[...] ma non sarebbe egli più ragionevole di credere, dietro il conosciuto carattere di quest'uomo, che la di lui timida coscienza spaventata dalle tentazione della carne, l'avesse deciso a disfarsi tutto ad un tratto e per sempre d'un formidabilissimo nemico *come ha fatto Origene per non aver bene interpretato le parole di S. Matteo?*'.

61   Ibid., 7: '[...] non commise Mattio alcuna stravaganza [...]', ibid., 5: '[...] senza aver mai dato alcun segno di pazzia [...]', ibid., 6: '[...] e fin allora fu sempre tranquillo [...]'.

62   Ibid., 5: 'Il suo modo di vitto e di vita in generale fu sì buono in ogni rapporto, a segno che veniva considerato per un uomo assai pio, perchè non parlava che di Chiesa, di prediche, di Santi, e di digiuno ec.'.

as if they were only a disruption until the next abnormal or insane act. In this way, Ruggieri's case narrative turns Lovat's life into a sequence of normal and abnormal conditions. It suggests that Lovat's behaviour and his actions before his self-crucifixion reflect in themselves a certain mental derangement that had developed in Lovat over time.[63]

Making his patient's case history even more complex, Ruggieri interweaves this particular narrative of a mental disorder with a second narrative of a disease, that of pellagra. He describes several physical symptoms that Lovat displayed while staying under his care at the Clinical School, and he relates these first-hand observations to the biographical data he had gathered from his inquiries. 'When Lovat grew older and always in springtime, he reputedly suffered from dizziness and skin eruptions in the face and on hands and feet. Am I allowed to conclude that these afflictions depend on a *diatesi pellagrosa* (i.e. a pellagrous syndrome)? [...] In fact, I observed that the hands and feet of this man were attacked by herpes which scaled off as a mealy white substance.'[64] When talking about Lovat's self-inflicted wounds and his apparent insensitivity towards pain in the final part of his narrative, he returns to this diagnosis and claims that pellagra must in fact be considered its main cause: 'Mattio seemed to have been affected by a pellagrous disease (*una labe pellagrosa*), in fact I do believe he was, and that we have to attribute to this disease the major part of his insensibility, as you know well that the *pellagrosi* (i.e. those suffering from pellagra) have reacted with indifference to fire and many other pains to which they have been exposed in order to awaken them from their lethargy'.[65]

At the time Ruggieri was writing, pellagra was a common phenomenon in the region. The symptoms that Ruggieri observed in his patient – dizziness, skin eruptions and desquamation, diarrhoea, insensibility and lethargy – formed part of a clinical picture that Italian physicians had depicted and labelled as pellagra since the second half of the eighteenth century. The term derived from

---

63   On the use of the same rhetoric device in the context of nineteenth century sexual pathology see P. Weber, *Der Trieb zum Erzählen. Sexualpathologie und Homosexualität 1852–1914*, Bielefeld, transcript, 2008, 142f.

64   Ruggieri, *Storia della crocifissione*, 4: 'Col crescere dell'età andò soggetto in primavera ai capo-giri, e ad eruzioni erpetiche sul viso, e sulle mani. Sarebbe permesso il sospettare, che tali mali dipendessero da una diatesi pellagrosa?' And ibid., 5: 'Difatti io osservai nell'uomo in questione che Egli aveva le mani ed i piedi attaccati di erpeti che si squammavano in un bianco farinaceo'.

65   Ibid., 17: 'Mattio altronde parve affetto d'una labe pellagrosa, anzi inclino molto a credere lo fosse, e che abbiasi ad attribuire a questa la maggior parte della sua insensibilità, e voi sapete che i pellagrosi hanno con indifferenza resistito ai bottoni di fuoco, ed a molti altri tormenti instituiti su d'essi per risvegliarli dal loro letargo'.

the Lombard dialect (*pelle agra*) and referred to the rough skin of the affected, which was regarded as one of the disease's first symptoms. From the 1770s a broad debate developed in which Italian medical authors debated the various symptoms of pellagra and suggested different theories about its possible causes, one of them being a maize-based diet.[66] As the disease appeared to be epidemic and 'was currently causing depopulation in the area',[67] as Ruggieri emphasised in the second edition of his case history in 1814, pellagra was one of the most important medical problems that troubled physicians as well as political authorities at the time in Northern Italy and beyond, and that would continue to concern them throughout the long nineteenth century.[68]

Ruggieri was interested in the medical debates concerning pellagra. When he translated an important French surgical dictionary between 1805 and 1810, he included his own long article on pellagra.[69] This article testifies that Ruggieri was familiar with the existent medical literature on the disease. In accordance with other authors, Ruggieri describes pellagra as

> a disease of the skin, also called dermatagra, which appears in springtime, normally becomes less apparent in autumn so that it seems overcome, and attacks mostly the poor peasants living in the villages of the mountains, producing a bothersome feeling of tenseness, itchiness and burning

---

66   On this early medical debate see D. Gentilcore, '"Italic Scurvy", "Pellarina", "Pellagra": Medical Reactions to a New Disease in Italy, 1770–1815', in K. Siena and J. Reinarz (eds.), *A Medical History of the Skin: Scratching the Surface*, London, Taylor&Francis, 2013, 57–69. See also M. Ginnaio, *La pellagre: Histoire du mal et de la misère en Italie. XIXe siècle – début XXe*, Paris, L'harmattan, 2014 and R. Mariani-Costantini and A. Mariani-Costantini, 'An Outline of the History of Pellagra in Italy', *Journal of Anthropological Sciences*, vol. 85, 2007, 163–171. Older works on pellagra are D.A. Roe, *A Plague of Corn. The Social History of Pellagra*, Ithaca, Cornell University Press, 1973; A. De Bernardi, *Il mal della rosa. Denutrizione e pellagra nelle campagne italiane tra '800 e '900*, Milan, Franco Angeli, 1984; A. De Bernardi, 'Malattia mentale e trasformazioni sociali. La storia dei folli', in A. De Bernardi (ed.), *Follia, psichiatria e società. Istituzioni manicomiali, scienza psichiatrica e classi sociali nell'Italia moderna e contemporanea*, Milan, Franco Angeli, 1982, 11–32.

67   Ruggieri, *Storia della crocifissione*, 4f.: '[...] e che altronde tali sono i charatteri in generali che accompagnano questa malattia, la quale fatalmente *sensim sine sensu* va spopolando molte di queste Contrade'.

68   See for instance E. Priani, 'Shrouded in a Dark Fog': Comparison of the Diagnosis of Pellagra in Venice and General Paralysis of the Insane in the United Kingdom, 1840–1900, *History of Psychiatry*, vol. 28, no. 2, 2017, 166–181 and literature cited below.

69   C. Ruggieri, 'Pellagra. Malattia della pelle chiamata anche da alcuni dermatagra [...]', in C. Ruggieri (ed.), *Dizionario enciclopedico di chirurgia. Tradotto dal francese in italiano ed accresciuto di aggiunte e note*, vol. 4, Padua, Nella Stamperia del Seminario presso Tommaso Bettinelli, 1808, 105–122.

at the back of hands and feet, followed by the peeling off of the skin [...].
The disease is not accompanied by fever from the beginning, but because
of the remarkable loss of energy, because of which the sick feel week, lazy,
tired, they experience disturbances of the stomach, anorexia, and, in the
following years, they feel tremor, dizziness, diarrhoea, and such a freezing
of all the nervous faculties, that, after they have been brought to exhaus-
tion by all the phenomena, they also become maniac, and try to commit
suicide, most often by throwing themselves into water.[70]

Ruggieri then works out the typical clinical picture of pellagra at the time by
citing leading authors in the field. Touching controversial questions, Ruggieri
is convinced that pellagra is a new disease and therefore should not be equated
with pre-existing diseases, neither with scurvy nor with leprosy, and especially
not with hypochondria.[71] As to its causes, Ruggieri refers to environmental factors such as bad air, bad living conditions, poverty, but also poor diet and hard
labour. Following Gaetano Strambio, he considers pellagra 'a disease of poverty'
(*malattia della miseria*).[72] Ruggieri believes that the disease is hereditary, but
not contagious, another controversial question at the time.[73] When describing
the course of the disease over time, he stresses that the internal symptoms are
generally more severe than the external symptoms.[74] He describes how the
disease first affects the skin, in particular where exposed to sunlight, and then
gradually extends to the whole internal system and the organs, affecting the

---

70   Ibid., 105f.: 'PELLAGRA. Malattia della pelle chiamata anche da alcuni Dermatagra, la
      quale si manifesta in primavera, si ammansa d'ordinario in autunno fino al segno di far
      supporre che sia guarita, ed attacca per lo più i poveri coloni che abitano i paesi montuo-
      si, producendo un senso molesto di stiramento, di prurito e di ardore al dorso delle mani
      e dei piedi, al qual senso succede lo screpolamento della cuticola, per cui cadendo sotto
      forma di squame furfuracee, resta denudata la dermide, la quale poi spesso presenta delle
      macchie irregolari, rossiccie e lucenti. La malattia dapprincipio non è accompagnata da
      febbre, ma sibbene da notabile abbandono di forze, per cui gli ammalati si trovan lan-
      guidi, pigri al moto, sonnolenti, accusano sdilinquimento di stomaco, anoressia, e negli
      anni susseguenti vanno incontro a mano a mano a tremori, vertigini, fatuità, diaree col-
      liquative, emaciazione, e ad un tale assideramento di tutta la potenza nervosa, che dopo
      essere stati a lungo vessati da tutti i fenomeni del più espresso languore, divengono anche
      maniaci, ed attentano per fino contro la propria vita cercando per la più d'estinguerla af-
      fogati nell'aqua'.
71   Ibid., 117ff.
72   Ibid., 112.
73   Ibid., 114.
74   Ibid., 109.

stomach, spleen, liver, the muscles, the nerves in the back, the urinary track, the genitals, the respiratory system, and, most fatally, the nervous system.[75]

Ruggieri also describes in detail the mental afflictions induced by pellagra, which is particularly revealing in view of his interest in Lovat's case. Under the headline 'notes upon the delirium', he sketches how those *pellagrosi* suffering from the typical delirium generally behave:

> [...] But the *deliranti* do not behave all the same: some are sad and distressed, they refuse food and drink, and do not answer a word if they are asked something; others are happy, jeer and gaggle; others murmur between their teeth and look grim; others even move their heads here and there, and make sounds like a belfry [...] In the first [delirium], the *pellagrosi* [...] laugh, cry; and in the second they are stupid, forgetful, and do not react to the impressions of any objects; the third [delirium], finally, which is the most frequent, is often religious, aghast, uncertain, sad, because of which the sick always desire to be close to ministers of religion; they believe that their imagination is disturbed by ideas to commit crimes that they probably never commit; and that domineer over them until total desperation; they are afraid of God's judgement, pray all night long; some meditate and immobile; if they are asked something, they would not respond; many flee from society, and walk around with an undecided anxiety. Under this condition of insuperable desolation they bawl, they strangle themselves with a cord, sometimes they throw themselves into a fire, but most often, they dive into fountains and rivers.[76]

---

75   Ibid., 109f.
76   Ibid., 11: '[...] Ma i deliranti non si portano tutti in pari modo; alcuni tristi ed attoniti ricusano il cibo e le bevande, nè interrogati rispondono alcuna parola; altri allegri, gridano e schiamazzano; altri mormorano fra denti con aspetto truce; altri finalmente agitando qua e là velocemente il capo mandano una voce simile al suono di un campanello. [...] Nella prima i pellagrosi [...] ridono, piangono; e nella seconda sono stupidi, smemorati, e neppure abbadano alle impressioni degli oggetti; la terza finalmente, che è la più frequente, spesso è religiosa, attonita, incerta, triste, per cui gli infermi bramano di aver sempre presenti e vicini i ministri della Religione, che rincorino la loro immaginazione turbata dall'idea di delitti, che forse non commisero, e che se li rappresentano per tiranneggiarsi fino alla disperazione; temono i giudizi di Dio, fan preci tutta la notte; alcuni meditabondi ed immobili, se vengono interrogati, non rispondono, moltissimi fuggono la frequenza degli uomini, e camminano qua e là con angoscia indecisione. Sotto questo stato d'invincibile scconfortamento inveiscono si strangolano appesi ad un laccio, qualche volta si gettano nel fuoco, ma più di frequente si slanciano ne' pozzi, e nei fiumi. Strambio chiama dromanio [sic!] questa tendenza, questa smodata cupidigia dei pellagrosi di precipitarsi nell'aqua'.

Compared with Ruggieri's few observations of Lovat's individual symptoms in the *Storia della crocifissione*, this description provided the reader with a general clinical picture and was obviously based on a number of cases. On the one hand, this implication of multiple observed cases corresponded to the genre of the dictionary which, in contrast to an individual case description, required to present general findings and doctrinal knowledge rather than single observations. On the other hand, it is likely that Ruggieri was in fact frequently faced with patients suffering from these symptoms: Before coming to Venice, Ruggieri had worked as a physician in several hospitals in the regions of Lombardy and Venetia, and Lovat's case was thus not the only one he had observed himself. However, that Ruggieri was able to depict such a detailed picture of the delirium induced by pellagra does not mean that he had solved the question of its causes. On the contrary, as Ruggieri recalled at the end of his article, '[...] the true nature of this disease is still an enigma, and this is why it is still arguable which cures are indicated, and the use of preventions, and of the various remedies that are proposed to cure it, are likewise dubious.'[77]

Considering the systematic discussion of pellagra published by Ruggieri in the *Dizionario cnciclopedico di chirurgia* in 1808 why did he not explain more clearly the connections between pellagra and Lovat's mental disorder in his case history? Other contemporary authors did connect their observations of the disease with new findings about mania. The physician Francesco Fanzago, for instance, explicitly referred to Philippe Pinel's study of mental diseases.[78] However, in the *Storia della crocifissione*, Ruggieri's concern was not to write a systematic study on pellagra, but to describe the empirical observations he had made in Lovat's particular case. As the genre demanded, he concentrated on what he had observed in Lovat's individual case, excluded the theoretical discussion to a great extent and only very cautiously provided some diagnostic explanations. By relating pellagra to mania and melancholy, Ruggieri invited the medical readers of his case history to further reflect upon the relations between mental disorder and pellagra – which only few of them would do.[79]

---

77   Ibid., 121: '[...] la vera natura adunque di questo morbo è ancora un enigma, e quindi ancora incerte faranno le indicazioni curative da seguirsi, e non sarà meno dubbiosa la convenienza de' provvedimenti, e dei varj rimedj suggeriti per guarirlo'.

78   F. Fanzago, *Sulle cause della pellagra. Memoria del Sig. Prof. Francesco Fanzago*, Padua, Tipografia del Seminario, 1809. The reference to Pinel is on 37f. The paper was already read in 1807 in the *Accademia di scienze, lettere ed arti di Padova*.

79   In particular German physicians were interested in pellagra as a new medical problem. Several reviews of German translations of Italian studies appeared in German enlightened journals. See for instance Anonymous, 'Michaeli Gherardini, Geschichte des Pellagra, aus dem Ital.', in F. Nicolai (ed.), *Neue allgemeine deutsche Bibliothek*, Kiel, Carl-Ernst

It was only in the 1930s, after long disputes over various theories of aetiology for the disease, that physicians declared pellagra a deficiency disease, caused by the lack of the vitamin B2. In the light of this knowledge, the causes of the nineteenth-century pellagra epidemic in Northern Italy retrospectively were understood in new terms. During the eighteenth century, the New World plant maize had replaced other cereals and had become the staple diet. As a consequence of the increasing consumption of maize, pellagra erupted in Northern Italy from the middle of the eighteenth century, in particular among the poor agrarian population. In the way people prepared maize in the Italian states in the form of the regional dish polenta, the grain lacked the niacin necessary to produce vitamin B2. A diet that was exclusively based on maize led to a deficiency of this vitamin and could cause severe physical and mental damage.[80]

Pellagra was the first diagnosis given for Lovat's case by Ruggieri in the *Storia della crocifissione*. Can we thus attribute Lovat's mental condition – and ultimately his self-crucifixion – to this particular disease, which still exists today in some areas of the Global South? Some modern historians of medicine and food have in fact cited Lovat's case as a famous example of the pellagra epidemic in nineteenth-century Italy.[81] But it is not the aim of this book to retrospectively diagnose Lovat. Disease concepts are historically contingent, and how physicians explain pellagra today is hardly identical with what the disease meant for Ruggieri and his contemporaries. In the long run, Ruggieri's initial diagnosis was only one of the many different readings of Lovat's case in the course of the nineteenth century, one that got lost quite early in the international discussion of Lovat's case, to be replaced by many alternative interpretations of the case.

6   A Unique Case?

Are there any other cases of self-crucifixion known in Italian or European history, before or after Lovat? And how did people respond to these cases? Like

Bohn, 1793, 90–91; Anonymous, 'Cajetan Strambio, Abhandlungen über das Pellagra', in F. Nicolai (ed.), *Neue allgemeine deutsche Bibliothek*, Kiel, Carl-Ernst Bohn, 1797, 157–158.

80   On the dispute over different pellagra aetiologies at the beginning of the twentieth century see D. Gentilcore, 'Louis Sambon and the Clash of Pellagra Etiologies in Italy and the United States, 1905–1914', *Journal of the History of Medicine and Allied Sciences*, vol. 71, no. 1, 2016, 19–42. See also Ch.S. Brian and Ch.R. Mull, 'Pellagra Pre-Goldberger: Rupert Blue, Fleming Sandwith, and The "Vitamine Hypothesis"', *Transactions of the American Clinical an Climatological Association*, vol. 126, 2015, 20–45.

81   D. Gentilcore, 'Peasants and Pellagra in Nineteenth-Century Italy', *History Today*, vol. 64, 2014, 32–38.

the other questions this chapter has dealt with, this is one that Lovat's case raised for the nineteenth-century commentators, but it is also one the historian has to deal with when exploring the history of Lovat's case. In his study on rituals of the Passion in Christendom, the anthropologist Peter Bräunlein has analysed the extraordinary role of crucifixion in Christian societies.[82] His ethnographic field is the Philippines, where collective self-crucifixion continues to be a form of a Catholic ritual even today. From the historical part of Bräunlein's study it is clear, however, that self-crucifixion was at no time officially recognized by the church as an orthodox religious practice, even if it was meant as such by those who tried it. On the contrary, the act was a rare exception and a controversial issue in Christian societies.

During the Middle Ages, the Cross became increasingly important in Christian belief. After it had lost its original use as an execution instrument in Roman law, it took centre stage as a symbol in high medieval Christian theology that focused strongly on the Passion of Christ. The visual representation of the Crucified and its cults were integrated into Roman liturgy, and several religious practices evolved that were directed at the imitation of the Passion, such as self-flagellation. The figure most often associated with such practices is St. Francis of Assisi, who formulated a mystical belief that concentrated on the physical imitation of Christ's Passion.[83] However, the imitation of the Passion has always been a tightrope walk between a socially accepted idea of *conformitas Christi* and heresy. While certain forms of martyrdom could be grounds for public devotion and, in the case of saints, even official recognition by the Church, others were not. The experience of physical stigmata, for instance, could be suspected to be the result of self-inflicted wounds and thus heresy, but it could also be admired as a divine sign. The few historical cases of self-crucifixion in Christian societies were generally seen as provocations. Depending on time and circumstances, self-crucifixion was understood either to be a work of the devil or as a criminal act. From the eighteenth century onwards, authorities increasingly looked at self-crucifixion from a medical perspective and, like in Lovat's case, considered it as an act of madness.[84]

While the publication of case narratives describing self-destructive actions motivated by religion abound in the eighteenth and nineteenth centuries,

---

82 P.J. Bräunlein, *Passion/Pasyon. Rituale des Schmerzes im europäischen und philippinischen Christentum*, Munich, Wilhelm Fink, 2010, see in particular his historical analysis 127–155.

83 Ibid., 138. On the crucial role of visual representations in the acceptance of S. Francis' stigmata, see A. Davidson, 'Miracles of Bodily Transformation, or, How St. Francis Received Stigmata', in C.A. Jones and P. Galison (eds.), *Picturing Science and Producing Art*, New York and London, Routledge, 1998, 101–124.

84 Bräunlein, *Passion/Pasyon*, 155.

reports on individual cases of self-crucifixion remained indeed rare.[85] One famous case from the nineteenth century is that of a Swiss woman called Margarethe Peter who believed to be destined to fight the devil. She forced her family and her adherents to join a cruel orgy of reciprocal torture and homicide, which culminated in her being crucified by the others.[86] Similar to Lovat's case, the narrative of Margarethe Peter's crucifixion circulated in nineteenth-century scientific and popular publications as an example of enthusiasm or religious madness, as described in Chapter 4.

Other known cases of crucifixion from the eighteenth and nineteenth centuries were collective enterprises that became an issue of public order. The most famous example of this kind are the so-called Convulsionists. These were a small group of adherents to Jansenism, a French Catholic movement considered heretical. In Paris in the 1730s, some adherents claimed that they experienced miraculous cures and convulsions at the tomb of one of the leaders of the group, and achieved broad public attention. The Catholic authorities did not recognise these putative miracles and, repressed by the police, a few men and women were said to have tried to crucify themselves as a means of gaining public attention.[87]

It would of course be misleading to equate the crucifixions of the Convulsionists or that of the Philippines with the self-crucifixion of one individual like Lovat. Whereas these were collective events happening within small social groups that gave meaning to them, Lovat's self-crucifixion was a singular case within a Catholic urban society that did not recognise such a practice as a legitimate expression of Christian belief. This does not mean, however, that at the beginning of the nineteenth century, religious interpretations of extraordinary events within the Venetian society did not persist. Other medical case histories published in Venice at the same time as Lovat's case suggest indeed that certain surprising phenomena such as a sudden healing, were sometimes

---

85   For examples of historical cases of crucifixion see C. Daxelmüller, 'Süße Nägel der Passion'. *Die Geschichte der Selbstkreuzigung von Franz von Assisi bis heute*, Düsseldorf, Patmos, 2001, 237–254 and P. Dinzelbacher, 'Diesseits der Metapher: Selbstkreuzigung und Stigmatisation als konkrete Kreuzesnachfolge', *Revue Mabillon*, vol. 7, 1996, 157–181.

86   The case is reported in I.H. Wessenberg, *Ueber Schwärmerei. Historisch-philosophische Betrachtungen mit Rücksicht auf die jetzige Zeit*, Heilbronn, Claßische Buchhandlung, 1835, 548–554.

87   On the convulsionists see C. Maire, *Les convulsionnaires de Saint-Medard. Miracles, convulsions et propheties à Paris au XVIIIe siècle*, Paris, Gallimard, 1985 and J. Goldstein, 'Enthusiasm or Imagination? Eighteenth-Century Smear Words in Comparative National Context', *Huntington Library Quaterly*, vol. 60, 1997, 29–49.

perceived as miracles, and were even attested as such by physicians.[88] But with Lovat's self-crucifixion, this was not the case. A medical view clearly prevailed, promoting the general understanding of Lovat's case as an extraordinary suicide resulting from insanity.

As this chapter has shown, this medical view was, first and foremost, the result of Lovat's admission to the Venetian hospitals, the Clinical School and the mental asylum San Servolo. The Venetian authorities clearly perceived Lovat's self-crucifixion as an extraordinary case, however, by hospitalising Lovat as a patient and by assigning broader disease categories, they also gave a clear signal as to how the case was to be understood and categorised – namely as a medical case. Appropriating Ruggieri's medical terms, the police, the Venetian tribunal of justice and the staff of San Servolo talked of mania or a melancholic delirium in order to refer to Lovat's mental disorder, but interestingly, they did not yet talk about pellagra – the notion that Lovat suffered from pellagra was firstly introduced and transmitted in Ruggieri's published case narrative. Although in this first correspondence on Lovat's case, the focus was on the man who crucified himself, Mattio Lovat himself remains largely obscure. We do have some personal statements from him, but even if we take them seriously, our understanding of his motives and his deeds remains limited. From the beginning, Lovat's case was therefore not so much constituted by his own voice, but by the framing of his self-crucifixion by other locals.

Implicitly more than explicitly, the different local commentators on the incident of the self-crucifixion asked what Lovat's case was essentially about: A suicide? A religious martyrdom? A case of madness? This framing of the case in the local context predetermined the production of a case *narrative* on Lovat's self-crucifixion. Ruggieri had a central role in shaping this narrative, by collecting the diverse local records, arranging them chronologically and suggesting possible disease explanations. He created a narrative sequence and put Lovat's case in the form of a medical case narrative, the *Storia della crocifissione*, which would soon travel in different guises from its place of origin, Venice, to new places in Europe.

---

88   See for instance the case history G.B. Savoldello, *Relazione della gravissima mortal malattia sofferta dalla neofita Elena Savorgnan e della sua perfetta guarigione istantanea ottenuta da Dio per intercessione de' Santi Martiri di Concordia estesa da Giovanni Battista Savoldello maestro e prefetto del pio luogo de' catumeni di Venezia e corredata di documenti autentici estratti dal processo istituito nella reverendissima cura patriarcale capitolare*, Venice, Nella Stamperia di Andrea Santini, 1807.

CHAPTER 2

The *Storia della Crocifissione* as an Epistemic Genre

This chapter studies the *Storia della crocifissione* as a medical publication in the local medical context of early nineteenth-century Venice. It aims to answer the broader questions of why Ruggieri wrote down and published Lovat's case history at all, and why he presented it in the specific narrative form it has. The chapter therefore examines various social spaces and debates in which Ruggieri participated in Venice, which affected the way that Ruggieri recorded and published Lovat's case. I suggest that the particularities of the *Storia della crocifissione* as a medical publication can best be understood if we consider it as an 'epistemic genre'. Gianna Pomata has introduced the notion of 'epistemic genres' as useful 'tools for the cultural history of knowledge'.[1] The concept is based on the premise that scientific texts should be distinguished from literary genres because of their particular purpose: epistemic genres are 'a specific kind of genre whose function is fundamentally cognitive, not aesthetic or expressive – that specific kind of genre whose primary goal is not the production of *meaning* but the production of *knowledge*'.[2] In contrast to literary genres, epistemic genres 'develop in tandem with scientific practices', and are 'directly related with the making and the transmission of knowledge'.[3]

In order to understand the *Storia della crocifissione*, the concept of epistemic genres is useful because as a medical case history, the text stands in the tradition of the *observationes*, an important epistemic genre of pre-modern medicine.[4] The *observationes* were collections of individual medical case histories, published in Latin by physicians and learned surgeons from the sixteenth century onwards.[5] They were used to communicate and to share practical knowledge,

---

1   G. Pomata, 'The Recipe and the Case: Epistemic Genres and the Dynamics of Cognitive Practices', in K. von Greyerz, S. Flurbacher, and P. Senn (eds.), *Wissenschaftsgeschichte und Geschichte des Wissens im Dialog – Connecting Science and Knowledge*, Göttingen, V&R unipress, 2013, 131–154.

2   Pomata, *The Medical Case Narrative*, 3.

3   Pomata, *The Recipe and the Case*, 133.

4   On the *observationes* as epistemic genre see G. Pomata, 'Observation Rising: Birth of an Epistemic Genre, ca. 1500–1650', in L. Daston and E. Lunbeck (eds.), *Histories of Scientific Observation*, Chicago, University of Chicago Press, 2011, 45–80.

5   Philologically, the genre originated from an ancient concept of observation in the context of astronomy and medicine, see G. Pomata, 'A Word of the Empirics: The Ancient Concept of Observation and its Recovery in Early Modern Medicine', *Annals of Science*, vol. 68, no. 1, 2011, 1–25. The *observationes* developed from the hybridisation of two other epistemic genres

that is, knowledge that derived from the physicians' medical practice and first-hand experience.[6] While the recording of cases goes back to Hippocratic medicine, the novelty of the *observationes* in Renaissance medicine was that for the first time in the history of medicine, physicians invented a genre that was dedicated solely to the description and communication of individual cases.[7] As Pomata writes, 'From late antiquity throughout the middle ages, cases could be found, as anecdotes or exempla, in a variety of medical texts, such as textbooks of practical medicine, biographies and autobiographies of physicians, treatises on specific diseases. But these narrative accounts of the treatment of single patients were to be found in the folds of the text, so to speak: they did not emerge as a genre on their own'.[8] The *observationes*, by contrast, brought the individual case to the fore. This chapter studies the ways in which Ruggieri interacted with this pre-modern tradition of the *observationes* when publishing the *Storia della crocifissione*. In order to publish Lovat's case in the form of an individual medical case history, he appropriated and adapted the genre according to his individual professional needs.

The notion of epistemic genres introduced by Pomata maintains not only that they are the 'vehicle of a cognitive project',[9] it is also based on the view that a genre is always a form of social action: 'As shared textual conventions, genres are intrinsically social. Contributing to a genre means consciously joining a community; indeed, some genres are eminently instruments of "community-building", tools for the establishment of a community of scholarly endeavour as a social and intellectual shared space'.[10] For this reason, studying the *Storia della crocifissione* as an epistemic genre means more than paying attention to its formal textual features: it requires to learn more about its author, Cesare Ruggieri, and to examine the concrete professional and social spaces to which he was associated in Venice and beyond. Which intellectual community did Ruggieri seek to join by publishing the *Storia della crocifissione*? What professional agenda did he pursue when publishing his case history? And which actors,

---

in medicine, the recipe and the commentary, and prospered within the medical science during the Early Modern Period, in close relation with a renewed emphasis on empiricism, see G. Pomata, '*Praxis Historialis*: The Uses of *Historia* in Early Modern Medicine', G. Pomata and N.G. Siraisi (eds.), *Empiricism and Erudition in Early Modern Europe*, Cambridge, MA and London, MIT Press, 2005, 105–146, 135; G. Pomata, '"Observatio" ovvero "Historia". Note su empirismo e storia in età moderna', *Quaderni storici*, no. 91, 1996, 175–198.

6   Pomata, *Sharing Cases.*
7   Pomata, *The Recipe and the Case,* 149.
8   Ibid.
9   Ibid., 134.
10   Pomata, *Sharing Cases,* 197.

institutions and ideas have in turn influenced Ruggieri's writing of Lovat's case in the Venetian medical context?

1   Cesare Ruggieri: A 'Scientific' Surgeon

As a Professor of Surgery at the beginning of the nineteenth century, Ruggieri embodied the new type of a learned surgeon. His academic career is emblematic for the rise of surgeons to medical specialists, a development, which happened in the course of the eighteenth century.[11] Before that time, surgery had for centuries been considered an inferior art in Western European medicine. Academic physicians tended to rely on the primacy of theory and doctrine above empiricism, and because they considered surgery a manual art, they denied surgery the status of a proper science. In a German encyclopaedic dictionary from the middle of the eighteenth century, for instance, the competences of surgeons are described as limited to interventions on external bodily parts: 'The task of a surgeon (*Wund-Arzt*) is (1) to bring together those parts that are separated; (2) to repair, to put in the right order and to heal those parts that are fractured and dislocated; (3) to artificially remove superfluous parts; (4) to replace what is lacking; (5) to rearrange what is malformed, buckled and stiff. In all this, the surgeon has to keep in mind three things: he has to heal (1) fast, (2) good and without pain, (3) and safely'.[12] In the same dictionary, the author of an article on 'the art of surgery' admits, however, that 'it is difficult to define

---

11   See T. Gelfand, *Professionalizing Modern Medicine. Paris Surgeons and Medical Science and Institutions in the 18th Century*, Westport, CT and London, Greenwood Press, 1980 and J. Doyle, 'The Spectre of the Scalpel: The Historical Role of Surgery and Anatomy in Conceptions of Embodiment', *Body and Society*, vol. 14, no. 1, 2008, 9–30. On the leadership of French surgery see C.C. Gillispie, *Science and Polity in France at the End of the Old Regime*, Princeton, Princeton University Press, 1980, 203–212. On the local context of Venice see N. Vanzan Marchini, *Dalla scienza medica alla pratica dei corpi. Fonti e manoscritti per la storia della sanità*, Venice, Neri Pozza, 1993, in particular the chapter 'La chirurgia europea e gli 'atti' dei Collegi Veneziani', 45–60.

12   Anonymous, 'Wund-Artzt', in J.H. Zedler (ed.), *Grosses vollständiges Universallexikon aller Wissenschaften und Künste*, vol. 59, Leipzig and Halle, Johann Heinrich Zedler, 1749, 1490–1511, 1490: 'Das Amt eines Wund-Arztes bestehet darinne, daß er suchen muß, (1) dasjenige, so von einander gesondert, zusammen zu bringen; (2) das Zerbrochene und Verrenckte einzurichten, zu rechte zu bringen, und wieder zu heilen; (3) das Ueberflüßige künstlich wegzunehmen; (4) das Mangelhaffte zu ersetzen; (5) das Uebel beschaffene, Krumme und Steiffe in eine, so viel möglich, andere Ordnung zu bringen. In diesen allen hat ein Wund-Arzt drey Dinge wohl zu beachten, als, daß er (1) geschwind, (2) gut und ohne Schmertzen, und (3) sicher heile'.

the actual competences of a surgeon of our days', because the surgeons would tend to transgress the sphere of physicians.[13]

Indeed, over the course of the eighteenth century, the status of surgery gradually changed. Many cities in Europe founded schools of surgery in hospitals, and surgeons increasingly gained academic reputation. As a consequence, learned surgeons set themselves apart from the purely practical surgeons who had traditionally belonged to the group of the barbers and other healing professions. The learned surgeons now sought to ally themselves with academic physicians and wanted their art to be recognised as a proper science, on a par with medicine. By 1800, the status of surgery had changed utterly. As Roy Porter put it, 'within a century, the surgeon had further risen in status to become, perhaps, the most fashionable of all the medical practitioners'.[14]

In Venice as elsewhere in Europe, the surgeons' call for more autonomy and recognition had led to conflicts and rivalry. Gradually, however, a new understanding of the surgeons' role was established. Criticising the traditional separation of surgery and medicine, medical authors emphatically called for an alliance of medicine and surgery. The Venetian physician Francesco Bernardi, for instance, published a detailed history of Venetian surgery in 1797.[15] In his double role of a *medico-fisico* and learned surgeon, Bernardi argued for a specialised academic education of surgeons, and stressed the distinction between 'scientific' surgeons on the one hand, and simple surgeons and barbers on the other. By distributing his works to medical colleagues beyond Venice, Bernardi sought to communicate the importance of Venetian surgery to an international audience.[16]

---

13 Ibid.: 'Es ist aber schwer zu bestimmen, was eigentlich für welche heutiges Tages zur Chirurgie gehören [...]'.

14 R. Porter, 'The Eighteenth Century', in L.I. Conrad et al. (eds.), *The Western Medical Tradition 800 BC to AD 1800*, Cambridge, UK, Cambridge University Press, 1995, 371–476, 439.

15 F. Bernardi, *Prospetto storico-critico dell'origine, facoltà, diversi stati, progressi, e vicende dell collegio medico-chirurgico, e dell'arte chirurgica in Venezia. Arricchito d'aneddoti interessanti l'italiana letteratura, utilissimo alla disciplina dell'arte medica ed alla comun salute*, Venice, Dalle stampe del cittadino Domenico Costantini, 1797.

16 In the appendix to Bernardi's printed work conserved in the *Biblioteca Marciana* in Venice, we find manuscript documents regarding his correspondence with European libraries. The sources Bernardi used for his compilation derived from the archive of the *Collegio medico* itself; this archive was destroyed in 1800 when the whole site of the Collegio Medico-Chirurgico together with the anatomical theater burned down, see the chapter 'Il teatro anatomico di S. Giacomo dell'Orio' in Vanzan Marchini, *Dalla scienza medica alla pratica dei corpi*, 61–70.

As a professor of Surgery, Ruggieri was a representative of the new 'scientific' surgeons.[17] He was deeply rooted in the medical culture of Northern Italy, in particular that of Venice and Padua.[18] Born on 12 November 1766 in Crema, a small town in the north Italian region of Cremona, he received a deep humanistic education.[19] After several years of medical training, he gained a first university degree in surgery from the University of Pavia in 1790 with a surgical dissertation.[20] Consequently, he went to Milan to deepen his knowledge in surgery and anatomy while working as an assistant in the city's main hospital.[21]

---

17   Ruggieri's biography has hitherto remained unstudied. To reconstruct Ruggieri's career, I use two main sources: first, an autograph of Ruggieri conserved in the archive of the University of Padua, that is a table that was produced on the occasion of Ruggieri's appointment as Professor at the University of Padova in 1815, listing the single steps of his academic career: Padova, Archivio Generale di Ateneo, Archivio dell'Ottocento, atti del rettorato, 1817, b. 17 (in the following referred to as *Autograph of Cesare Ruggieri*). The second source is a glorifying description of Ruggieri's life, the funeral speech held by the physician Floriano Caldani on the occasion of Ruggieri's death: F. Caldani, *Discorso funebre recitato nella chiesa di Santa Maria de' servi di Padova il giorno xv di febbrajo dell'anno MDCCCXXVIII nelle solenni esequie del Professore Cesare Ruggieri professore di clinica chirurgia nell'I.R. università colla descrizione della sezione anatomica del suo cadavere*, Padua, Coi Tipi della Minerva, 1828. An almost complete copy of the speech is contained in: M.G. Levi, *Ricordo intorno agli incliti medici chirughi e farmacisti che praticarono loro arte in Venezia dopo il 1740 raccolti aumentati e pubblicati da M.G. Levi...*, Venice, Tipografia di Giuseppe Antonelli, 1835, 56–59. Scattered information on Ruggieri can be found in G. Dandolo, *La caduta della repubblica di Venezia ed i suoi ultimi cinquant'anni*, Venice, Coi tipi di Pietro Naratovich, 1855, 231–233; F. Sforza Benvenuti, 'Ruggieri Cesare', in F. Sforza Benvenuti (ed.), *Dizionario biografico cremasco*, Crema, Forni, 1888, 247f., cited after Bandirali, *Storia della crocifissione*, 43–44.

18   On Venetian medical culture see N. Vanzan Marchini, 'La politica sanitaria e i medici riformatori', in N. Vanzan Marchini (ed.), *I mali e i rimedi della serenissima*, Venice, Neri Pozza, 1995, 157–194; N. Vanzan Marchini, *La memoria della salute. Venezia e il suo ospedale dal xvi al xx secolo*, Venice, Arsenale, 1985; Archivio di Stato di Venezia (ed.), *Difesa della sanità a Venezia, secoli XIII–XIX, catalogo della mostra documentaria*, Venice, Ministero per i beni culturali e ambientali, 1979; U. Stefanutti, *Documentazioni cronologiche per la storia della medicina, chirurgia e farmacia in Venezia*, Venice, Ongania, 1961. On the Italian medical context in general see F. della Peruta (ed.), *Storia d'Italia. Annali. Vol. 7: Malattia e medicina*, Turin, Einaudi, 1984.

19   Caldani, *Discorso funebre*, 9.

20   See A. Maggiolo, *I soci dell'academia pataviana dalla sua fondazione (1599)*, Padua, Accademia Padavina di scienze, lettere, ed arti, 1983, 285. The title of Ruggieri's doctoral dissertation was *De capitis humeri luxatione, et de colli ejusdem fractura simultanea. Diss. anat. chir. Cremae, 1790*, see *Autograph of Cesare Ruggieri*. Strangely, the title is almost identical with a French doctoral thesis published in Paris in 1786: P. Gallée, *De capitis humeri luxatione et colli ejusdem fractura simultanea. Dissertatio anatomico-chirurgica*, Paris, Typis Michaelis Lambert, 1786.

21   Caldani, *Discorso funebre*, 9.

In the following years, Ruggieri travelled around in Europe for educational purposes spending some time in Spain where he became a member of the Royal Academy of Science in Madrid.[22] In 1789, he undertook journeys to London and Paris in order to be instructed by important professors of medicine and surgery.[23] After having refused a job offer from the main hospital of Genoa, Ruggieri temporarily turned back to his hometown Crema to replace the chief surgeon of the local hospital.[24]

Thanks to his increasing professional reputation, Venetian authorities invited Ruggieri to be employed in the service of the city of Venice. He arrived in Venice in 1798, thus one year after the fall of the Venetian Republic,[25] and settled in the neighbourhood of *San Marco* together with his wife and his younger brother Gaetano Ruggieri, who was a physician as well.[26] By that time, it was indispensible for physicians to have a degree from the University of Padua or from the Venetian schools to be allowed to practise medicine in Venice: in 1791, the *Magistrato alla Sanità*, the Venetian magistracy responsible for sanitary matters, had even re-enacted an old law in this regard.[27] This explains why Ruggieri hastened to receive his second degree as a *medico fisico* in Padua in 1800.[28]

---

22   Ibid., 10.

23   This date of his journey to Paris is mentioned in a pathography of Ruggieri, published as an appendix to the funeral speech by Caldani: 'Lettera del Signore Dottor Vittore Fabris Membro della facoltà di medicina nell'I.R. università di Padova chirurgo onorario municipale della pia casa di Ricovero e del pio ospitale degl'infermi al chiarissimo Signore Professore F. Caldani intorno alla sezione anatomica eseguita sul cadavere del Professore Ruggieri', ibid., 27.

24   Ibid., 10.

25   Ibid., 10f. He had received this invitation already during the time of the Venetian Republic by a certain Francesco Pesaro who held the important office of a *Procuratore di S. Marco*, see ibid., 10.

26   Ruggieri was married to a certain Antonia Bonaldi Fogaroli from Milan, see Caldani's dedication of the speech in ibid. Ruggieri was Antonia's second husband, as indicated by the inscription of Ruggieri's funeral stone on the cimetary, see the appendix to ibid. According to a register which records the inhabitants of Venice in the year 1805 they lived in the area of *San Marco*, contrada S. Basso, in the Street Corte de la Trevisan No. 344, see Archivio Comunale di Venezia, Serie Anagrafe, Prima Dominazione Austriaca, anagrafi generale 1805, letters RA-RE. Ruggieri's social status is denoted 'civile' and his profession 'chirurgo'. On Gaetano Ruggieri see M.G. Levi, *Biografia di Gaetano Alfonso Ruggieri, medico e letterato veneziano. Scritta da Mosè Giuseppe Levi, medico e letta nel veneto ateneo la tornata del giorno 19 Dicembre 1836*, s.l., s.n., 1836.

27   See the transcripts in N. Vanzan Marchini (ed.), *Le leggi di sanità della repubblica di Venezia*, vol. 1, Venice, Neri Pozza, 1995, 422 and 392. The first time that a law in this matter was enacted was already in the fifteenth century, see Vanzan Marchini, *La politica sanitaria*, 163.

28   *Autograph of Cesare Ruggieri*: 'Dottore in Medicina e Chirurgia laureato nell'I.R. Università di Padova nell' 1800 giugno'.

The following years were characterised by political upheaval leading to changing governments of the city of Venice. During the period of the first Austrian Government (1798–1806), the traditional medical hierarchies were shaken up, and sanitary structures in Venice were completely reorganised.[29] Working his way up, Ruggieri profited from these structural reorganisations. He took over one medical post after another within the Austrian and later the French magistracies (1806–1814). His medical specialty gradually expanded: Ruggieri's first job in 1798 was to control the production of Venetian pharmacies, and to advise the government in questions of medical-surgical policy and reform.[30] In 1801, the Austrian *Governo Generale* also put him in charge of the inoculation of the public against the pox (*Delegato Generale al Pubblico Innesto Vajolo*).[31] Two years later, he was nominated as the official surgeon of the *Direzione Generale di Polizia* as well as a medical consultant of the *Tribunale di Giustizia*.[32] He also served as the secretary of an interim medical commission established to advise the government in all matters of sanitary reform regarding the city of Venice and the broader region of Venetia.[33] Still in 1803, he was appointed Professor of Surgery (*Pubblico Professore di Clinica Chirurgia*) in a newly established clinical school for surgery, the *Scuola Clinica di Chirurgia*.[34] This was the very place where he treated Lovat after his self-crucifixion in 1805.

Ruggieri managed to pursue his career successfully under French rule, too. After Venice had been taken over by Napoleon's *Regno d'Italia* in 1806, Viceroy Eugene Napoleon nominated him a member of the *Commissione Dipartimentale di sanità dell'Adriatico*, the newly established sanitary commission.[35] At the same time, his former post related to vaccination was renewed, which he kept until 1815.[36] Ruggieri finally received a Professorship at the University of Padua, the most important step in the career of any Venetian physician. In 1815, he was appointed provisional Professor,[37] and was definitively elected

---

29   See Gottardi, *L'Austria a Venezia*, 24–77 and J.A. Davis, 'Health Care and Poor Relief in Southern Europe in the 18th and 19th Centuries', in O.P. Grell, A. Cunningham, and B. Roeck (eds.), *Health Care and Poor Relief in 18th and 19th Century Southern Europe*, Aldershot, Ashgate, 2005, 10–33.

30   *Autograph of Cesare Ruggieri.*

31   Ibid. Ruggieri kept this office also during the French government (1806–1814), see the documents in ASV, Prefettura dell'Adriatico (1806–1814), b. 85 (= anno 1807), fasc. 13.

32   *Autograph of Cesare Ruggieri.*

33   Ibid.

34   Ibid.

35   See the document of the official appointment in ASV, Prefettura dell'Adriatico (1806–1814), b. 85 (= anno 1807), fasc. 83.

36   *Autograph of Cesare Ruggieri.*

37   Ibid.

Professore di Chirurgia Pratica e Clinica in 1817.[38] He kept this post until he died in Padua on the 13 February 1828.[39]

With his double university degree in medicine and surgery, Ruggieri stood at the top of the hierarchy of the health professions in Venice. During the time of the old Republic, the Venetian sanitary market had been characterised by the competition of many different professional groups, such as the *barbieri* (barbers), *spezieri* (pharmacists) and *charlatani* (quacks).[40] The physicians and surgeons were organised in the *Collegio Medico-Fisico* and the *Collegio Medico-Chirurgico* respectively. While the *medici-fisici* had full rights to make diagnoses and to decide about therapies and surgical interventions, the *medici-chirurgici* were only allowed to practise after a special exam and by order of a *medico-fisico*.[41] Since the fourteenth century and up to its dissolution in 1806, the *Collegio Medico-Fisico* controlled the medical practice and organised the medical provision for the city of Venice,[42] and every physician practising in Venice had to be registered with this organisation.[43]

While other resident doctors in Venice were either employed as *medici di contrada* or *medici delle fraterne* (also called *medici condotti*), or had to look for their clients on the free market as *ventuniere*,[44] Ruggieri made his career as an employee of changing governments in universities and hospitals. He was part of juridical processes in which medical expertise was required. For instance,

---

38 Ibid. See also the *Ausweis über alle bei der königlichen Universität in Padua angestellten Professoren, ausgestellt von der Königlichen Polizei...Kommissariat Padua, 27. April 1817,* contained in the manuscript collection of documents of the *Direzione Generale di Polizia* conserved in the Biblioteca Correr: BMC, Direzione Generale di Polizia, Documenti, 1–146, 1799–1823.

39 Ruggieri was buried in Padua, see Sforza Benvenuti, *Dizionario biografico cremasco*, 148. It does not lack irony that after his death, he was the subject of an anatomical case history himself, which is included as an appendix in Caldani's funeral speech. The *Lettera del Signore Dottor Vittore Fabris* [...] *intorno alla sezione anatomica eseguita sul cadavere del Professore Ruggieri* was written by an assistant of Caldani, a certain Vittore Fabris, who had carried out the dissection of Ruggieri's body. The description combines a pathography of Ruggieri's life with a detailed report of the post mortem examination of Ruggieri's cadaver, see Caldani, *Discorso funebre*, 23–28.

40 See Vanzan Marchini, *La politica sanitaria*, 162–165.

41 See the respective laws from the year 1321 and the year 1608 edited in: Vanzan Marchini, *Le leggi di sanità della repubblica di Venezia*, 377 and 379.

42 See V. Giormani, *I collegi dei medici fisici e dei medici chirurghi a Venezia nel settecento*, Pisa and Rome, Fabrizio Serra, 2007.

43 V. Giormani, 'I rapporti tra i due collegi veneziani, dei filosofi e medici e dei chirurghi, con l'università di Padova nel settecento', in G.P. Brizzi and J. Verger (eds.), *Le università minori in Europa (secoli XV–XIX)*, Soveria Mannelli, Rubbettino, 1998, 169–181, 181.

44 On these figures see Vanzan Marchini, *I mali e i rimedi*, 166–168.

Ruggieri was involved in the so-called *processo al moro*, a tragic Venetian criminal case. In 1811, a black man had killed his white pregnant girlfriend because
the Napoleonic laws prohibited a marriage between black and white people.
Both were servants in the same *palazzo* of a noble Venetian family. Together
with his colleague Francesco Aglietti, Ruggieri was an expert witness during
the trial. He had to judge whether the murderer of the Venetian servant suffered from a physical disease or from a mental disorder.[45] Lovat's case was thus
not the only occasion in which Ruggieri had to evaluate mental conditions of
patients. Indeed, he had a particular interest for legal cases which involved a
psychological dimension – an interest which he shared with many contemporary physicians who tried to advance medical expertise in the domain of law.

In line with his academic career, Ruggieri's self-understanding was that of
an academic surgeon who, in terms of professional hierarchy, was on a par if
not above physicians. This becomes clear when reading his inaugural lecture
Prolusione intorno ai progressi ed avvanzamenti della chirurgia (on the advancement of surgery over the centuries), which Ruggieri gave at the occasion
of the opening of the Clinical School in 1803.[46] Outlining the history of surgery
since Antiquity, Ruggieri stressed the chronological anteriority of surgery with
respect to medicine, and the equal practice of surgery and medicine by the
first surgeons up to Hippocrates.[47] Following Ruggieri's account, it was due to
Christian reservations against a bloody trade that surgery then came to be considered an inferior art and was to remain so for many centuries.[48] Thanks to

---

45   See the edition of the trial by G. Scarabello and V. Gusso, *Processo al moro. Razzismo, follia,
      amore e morte*, Rome, Jouvence, 2000. See especially the chapter called 'Il problema della
      "malattia morale"', 37–44, and the 'Verbale del processo' on 91–180; Ruggieri's contribution
      is on 132f.

46   C. Ruggieri, *Prolusione intorno ai progressi ed avvanzamenti della chirurgia recitata nel sa-
      cro collegio de' medici fisici di Venezia per l'apertura della scuola di clinica chirurgica dal
      Dr. Cesare Ruggieri medico fisico, e R. Prof. della scuola suddetta, il giorno 25. agosto 1803*,
      Venice, Per Gio, Antonio Perlini, 1803, III-XXXVII. Francesco Aglietti also gave a lecture
      in which he talked about the art of clinical observation as the core instrument of the
      medical science, see F. Aglietti, *Saggio sopra la costanza delle leggi fondamentali dell'arte
      medica. Discorso accademico di Francesco Aglietti P.P. di Clinica*, Venice, Dalla Stamperia
      Palese, 1804. Usually, all the normal teaching lessons took place in the Ospitaletto, see
      P.L. Bembo, *Delle istituzioni di beneficenza nella città e provincia di Venezia. Studii storico
      economico-statistici*, Venice, Nella Tipografia di P. Naratovich, 1859, 270. The inaugural lec-
      tures were held in the Collegio dei Medici on the campo S. Giacomo dell'Orio. This is the
      place were also the Venetian anatomical theatre, called *Teatro anatomico di S. Giacomo
      dell'Orio*, was situated. On this institution see Vanzan Marchini, *Dalla scienza medica alla
      pratica dei corpi*, 61–70.

47   Ruggieri, *Prolusione intorno ai progressi ed avvanzamenti della chirurgia*, VII.

48   Ibid., IX.

the breakthroughs in anatomy, surgery then regained its reputation.[49] In his speech, Ruggieri emphatically lamented the negative effects of the long separation of medicine and surgery, and recalled the contributions that surgery had made to other branches of medicine, such as midwifery and the treatment of eye diseases.[50] For Ruggieri, surgeons possessed the greatest power of saving human lives, and therefore deserved people's respect.[51]

Ruggieri's effort to enhance the status of surgery as a medical specialty is also evidenced by what was probably his most time-consuming publication. Between 1805 and 1810, he translated an important French encyclopaedia of surgery into Italian, the *Encyclopédie méthodique chirurgie*.[52] The six Italian volumes included many additional articles written by Ruggieri.[53] Clearly, this work had made him familiar with the advanced status of surgery in French medicine as well as with the rhetoric used to fight for an alliance of surgery and medicine. In their foreword to the first volume, the French editors of the *Encyclopédie méthodique chirurgie*, Petit-Radel and De la Roche, claimed that the old separation should be abolished because 'medicine and surgery are sisters' with the equal right to be considered 'sciences'.[54]

Clearly, Ruggieri's professional and intellectual community was that of the new 'scientific' surgeons. His understanding of their social role went even beyond the realm of medicine. This becomes clear when reading the published inaugural speech which he gave on the occasion of his appointment as professor of surgery at Padua in 1823.[55] Here, Ruggieri depicted the physician – and

---

49   Ibid.

50   Ibid., xxivf.

51   Ibid., xxv.

52   D. de la Roche and P. Petit Radel (eds.), *Encyclopédie méthodique, chirurgie, publié par une société de médecins*, vols. 1 and 2, Paris, Panckoucke, 1790–1792; vol. 3, Paris, H. Agasse, 1798–1799.

53   C. Ruggieri, *Dizionario enciclopedico di chirurgia, tradotto dal francese in italiano ed accresciuto di aggiunte e note di Cesare Ruggieri medico fisico e chirurgo e regio pubblico professore di clinica chirurgica in Venezia*, Padua, Nella Stamperia del Seminario presso Tommaso Bettinelli, 1805–1810.

54   Ruggieri, *Dizionario enciclopedico di chirurgia*, vol. 1, VII: '[...] la medicina e la chirurgia sono sorelle [...]' and IX: '[...] Il sapere del medico non merita meglio il nome di scienza di quello del chirurgo bene istrutto delle funzioni dell'economia animale [...]'. This metaphor was also used by other contemporary medical writers, see for instance G.A. del Chiappa, *Della stretissima unione della medicina e della chirurgia. Lezione accademica tenuta nella grand'aula dell'imp. r. università di Pavia il dì 14 Dicembre in occasione di laure dottorale*, Pavia, Nella Tipografia di Pietro Bizzoni successore di Bolzani, 1820, 27: '[...] e che e medici e chirurghi si riunischino insieme, anzi quasi sotto un medesimo tetto raccolgansi, siccome membri e figli di una istessa famiglia'.

55   C. Ruggieri, *Dei doveri di chi studia e di chi esercita la medicina. Discorso inaugurale letto nella grande aula dell'imp.reg.università di Padova nel giorno XXX novembre MDCCCXXIII*

he included surgeons – as deeply involved in various aspects of civic life. He reminded his students that the medical science, including surgery, was the most universal of all sciences.[56] The physician's expertise would often reach beyond medicine, especially into the domain of law and religion.[57] Practising medicine would therefore not only require a broad humanistic education,[58] but its representatives, in particular forensic doctors, would also have to play an important social and moral role.[59] In Ruggieri's words, the ideal physician would have to serve 'simultaneously as instructor, as magistrate, as priest; in one word, he becomes the guardian angel (*angelo tutelare*)' who triumphs over societal subversion.[60] As we shall see in the course of this chapter, this self-understanding of Ruggieri shines not only through the *Storia della crocifissione*, but also characterises his other publications.

2   Observing the Case: Making Empirical Knowledge

Right after Lovat's self-crucifixion, Ruggieri had arranged for Lovat to be brought to the Venetian Clinical School for Surgery.[61] Several hints in the *Storia della crocifissione* suggest that Ruggieri's intention was not only to render first aid and to heal Lovat's self-inflicted injuries, but that it was in his personal interest to treat Mattio Lovat in order to make him an object of further medical study. During his visits at Lovat's bedside, students always surrounded Ruggieri: 'I observed him constantly, and I made my students observe him [...]'.[62] Concerned that Lovat would not like to speak in front of his students, Ruggieri also spent some time alone at Lovat's bedside to inquire about the reasons for his self-crucifixion.[63] When compiling Lovat's case history one year after the incident, Ruggieri drew on these inquiries and first-hand observations he had made at Lovat's bedside during the weeks when Lovat was under his care in the autumn of 1805. The Venetian Clinical School is therefore the place that

dal Dott. Cesare Ruggieri p.o. prof. di clinica, terapia speciale e di operazioni chirurgiche, Padua, Nella tipografia del seminario, 1824. This date is mentioned in Caldani, *Discorso funebre*, 8.

56   Ruggieri, *Dei doveri di chi studia e di chi esercita la medicina*, 5.
57   Ibid., 7.
58   Ibid., 8f.
59   Ibid., 30.
60   Ibid., 31: '[...] esercita in un sol tempo le funzioni d'istruttore, di magistrato, di sacerdote, in una parola diventa l'angelo tutelare, che trionfa del flagello sterminatore'.
61   Ruggieri, *Storia della crocifissione*, 10.
62   Ibid., 15: 'Osservai costantemente, e lo feci osservare a' miei pratici [...]'.
63   Ibid., 13.

links the genre of the *Storia della crocifissione* to medical practice. Ruggieri's text documents the epistemic practice of observing as well as the empirical knowledge he gained from working with Lovat's case in this institution.

The *Scuola di Clinica Chirurgica* had been created by decree of the Austrian government in the summer of 1803, as part of the Venetian hospital *Derelitti*, called *Ospedaletto* by the locals.[64] The new institution was advertised in an announcement to the Venetian public which criticised the lack of possibilities for medical students to gain practical experience after their graduation, and claimed that the new provisional institution would compensate for this:

> We have had the experience that many students of medicine and surgery do not have sufficient practice in the art of healing diseases [...]. This is why the General government has decided to provisionally establish a clinical school in Venice in which they can, at the bedside of the patient, improve their skills in the scientific practice of healing, under the instruction of the two famous professors doctor Aglietti for medicine and doctor Ruggieri for surgery [...].[65]

The Venetian Clinical School had about 30 patients, with a majority of surgical cases.[66] The patients were either selected from the main hospital, or admitted directly when the professors deemed them to be interesting and useful enough to instruct the students in the 'scientific practice of healing'. According to their ailments, the patients were placed either in the medical section under the care of Francesco Aglietti, or Cesare Ruggieri treated them in the surgical section. The two professors instructed six medical attendants. Using the method of

---

64   ASV, Deputazione alle cause pie, b. 33 (=anno 1803), n. 264 ('Decreto del governo generale n. 12199/227', 1803, 15 luglio). The document is signed by the head of the *Governo generale* in this period, Conte Ferdinand von Bissingen-Nippenburg, a Tirolese with German origins.

65   Bembo, *Delle istituzioni di beneficenza nella città e provincia di Venezia*, 269f.: 'Avendo l'esperienza fatto conosccre [sic!] che molti studenti in medicina ed in chirurgia non riescono valenti nell'arte di curare le malattie, quali essere dovrebbero in grazia dei loro talenti, perchè dopo ottenuto il grado accademico non vengono educati a dovere nello studio pratico; perciò l'Imp. Regio Governo generale è venuto in deliberazione d'istituire interinalmente una Scuola Clinica anche in Venezia, mediante la quale possano istruirsi al letto dell'ammalato nella pratica scientifica del medicare, sotto la disciplina dei due riputati Professori, dottore Aglietti per la Medicina e dottore Ruggeri [sic!] per la Chirurgia. [...]'. The document dates from the first August 1803 and is signed by a certain Piccioli who belonged to the medical advisors of the government.

66   I have deduced the following details from an account of costs of the *Ospedaletto* dating from 1804 in: ASV, Deputazione alle cause pie, b. 33 (=anno 1803), n. 317/864 ('26. Genn. 1804, Voto del N.H. Aggiunto sopra supplica dell'agente dell'ospedale dei derelitti accompagnante spesa della scuola clinica').

bedside teaching, they taught them how to observe and treat patients, that is, how to transform theoretical knowledge into practice. Due to a lack of funding, however, the institution was shut down already by the end of 1805.[67]

As a special division of a general hospital that served the practical education of medical students, the Venetian Clinical School mirrors a broader development in European medicine at the time: a renewed emphasis on medical practice, and, as a consequence, the introduction of systematic medical teaching in hospitals. Revising Michel Foucault's famous argument about 'the birth of the clinic' around 1800,[68] Othmar Keel has argued that rather than being a sudden invention of Parisian physicians only, this 'clinical medicine' developed at various medical institutions in European cities in the period between roughly 1750 and 1815.[69] In the Italian states, the idea of establishing a clinical school where students were to be instructed at the bedside of patients even had pre-modern roots. The hospital of San Francesco in Padua is said to have already introduced bedside teaching and the recording of individual cases in the sixteenth century.[70] In the context of a Europe-wide revaluation of medical practice at the end of the eighteenth century, many physicians considered clinical schools to be the most reliable source for the production and transmission of empirical knowledge gained through first-hand observation.[71]

Only this broader context explains why, in the years following the fall of the Venetian Republic in 1797, the first Austrian Government in Venice (1798–1806) was eager to establish a medical school in Venice. Within the Austrian Empire, to which Venice then belonged, the Vienna hospitals provided a model. Under the reign of Joseph II, the Vienna medical school had systematised and

---

67   A. Pelizza, 'Da "alberghi informi di ammalati" a "fortunati nosocomiali ritiri". Gli ospedali maggiori veneziani tra la fine della repubblica veneta e le riforme italiche', *Studi veneziani*, vol. 60, 2010, 415–486, 454. See also P. Zannini, *Biografia di Francesco Aglietti*, Padua, Coi tipi della Minerva, 1836, 20.

68   M. Foucault, *La naissance de la clinique. Une archéologie du regard medical*, Paris, Presses universitaire de France, 1963. On 'Paris medicine' see C. Hannaway and A. La Berge (eds.), *Constructing Paris Medicine*, Amsterdam, Rodopi, 1998; E.H. Ackerknecht, *Medicine at the Paris Hospital, 1794–1848*, Baltimore, Johns Hopkins University Press, 1967; E.H. Ackerknecht, 'Die Pariser Spitäler von 1800 als Ausgangspunkt einer neuen Medizin', *Ciba-Sympoisum 7*, 1959, 98–105.

69   O. Keel, *L'avènement de la médecine clinique moderne en Europe 1750–1815*, Montreal, Presses de l'Université de Montréal, 2001.

70   Pomata, *Praxis Historialis*, 128f. Nineteenth-century medical writers emphasise the hospitals of Leiden, Edinburgh, Vienna, Pavia and Genua as other early examples for clinical teaching, see for instance E. Isensee, *Neuere und neueste Geschichte der Heilwissenschaften und ihrer Literatur*, Berlin, Albert Nauck & Comp., 1834, 519ff.

71   On this turn to 'practical medicine' see P. Rieder, 'La médecine pratique: Une activité heuristique à la fin du 18e siècle?', *Dix-huitième siècle*, vol. 47, 2015, 135–148.

integrated bedside teaching as part of the syllabus in 1785. This impacted on the development of other hospitals in the Austrian Empire.[72] Most likely, the specific model for the Venetian *Scuola Clinica* was the Clinical School of Padua. In close proximity to Venice, Padua was the most important place of education for prospective Venetian physicians. For centuries it had been considered a model of quality in medical practice and learning.[73] Because so little is known about the Venetian Clinical School, a brief look at the Clinical School of Padua helps to get an idea about the role of case recording in the Venetian Clinical School.

In 1793 Andrea Comparetti (1745–1801), Professor of Medicine at the *Scuola Clinica di Padua* from 1764 onwards, published a detailed description of this institution in the years before the end of the Venetian Republic.[74] His book provides a general history as well as an ideal sketch of future clinical schools, promoting them as 'schools of medical observation' and as an instrument of medical progress.[75] Comparetti describes in detail how, in the Clinical School of Padua, students were instructed to observe and to record individual cases according to the model of the Hippocratic case histories.[76]

As in the Venetian clinical school, the professor in charge first selected those patients from the general hospital that he considered 'the most valuable for observation and most adapted for clinical instruction'. The patients were then distributed to separate divisions, according to the nature of their diseases.[77] The professor observed them constantly, and instructed his students at their bedside. Comparetti was convinced that this was the best way to teach and learn the practice of medicine:

---

72   See E. Lesky, 'The Development of Bedside Teaching at the Vienna Medical School from Scholastic Times to Special Clinics', in C.D. O'Malley (ed.), *The History of Medical Education: An International Symposium*, Berkeley, University of California Press, 1970, 217–234, 224f.

73   See Vanzan Marchini, *La politica sanitaria*, 163. On the relations between the medical cultures of Padua and Venice, see V. Giormani, 'Contrasti tra l'università di Padova e il collegio dei medici di Venezia nel '700', *Quaderni per la storia dell'università di Padova*, vol. 28, 1995, 23–87; Giormani, *I rapporti tra i due collegi veneziani, dei filosofi*.

74   A. Comparetti, *Saggio della scuola clinica nello spedale di Padova*, Padua, Nella Stamperia Penada, 1793. See also his later publication *Riscontro clinico nel nuovo spedale. Regolamenti medico-pratici*, Padua, Nella Stamperia Penada, 1799. On Comparetti see G. Corniani, *I secoli della letteratura italiana dopo il suo risorgimento*, vol. VII, Turin, Unione Tipografico-Editrice Torinese, 1855, 110f.

75   Comparetti, *Saggio della scuola clinica*, 11: 'La Scuola di Clinica, introdotta negli Spedali in questi ultimi tempi, e trattata con un metodo analitico per la via sperimentale, e ragionata, prometter deve il più grande progresso alla disciplina medica, che dalla varia osservazione trasse il vero suo origine'.

76   Ibid., 83.

77   Ibid., 88f.

There is no doubt that the right way to teach the practical medicine is the bedside of the sick. In this way, instruction passes directly and through several senses from the master to the student. The presence of the sick person allows the eyes to discover the smallest particularities of every phenomenon, and it touches in different ways the physical senses, the spirit of the observer and the auditor, and it prepares him for every examination and interrogation. It makes every doubt and obscurity disappear, and becomes the touchstone, which shows the true condition of the object one is trying to understand.[78]

Comparetti proposed that clinical schools should use two structured forms to record observations, the *foglio di visita* and the *foglio di osservazione*.[79] The *foglio di visita* was a protocol of the medical treatment and contained prescriptions directed to hospital staff. It served primarily administrative purposes, recording the number of the bed, the name and the beginning of the disease, the symptoms of the sick as well as the remedies and the diets prescribed. It was filled in by the assistant and was kept in a special place accessible to the staff.[80] In the *foglio di osservazione*, by contrast, the professor recorded his daily medical observations of the patient and the course of the disease over time. He included observations about how the disease changed in consequence of medical treatment as well as meteorological observations. In case the patient died, he noted the results of the anatomical dissection.[81] This *foglio di osservazione*, also called *foglio d'Ippocrate*,[82] was fixed to the patient's bed during the whole treatment.[83]

Produced directly at the patients' bedside, these two forms later provided the material base for the compilation of more elaborated narrative case histories, called *storie* in Italian. They formed an important part of the student's examination in the Clinical School:

---

78   Ibid., 104f.: '§. LXXXIX. Non vi deve essere alcun dubbio, che la vera maniera d'insegnare la Medicina pratica non sia al letto dell'Ammalato, dovendo in tal modo direttamente e per varj sensi passare l'istruzione del Maestro all'Allievo. La presenza dell'infermo, che fa risaltare agli occhi la più minima circostanza d'ogni fenomeno, e ferisce vivamente in più modi, ed a più colpi li sensi, e lo spirito dell'osservatore, e dell'uditore, e lo rende pronto ad ogni esame, ed inquisizione, giugne prontamente a dissipare ogni dubbio, ed oscurità, e diviene la pietra di paragone, che mostra il vero stato dell'oggetto, che si cerca di conoscere'.

79   At the end of his book, Comparetti includes reprints of these forms.

80   Ibid., 119.

81   Ibid., 114 and 118.

82   Ibid., 117: '§. XCVII: '[...] Fogli di osservazione d'Ippocrate'.

83   Ibid., 119f.

> After the disease has come to an end, one begins to compile the *storia* by taking into account both the *fogli di Visita* and the *fogli di Osservazione*. The student who was the first assistant reads the *storia* out loud in front of the public in the teaching room, together with some of his considerations. The professor completes it with some more reflections and illustrations. This *Storia completa* is kept in a case in the manner that altogether, they build a collection, so that after a while, they can be published in the annual records of the clinical school; at the same time testifying to the value of the students producing *storie* [...].[84]

As Comparetti's book confirms, by the end of the eighteenth century Italian clinical schools had introduced the systematic recording of cases with the help of pre-structured forms. In comparable ways, such a bedside teaching was integrated in the syllabus of many other contemporary clinical schools in Europe, where the teaching of observation went hand in hand with the instruction of techniques of documentation, as Volker Hess has shown.[85]

According to the historian of Venetian medicine Vanzan Marchini, Comparetti's ideas are representative for the Austrian model of health policy in so far as he defended the systematic registering, treatment and isolation of patients in hospitals, while criticising the treatment of patients at home.[86] She rightly observes that Comparetti's concept of case histories was contrary to those of contemporary Venetian physicians who worked outside hospital structures. While some of them tended to emphasise the importance of case histories for the patients and their families as well as for the better communication between physicians,[87] for Comparetti, case histories were a product of administrative procedures and were systematically used as an epistemic tool for the instruction

---

84   Ibid., 130f.: '§. CX. Terminata in qualunque maniera la malattia, riscontrando sin dapprincipio li registri de' Fogli di Visita con quello di Osservazione si estende ordinatamente la Storia, e la si legge pubblicamente nella camera della Lezione dall'Allievo, che ne fu di essa il primo Assistente con alcune riflessioni, che e'vi fece. Il Professore di poi vi aggiunge qualche altra riflessione, ed illustrazione. Questa Storia completa, ponendo ne' cancelli per formarvi una racolta, dopo certo tempo può dimostrare gli atti della Scuola di Clinica annui, ed insieme il valore degli Allievi nel formarvi le Storie [...]'.

85   Volker Hess has shown how in Paris and Berlin a kind of 'formalised observation' was taught, which produced different forms serving to record and to organize medical observation. The forms described and reprinted by Comparetti for Padua look very similar to those produced in the hospitals studied by Hess, see V. Hess, 'Formalisierte Beobachtung. Die Genese der modernen Krankenakte am Beispiel der Berliner und Pariser Medizin (1725–1830)', *Medizinhistorisches Journal*, vol. 45, 2010, 293–340, 306f.

86   Vanzan Marchi, *La memoria della salute*, 161. See also Vanzan Marchi, *La politica sanitaria*, 187f.

87   Ibid., 175.

of students. In this sense, Comparetti's work stands for the general specialisation of medical knowledge and the extension of hospital structures at the end
of the eighteenth century.[88]

In view of this Paduan model, it is very likely that in the Venetian Clinical
School between 1803 and 1805, Ruggieri and Aglietti used similar methods to
instruct their students in medical and surgical practice. Mattio Lovat was apparently one of those selected surgical cases that Ruggieri considered particularly interesting and useful for teaching. When he observed and treated him
together with his assistants, they probably recorded the treatment as well as
their daily observations with the help of structured forms. Unfortunately, these
forms are not conserved, as it is generally very rare that unpublished material
behind published case histories survives.[89] It is clear, however, that Lovat's stay
in the Clinical School in Venice did provide the material base for Ruggieri's
published case history: Compiling the *Storia della crocifissione* more than a
year after he had treated Lovat, Ruggieri must have reviewed some of the forms
produced in the Clinical School during the time of Lovat's recovery. This also
explains how he was able to remember so many details about Lovat's behaviour, the remedies applied and the discussions he had with his patient when
writing down his case history. The *Storia della crocifissione* was a retrospective
narrative account of the formalised production of empirical knowledge in the
Venetian Clinical school.[90]

3   Printing and Publishing the *Storia della crocifissione*: Appropriating
       a Genre

According to Pomata, epistemic genres are '[...] highly structured and clearly
recognizable textual conventions – textual tools, we may call them – handed

88   Ibid., 187.
89   See K. Nolte, 'Vom Verschwinden der Laienperspektive aus der Krankengeschichte: Med-
      izinische Fallberichte im 19. Jahrhundert', in S. Brändli, B. Lüthi, and G. Spuhler (eds.),
      *Zum Fall machen, zum Fall werden. Wissensproduktion und Patientenerfahrung in Medizin
      und Psychiatrie des 19. und 20. Jahrhunderts*, Frankfurt, campus, 2009, 33–61, 36. The rea-
      son for this is that in many cases physicians used to take their observations home when
      they left the institutions they had worked in, see Hess, *Formalisierte Beobachtung*, 326.
90   On the complex process of transforming and 'translating' clinical patient records into
      (published) case narratives see V. Hess and J.A. Mendelsohn, 'Case and Series: Medical
      Knowledge and Paper Technology, 1600–1900', *History of Science*, vol. 48, 2010, 287-314 and
      S. Ledebuhr, 'Schreiben und Beschreiben. Zur epistemischen Funktion von psychiatrisch-
      en Krankenakten, ihre Archivierung und deren Übersetzung in Fallgeschichten', *Berichte
      zur Wissenschaftsgeschichte*, vol. 34, no. 2, 2011, 102–124.

down by tradition for the expression and communication of a particular content [...]'.[91] What were the recognisable textual conventions of the *Storia della crocifissione* which helped Ruggieri to describe Lovat's case? Ruggieri published his narrative in three different formats and at different points in time. Considering the physical particularities of these three publications reveals different ways that Ruggieri appropriated the *observationes* genre with the purpose of communicating the case to the medical community, and to thereby transmit the empirical knowledge he deduced from it. It also helps us to understand how the specific materiality of the *Storia della crocifissione* determined its later distribution.

In 1806, the first version of Ruggieri's case history appeared in the *Nuova scelta di opuscoli interessanti sulle scienze e sulle arti*, a collection of articles published by the Milan librarian and polymath Carlo Amoretti.[92] In the tradition of natural history, Amoretti collected, translated and published texts in it from different scientific fields.[93] He aimed at publishing works which otherwise 'would never come to light or would remain in the files of scientific societies, read only by a few, or in small brochures difficult to purchase'.[94] The single

---

91   Pomata, *Sharing Cases*, 197.

92   Ruggieri, *Storia della crocifissione di Matteo Lovat*, ed. Amoretti, 403–412. As results from a
      list of new books (*Libri nuovi*) at the end of vol. 1 of the *Nuova scelta di opuscoli interessan-
      ti* (1–44), this first volume includes six parts that were also published separately. Part I to
      IV were published in 1804, whereas Part V and VI were published in 1806. Thus, Ruggieri's
      text was published in 1806, even if on the cover-page of volume 1 it says 'Milano 1804', see
      ibid., 41 and 438. A Milan copy of this edition is reprinted in: Bandirali, *Ruggieri*, 30–42.

93   Carlo Amoretti (1741–1816), librarian of the Milan *Ambrosiana* library from 1797 until 1816,
      was a lay priest and learned man interested in different areas of knowledge including
      ecclesiastical law, mineralogy, palaeography, art history, and geography. He had already
      collected and published articles from different scientific areas already in a previous work
      entitled *Opuscoli scelti sulle scienze e sulle arti, tratti dagli atti delle accademie e dalle altre
      collezioni filosofiche e letterarie dalle opere più recenti inglesi, tedesche, francesi, latine, e
      italiane, e da manoscritti originali, e inediti*, Milan, Presso Giuseppe Marelli, 1778–1803.
      The *Nuova Scelta* series was a sequel of these volumes, see Anonymous, 'Amoretti, Karl', in
      C. von Wurzbach (ed.), *Biographisches Lexikon des Kaiserthums Österreich*, vol. 1, Vienna,
      L.C. Zamarsti, 1856, 31–32. An even earlier model for this editorial project was G. Galeazzi
      and G. Marelli (eds.), *Scelta di opuscoli interessanti tradotti da varie lingue*, Milan, Marelli,
      1775–1777.

94   C. Amoretti, 'Ai leggitori. L'editore', in C. Amoretti (ed.), *Nuova scelta di opuscoli interessanti
      sulle scienze e sulle arti tratti dagli atti delle accademie, e dalle altre collezioni filosofiche e
      letterarie, dalle opere piu recenti inglesi, tedeschi, francesi, latine, e italiane, e da' manoscrit-
      ti originali, e inediti*, vol. 1, no. 6, Milan, Presso Giacomo Agnelli successore Marelli Librajo-
      Stampatore in S. Margherita, 1804–1807: '[...] destinata a raccogliere originali o tradotta le
      memorie, che senza essa non vedrebbono mai la luce, o rimarebbono, lette solo da' pochi,
      negli Atti Accademici, o in piccoli libretti di non facile, e non esteso commercio [...]'.

contributions contained in the *Nuova scelta* were either extracts from publications of scientific academies, from philosophical and literary works, from recent English, German, French, Latin and Italian publications, or printed versions of original manuscripts. Amoretti included Ruggieri's case history in the section entitled 'medicine and anatomy', where it appeared in the form of an article under its full title *Storia della crocifissione di Mattio Lovat da se stesso eseguita. Comunicata in lettera da Cesare Ruggieri medico fisico, e p.p. di clinica chirurgica in Venezia ad un medico suo amico* (see illustration 2).

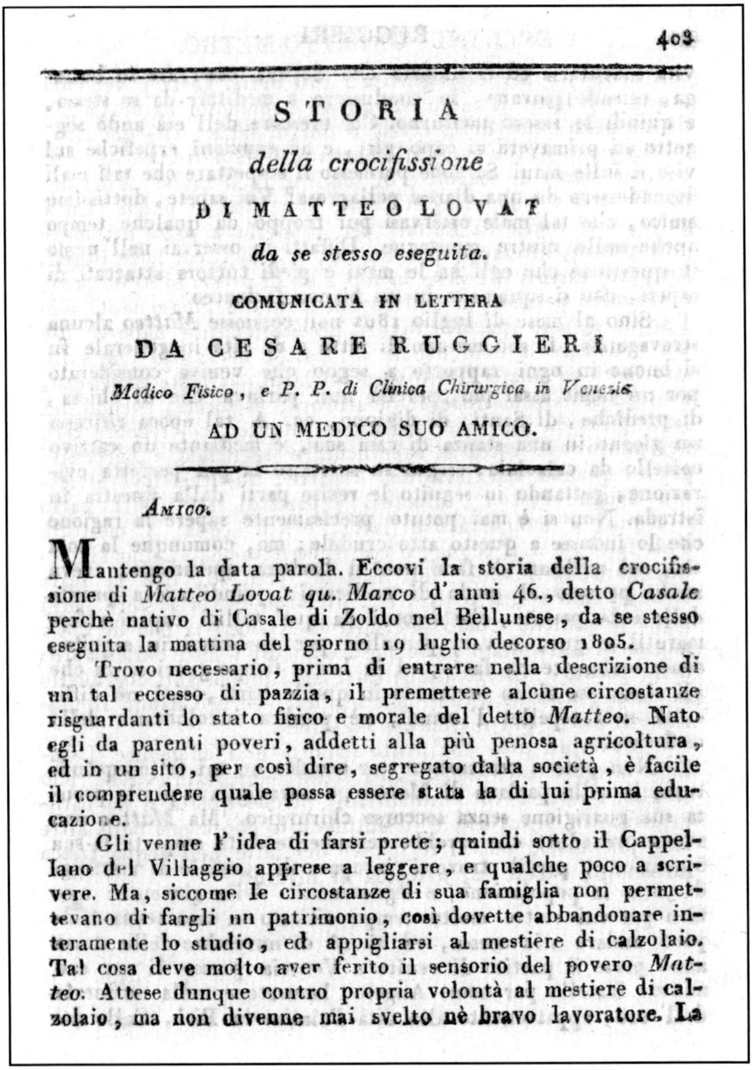

403

STORIA

della crocifissione

DI MATTEO LOVAT

da se stesso eseguita.

COMUNICATA IN LETTERA

DA CESARE RUGGIERI

Medico Fisico , e P. P. di Clinica Chirurgica in Venezia

AD UN MEDICO SUO AMICO.

Amico.

Mantengo la data parola. Eccovi la storia della crocifissione di *Matteo Lovat* qu. *Marco* d' anni 46., detto *Casale* perchè nativo di Casale di Zoldo nel Bellunese, da se stesso eseguita la mattina del giorno 19 luglio decorso 1805.

Trovo necessario, prima di entrare nella descrizione di un tal eccesso di pazzia, il premettere alcune circostanze risguardanti lo stato fisico e morale del detto *Matteo*. Nato egli da parenti poveri, addetti alla più penosa agricoltura, ed in un sito, per così dire, segregato dalla società, è facile il comprendere quale possa essere stata la di lui prima educazione.

Gli venne l' idea di farsi prete; quindi sotto il Cappellano del Villaggio apprese a leggere, e qualche poco a scrivere. Ma, siccome le circostanze di sua famiglia non permettevano di fargli un patrimonio, così dovette abbandonare interamente lo studio, ed appigliarsi al mestiere di calzolaio. Tal cosa deve molto aver ferito il sensorio del povero *Matteo*. Attese dunque contro propria volontà al mestiere di calzolaio, ma non divenne mai svelto nè bravo lavoratore. La

ILLUSTRATION 2   Ruggieri, *Storia della crocifissione di Matteo Lovat*, ed.
                   Amoretti, 1806.

In Amoretti's volume, Ruggieri's text was twelve pages long. It included a reference to a copperplate engraving that could be found in an appendix to the volume, among several other scientific illustrations, which belonged to the other articles in the volume and represented various objects of natural history. The engraving displayed two pages of the same size next to each other: the left page showed a full-page drawing of a man fixed with nails, a net and cords to a wooden cross, hanging out of a window. The right page featured on white paper some single artefacts that were contained in the first illustration in greater detail: the wooden cross, the nails and a crown of thorns (see illustrations 1A and 1B in the Introduction).[95] As can be concluded from the inscriptions on the plate ('T. Matteini dis./G. Rosaspina scul'.), Ruggieri had instructed the painter Theodoro Matteini to sketch the illustrations and the illustrator and engraver Giuseppe Rosaspina to draw them up.[96]

Considering the fact that Ruggieri had these illustrations produced for publication and that they played an important role in the reception of Lovat's case, it is important to briefly reflect on their status. At first sight, because of their subject, the illustrations evoke with the observer two famous iconographic traditions in European painting: that of the Crucified and that of the *arma Christi*, the instruments of Jesus' martyrdom, which was a favourite subject of medieval representations.[97] In this perspective, the two plates join the long tradition of visual representations of Christ's passion in art history. Therefore, with contemporary observers, the illustrations probably raised the expectation that this was a religious text rather than a scientific one.

However, taking a closer look at the first plate, one observes a rather untypical iconography of Christ: the crucified man is depicted from the side and not, as usual for the crucifix and other devotional pictures, in frontal view. It seems indeed that this realistic posture of the hanging body aims at avoiding

---

95   The engravings are placed at the end of the volume after 440, entitled Tav. XII. Bandirali cites an edition of Amoretti's volume that is conserved in the private library of Alessandro Manzoni in the villa of Brusuglio. She says that despite the reference to the engravings in the text, the pictures only appeared in the French edition and the second Italian edition of 1814, see Bandirali, *Ruggieri*, 8. This is false; it seems that either she did not look at the back of the volume, or that in the Milan copy the engravings are in fact lacking.

96   On the original illustration see N. Gori Bucci, *Il pittore Teodoro Matteini (1745–1831)*, Venice, Istituto Veneto di Scienze Lettere ed Arti, 2006, 260. A reprint is on 414. The original engraving (210×132 mm) is conserved in Milan, Castello Sforzesco, Civica Raccolta di Stampe Bertarelli. Matteini was not a specialist of scientific representations but had gained a reputation primarily with portraits of noblemen and -women, still life for private use and, significantly, images representing religious topics.

97   See M. Rimmele, 'Geordnete Unordnung. Zur Bedeutungsstiftung im Zusammenhang der Arma Christi', in David Ganz and Felix Pürlemann (eds.), *Das Bild im Plural. Mehrteilige Bildformen zwischen Mittelalter und Gegenwart*, Berlin, Reimer, 2010, 219–242.

an idealistic interpretation of the Crucified, that is to say it avoids the equali-
sation of Lovat with Christ by diverting attention from the wounded body to
the technical dimension of the act. Correspondingly, the traces of pain seem
reduced: there is little blood coming out of the wounds, and the body appears
clean and even. In particular, the net covering Lovat's body is eye-catching.
This element differs the most from the traditional iconography of the Crucified.[98] It thus seems that the painter Matteini, most probably in agreement
with Ruggieri, tried to reduce the iconic power of his paintings, considering
that they were to appear in a scientific publication.[99]

    And in fact, due to their inclusion in a scientific publication, a medical case
history, the pictures also correspond with a long tradition of using illustrations
as a means of producing evidence in natural history, where remarkable and wondrous events were frequently published with illustrations in order to authenti-
cate the unbelievable.[100] And, maybe even more evident, the illustrations are
also shaped by a specifically medical visual tradition. Since the fourteenth century, surgical publications visualized all kinds of possible wounds in order to instruct surgeons how to treat these wounds; in particular, this was an important
didactive means in the realm of military medical care. One typical figure in this
context was the so-called 'man with wounds' (*Wundenmann*), the representation of a naked male figure covered with all possible kinds of medieval weapons
sticking in the body.[101] The individual arms and the respective wounds caused
by them were explained in a legend, often in vernacular language, indicating
that these figures especially served surgeons who lacked specialist knowledge. Due to their harmed bodies attacked with arms, figures of the wounded
man shared certain features with the iconography of martyrs, or even resembled the religious iconography of the man of sorrows. As a learned surgeon,

98   Beyond the iconography of Christ, the first plate alludes to another traditional repre-
      sentation, which is a specific form of execution that was frequent in late medieval Italy.
      Delinquents were hanged out of the windows of representative state buildings. In their
      disgrace, they should represent the appropriate punishment and the state's justice. See
      for this aspect H. Bredekamp, *Repräsentation und Bildmagie in der Renaissance als Form-
      problem*, Munich: Carl Friedrich von Siemens Stiftung, 1984.

99   On the relation between science and art in iconography see C.A. Jones and P. Galison,
      'Introduction. Picturing Science, Producing Art', Idem (eds.), *Picturing Science and Pro-
      ducing Art*, New York and London, Routledge, 1998, 101–124.

100   P.F. da Costa, 'The Making of Extraordinary Facts: Authentication of Singularities of Na-
      ture at the Royal Society of London in the First Half of the Eighteenth Century', *Studies in
      History and Philosophy of Science*, vol. 33, 2002, 265–288, see esp. the chapter 'The Depic-
      tion of Singularity', 270–277.

101   On the tradition of this figure see K. Neuhaus, *Der Wundenmann: Tradition und Struktur
      einer Abbildungsart in der medizinischen Literatur*, Münster, Diss. med., 1981.

Ruggieri was familiar with ancient and contemporary scientific conventions of representing surgical knowledge. In the same period in which he published Lovat's case, he also published a whole volume with surgical illustrations: the last volume of the French surgical dictionnary that he translated between 1805 and 1810 contained visual representations of the described tumours, wounds and fractures. Looking at these illustrations, one realizes that two important features of the illustrations in the *Storia della crocifissione* – the representation of weapons or surgical instruments as well as the indication of measuring units (at the bottom of the second plate) – were a common means used in surgical publications to indicate the real proportions of a depicted surgical problem.[102]

Still in 1806, an enlarged French edition of Ruggieri's case history appeared, entitled *Histoire du crucifiement éxécuté sur sa propre personne par Mathieu Lovat, communiqué au public dans une lettre de César Ruggieri docteur en médecine et professeur de chirurgie clinique à Venise. A un médecin son ami* (see illustration 3).[103] In contrast to Amoretti's edition, in which Ruggieri's case history appeared as one among many contributions, the French edition was a monograph of 24 pages. Making the text several pages longer, it included several passages that were not contained in the first Italian edition. Underlining its book-like appearance, the French edition included the identical two illustrations that were printed in Carlo Amoretti's edition, but with an important difference: the pictures were no longer hidden in the appendix; now, they prominently framed the text, one at the front, the other one at the back.

In 1814, Ruggieri published a second Italian edition in Venice with an enlarged title.[104] The Venetian printer, Fracasso, did not specialise in publishing medical writings. In the same year, for instance, he published political treatises, texts concerning the religious life in Venice, legal texts, panegyrics for weddings of Venetian noblemen, novels as well as several translations of

---

102   C. Ruggieri, *Dizionario enciclopedico di chirurgia. Tradotto dal francese in italiano ed accresciuto di aggiunte e note, Spiegazione delle tavole del dizionario enciclopedico di chirurgia dei signori Petit-Radel, e Allan*, vol. 4, Padua, Nella Stamperia del Seminario presso Tommaso Bettinelli, 1810, see in particular plate 12.

103   Ruggieri, *Histoire du crucifiement*. I worked with the copy conserved in the Biblioteca Nazionale Marciana di Venezia (in the following: BNMV). The brochure is included in the miscellanea MISC 0664. 011 as well as in the MISC 3526. 006. The miscellanea are collections of monographic brochures and articles grouped together by the library in the nineteenth century without indication of their origin.

104   Ruggieri, *Storia della crocifissione*. I worked with the copy conserved in the BNMV, miscellanea 268. Like the French version, this one was put together with other publications by the library. Note: This copy is not included in the online catalogue but only in the old alphabetical card box under the name Cesare Ruggieri.

HISTOIRE
DU CRUÇIFIEMENT
ÉXÉCUTÉ SUR SA PROPRE PERSONNE

PAR

MATHIEU LOVAT

COMMUNIQUÉ AU PUBLIC

DANS UNE LETTRE

DE

CESAR RUGGIERI

*Docteur en Medicine et Professeur de Chirurgie
Clynique à Venise.*

A UN MEDECIN SON AMI.

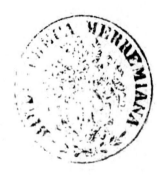

a

ILLUSTRATION 3   Ruggieri, *Histoire du crucifiement éxécuté sur sa propre personne par
Mathieu Lovat*, 1806.

French publications.[105] The 1814 edition of the *Storia della crocifissione* was also a book-like publication of about twenty pages and displayed the identical copperplate engravings as the other two editions. Except from some smaller adjunctions, the text corresponded to the French edition.

How can we account for the existence of these three different editions of the same case history? Why was Ruggieri eager to publish the *Storia della crocifissione* not one, but several times? And what did he expect from publishing Lovat's case at all? In the case of the first Italian edition, Ruggieri himself had probably sent his text by letter to Carlo Amoretti, hoping that the Milan librarian would publish it in his miscellanea so that it could be read by an Italian readership. With this way of publishing Lovat's case, Ruggieri closely followed the habit of early modern physicians who frequently shared cases via letters and publications, thereby contributing to the construction of a *res publica medica*, as described by Pomata.[106] In the case of the French booklet dating from the same year, the missing typographic details indicate that this edition was not distributed by an official publisher but circulated in print in unofficial ways. As we will see in the next chapter, Ruggieri indeed produced this edition in order to personally hand it over to several foreign colleagues, thereby ensuring that it would reach an international readership. Finally, the 1814 Italian edition proves that Ruggieri attentively followed the career of his published case history. In a footnote, he remarked that since its first publication in 1806, the *Storia della crocifissione* had been translated into German and English.[107] It was thus the rising international attention to Lovat's case which encouraged Ruggieri to publish a third edition of his case history in 1814. Tellingly, the enlarged title of this edition referred to his multiple memberships in scientific societies in various European capitals (namely Vienna, Madrid and Paris) and thus to the international academic reputation Ruggieri had gained in the years between 1806 and 1814 (see illustration 4). Ruggieri's publishing policy thus confirms what historians of the book have reminded us of: publishing a text is always a conscious action, involving the author as agent and the public as adressees of a publication.[108]

Neither the title nor the pictures of the *Storia della crocifissione* at first sight implied a medical subject. Rather, they suggested that the publication dealt with a religious subject, namely an act of *imitatio Christi*. Given the fact that the word *observatio* did not appear in the title of the *Storia della crocifissione*,

---

105   This results from a simple name search in the Venetian library catalogue: http://polovea.
         sebina.it.
106   Pomata, *Sharing Cases*, 199.
107   Ruggieri, *Storia della crocifissione*, 3.
108   See for instance C. Jouhaud and A. Viala (eds.), *De la publication entre renaissance et lumières*, Paris, Fayard, 2002.

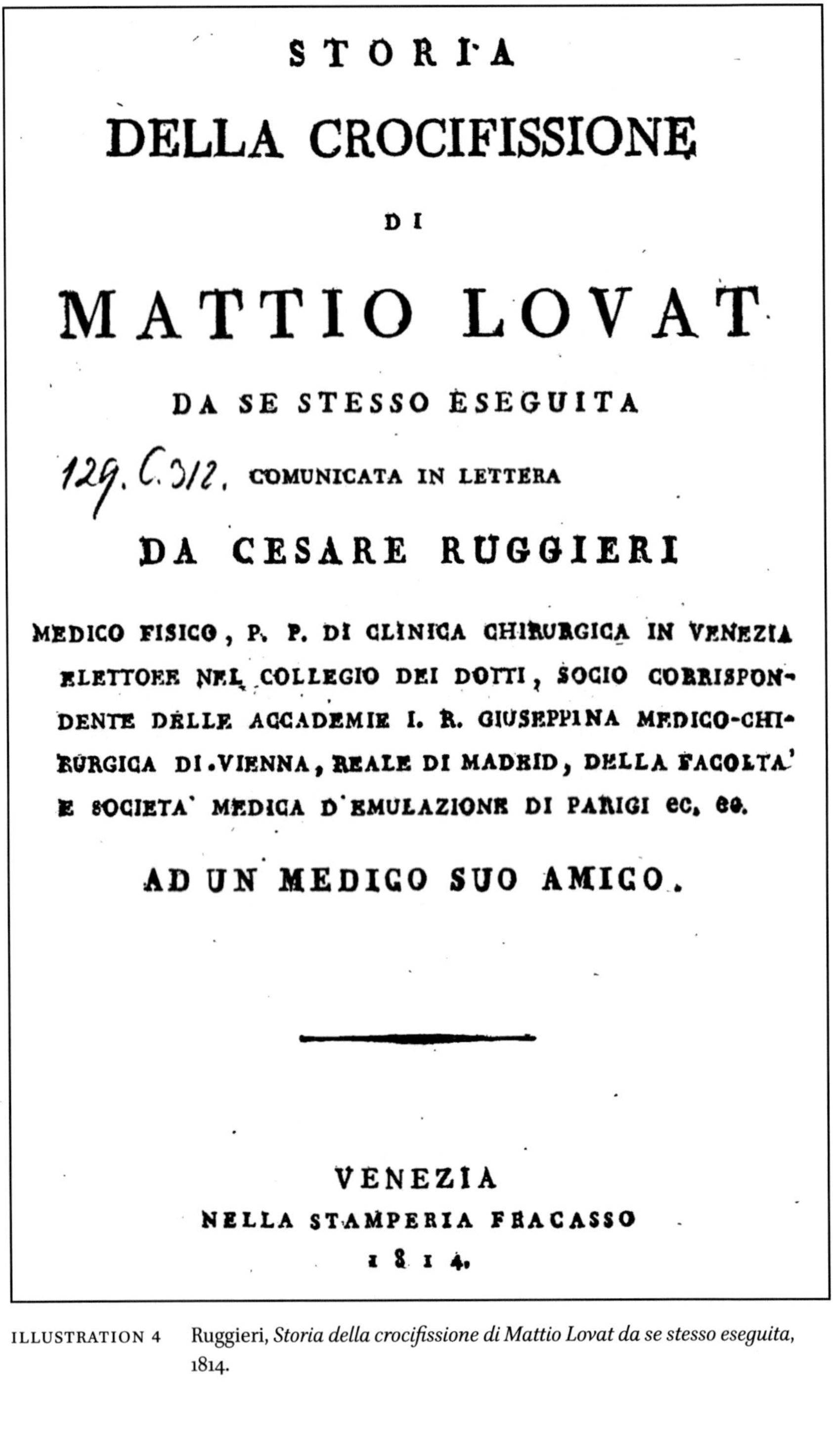

STORIA

DELLA CROCIFISSIONE

D I

MATTIO LOVAT

DA SE STESSO ESEGUITA

129. C.312. COMUNICATA IN LETTERA

DA CESARE RUGGIERI

MEDICO FISICO, P. P. DI CLINICA CHIRURGICA IN VENEZIA
ELETTORE NEL COLLEGIO DEI DOTTI, SOCIO CORRISPON-
DENTE DELLE ACCADEMIE I. R. GIUSEPPINA MEDICO-CHI-
RURGICA DI VIENNA, REALE DI MADRID, DELLA FACOLTA'
E SOCIETA' MEDICA D'EMULAZIONE DI PARIGI ec. ec.

AD UN MEDICO SUO AMICO.

VENEZIA

NELLA STAMPERIA FRACASSO

1814.

ILLUSTRATION 4   Ruggieri, *Storia della crocifissione di Mattio Lovat da se stesso eseguita*, 1814.

how could contemporary readers know that this was a medical case history in the genre of the *observationes*? What were the 'recognizable textual conventions'[109] of the three editions? The most obvious indicator is two words in the main title and in the subtitle title of the publication: history (*Storia*) and letter (*lettera*). To begin with the second, the text had all elements of a letter: it was a first-person narrative, it addressed a second person in polite form, and it ended with a closing statement. But the *Storia della crocifissione* was not a letter in a private sense. Rather, the subtitle was a rhetorical device indicating Ruggieri's intention to communicate Lovat's case to a broader medical public. The same device was a typical feature of early modern *epistolae medicae*, a tradition of medical writing that was closely connected with the communication of the *observationes*. During the early modern period, physicians all over Europe communicated and published their observations of single cases in letters, thereby building up broad networks of correspondents and contributing to scholarly communication – 'epistolary medicine', as Nany Siraisi has called it.[110] In particular, physicians used letters to communicate rare and extraordinary cases, something that they shared with many botanists and naturalists.[111] Titles of seventeenth-century medical publications reflect the hybrid form of the *epistolae medicae* and the medical *observationes*.[112]

Even more than the subtitle of the *Storia della crocifissione*, the title's first term *storia* revealed the text's connection to the *observationes* genre. It did not simply suggest that Ruggieri intended to tell the 'history' of Lovat's self-crucifixion; rather, with that term he referred to a specific tradition of writing case histories in medicine, called *historiae*. By Ruggieri's time, the term *historia* had a long career.[113] As the eponym of early modern empiricism, it had moved into the context of medicine at the beginning of the sixteenth century.[114] Consequently, the term became central in the language of Humanist physicians who used it to denote 'knowledge based on sense perception or observation'.[115]

---

109 Pomata, *Sharing Cases*, 197.

110 Ibid., 196; Siraisi, *Communities of Learned Experience*. On medical correspondence, see also I. Maclean, 'The Medical Republic of Letters before the Thirty Years War', *Intellectual History Review*, vol. 18, 2008, 15–30 and H. Steinke and M. Stuber, 'Medical Correspondence in Early Modern Europe. An Introduction', *Gesnerus*, vol. 61, 2004, 139–160.

111 Pomata, *Sharing Cases*, 222.

112 See the list of *curationes* and *observationes* in ibid., 223–236.

113 See A. Seifert, *Cognitio Historica: Die Geschichte als Namengeberin der frühneuzeitlichen Empirie*, Berlin, Duncker & Humblot, 1976.

114 Pomata, *Praxis Historialis*, 105f. On the broader meaning of *historia* in the field of medicine see N.G. Siraisi, *History, Medicine and the Traditions of Renaissance Learning*, Ann Arbor, University of Michigan Press, 2007.

115 Pomata, *Praxis Historialis*, 111.

Two major formats emerged, the *historia medica* and the *historia anatomica*.[116] According to Pomata, '[b]y the first half of the seventeenth century medical *observationes* and *historiae* were interchangeable terms, both indicating a condensed report of firsthand observation and meant as a cumulative contribution to a Europe-wide network of information exchange among scholars'.[117] This explains why in Italian language, *storia* was the term that physicians typically used in the title of their vernacular case histories.

In the course of the seventeenth century, the *observationes* developed into the 'primary medium for the circulation of information in the res publica medica'.[118] It became the favourite genre for publications of scholarly societies as well as for medical journals, a development that Pomata has called the genre's 'mainstreaming'.[119] The *observationes* became part of the programmatic attempt of eighteenth-century physicians to turn away from theory and doctrine as it was embodied in scholastic medical teaching, and to direct medicine towards an empirical science. The prominence of printed *observationes* in eighteenth-century medical publishing demonstrates that knowledge gained from practice was more esteemed than doctrinal knowledge.[120]

This explains why Ruggieri, when writing down Lovat's case at the beginning of the nineteenth century, opted for the *observationes* genre: Lovat's was a case that he had encountered during his medical practice, and which he had himself carefully observed in his clinical school. In Ruggieri's eyes, it was an extraordinary case that was worth publishing, not only because of the surprising subject, the self-crucifixion, but also because it dealt with an urgent medical problem in the Italian states, namely that of pellagra and its related insanity. To share his observations with international colleagues, the long-established authority of the *observationes* was the ideal tool. As the three different editions of the *Storia della crocifissione* demonstrate, Ruggieri appropriated the genre according to his own purposes: to reach an Italian readership, he first included the case in an Italian encyclopaedic collection, Carlo Amaretti's *Nuova scelta*; to reach a broader international audience, he published it in French, another vulgar language and at that time the *langue universelle*. And for a greater

---

116   On the differences between the *historia anatomica* and the *historia medica* see ibid., 114–137.

117   Ibid., 134f.

118   Pomata, *Sharing Cases*, 225.

119   Ibid.

120   On the role of medical case histories within the broader reform of knowledge in the seventeenth and eighteenth centuries see J. Geyer-Kordesch, 'Medizinische Fallbeschreibungen und ihre Bedeutung in der Wissensreform des 17. und 18. Jahrhunderts', *Medizin, Gesellschaft und Geschichte*, vol. 9, 1990, 7–19. Geyer-Kordesch analyzes two collections of case histories, published in 1733 by the German physicians Friedrich Hoffmann and Georg Ernst Stahl.

visibility on the Italian bookmarket, he published it eight years later again as an individual publication with a Venetian printer as a booklet. Clearly Ruggieri sought to make Lovat's case travel beyond Venice, and he therefore trusted the potential of an autonomous publication more than that of a collective volume. He also believed in the power of translations as an effective means of communicating medical knowledge to a broader international audience.

4   Sharing Cases in Venice and Beyond

Lovat's case was not the only one for which Ruggieri chose the genre of the *observatio* or *storia*. In order to communicate surgical and medical observations of individual patients, which he had encountered during his medical practice, he published several other texts in the same format. As a physician specialising in surgery, Ruggieri's interest was less in medical theory and doctrine, but in medical practice in general, and surgical techniques in particular. For this reason, the publication of case histories allowed him to share the practical knowledge that he gained from his first-hand observations with medical colleagues, thereby participating in both a local and an international medical community.

Two of Ruggieri's published case histories bear striking similarities with the *Storia della crocifissione*: the *Storia di una blennorea prodotta da lambimento canino associata ad ulceri, ec.* ('history of an ulcer produced by a dog's licking'), and the *Storia ragionata di una donna avente un gran parte del corpo coperta di pelle e pelo nero* ('rational history of a woman which had a great part of her body covered with pelt'). These texts resemble the *Storia della crocifissione* not only because of their format and style, but also because they deal with extraordinary and rare subjects: a case of bestiality, and a case of a hairy 'monstrous' woman. So they also dealt with problems that went beyond medical and surgical expertise in the strict sense and touched on delicate social and moral issues. Because of their psychological, social, legal and moral contents, these two other *storie* met the interests of different specialists as well as of a broader literate public. Like the *Storia della crocifissione*, they went through a second edition, were translated into other languages, and were received by an international readership.

In the *Storia di una blennorrea*, first published in 1809, Ruggieri reported a medical examination of two female patients he had treated in Venice in 1807.[121]

---

121   C. Ruggieri, *Storia di una blennorea prodotta da lambimento canino associata ad ulceri, ec. di Cesare Ruggieri, medico fisico, p.p. di clinca chirurgia in Venezia, elettore nel collegio dei dotti, socio corrispondente delle accademie i.r. giuseppina medico-chirugica di Vienna, reale di Madrid, della facoltà e società medica d'emulazione di Parigi ec.ec.*, Venice, Nella Stamperia Fracasso, 1814.

According to his account, he was called by two sisters who lived together in the same place and claimed to suffer from pain in the region of the genitals. Ruggieri first listened to the 'history' that one of the sisters told him about their sufferings,[122] and then undertook a physical examination of the lower parts, which the sisters first refused because they were ashamed. Initially, Ruggieri expected to be confronted with a venereal disease, because the two women suffered from genital ulcers.[123] After several home visits, he discovered, however, that the disease was caused by sexual intercourse with a dog. The sisters used to alternately keep a poodle in their bed, and to receive sexual satisfaction through the poodle's licking their genitals.[124] Despite the protest of the two sisters, Ruggieri gave orders to remove the dog and prescribed some external remedies for the lower parts concerned.

Implicitly more than explicitly, the *Storia di una blennorea* described a case of bestiality and raised delicate questions of sexual behaviour that conflicted with social norms.[125] Therefore, Ruggieri was eager to present the case as a medical rather than a moral problem. He emphasised that he considered the case singular not because it was 'curious and shocking', but because of the extraordinary way in which the disease in question was produced.[126] Remarkably, he also insisted that the two sisters were not vicious but respectable and prudent women, who had been victims of the dog's natural instinct.[127] In a long theoretical part of his text, Ruggieri presented a medical discussion about the similarity of the disease in question to other venereal diseases. Because of its comparable symptoms, he considered it to be a venereal disease produced by animal poison and the mixture of animal and human fluid.[128] From a medical viewpoint, the case history thus contributed to the current debate on syphilis and its treatment with mercurial substances, a controversial subject in European medicine at that time. Consequently, the *Storia di una blennorea*

---

122 Ibid., 5: 'Finalmente, la più giovane cominciò a parlare, ed a tessermi con una seccantissima cantilena la seguente storia. [...]'.

123 Ibid., 10f.

124 Ibid., 13.

125 On the problem of obscenity and pornography see L. Hunt, 'Introduction: Obscenity and the Origins of Modernity, 1500–1800', in L. Hunt (ed.), *The Invention of Pornography. Obscenity and the Origins of Modernity, 1500–1800*, New York, Zone Books, 1993, 9–45.

126 Ruggieri, *Storia di una blennorea*, 23: 'Avvertite soltanto che se nel principio ho detto di trattenervi su d'una malattia singola, nol dissi perchè presentasse dei curiosi ed inauditi fenomeni, ma per la singolarità della maniera, con cui fu essa prodotta'.

127 Ibid., 24f.

128 See ibid., 17ff.

was received in international debates on this topic.[129] As with the *Storia della crocifissione,* Ruggieri was proud that his case history was discussed in international medical debates, and this success encouraged him to publish a second edition in 1814.[130]

The *Storia ragionata di una donna avente gran parte del corpo coperta di pelle e pelo nero,* published in 1815[131] and 1822,[132] was likewise received by authors in several European countries.[133] In this case, Ruggieri was asked to perform his medical expertise in a legal matter. In question was the validity of a marriage between a young nobleman and a young noblewoman. On the wedding night, the man discovered that half of his bride's body was covered in black fur. Because of the disgust the husband felt towards his wife, the couple's families agreed that the marriage should be annulled. They sought to find rational reasons in order to receive the legal and religious permission for the annihilation of the marriage. To this end, they requested the expertise of theologians and lawyers. Those specialists, in turn, asked Ruggieri for his expert opinion regarding the physical condition of the woman. Ruggieri insisted on carrying out a

---

129 For a contemporary French discussion of the case see Anonymous, 'Blennorée produite par une cause singulière', *Journal général de médecine, de chirurgie et de pharmacie, françaises et étrangères; ou recueil périodique de la société de médecine de Paris,* vol. 60, 1817, 94–98. Still in the 20th century, the case history was cited, for instance in a German translation of an Italian work: C. Taruffi, *Hermaphrodismus und Zeugungsunfähigkeit. Eine systematische Darstellung der menschlichen Geschlechtsorgane von Prof. Cesare Taruffi, autorisierte deutsche Ausgabe von Dr. med. R. Täuscher mit Abbildungen,* Berlin, Verlag von H. Barsford Tissier, 1903, 224f.

130 In the 1814 edition of this case history, Ruggieri remarks that in the meantime, his text had been translated in German as well as in French and English, see Ruggieri, *Storia di una blennorrea,* 3.

131 C. Ruggieri, *Storia ragionata di una donna avente gran parte del corpo coperta di pelle e pelo nero,* Venice, Tipografia Picotti, 1815.

132 In the following, I cite the second edition: C. Ruggieri, *Storia ragionata di una donna avente gran parte del corpo coperta di pelle e pelo nero di Cesare Ruggieri medico fisico p. o. p. di clinica, terapia speciale ed operazioni chirurgiche nell'i. r. università di Padova, già elettore nel collegio dei dotti, socio corrispondente delle accademie imp. r. giussepina medicochirurgica di Vienna, reale di Madrid, della facoltà e società medica d'emulazione di Parigi, ec. ec. ec. Edizione seconda,* Padua, Dalla Tipografia della Minerva, dalla Nuova societa tipografica in ditta N. Zanon Bettoni e compagni, 1822.

133 The case was, for instance, cited briefly in E. Horn (ed.), *Vollständiges Universal-Register des Archivs für medizinische Erfahrung im Gebiete der praktischen Medizin und Staatsarzneikunde,* vol. 58, Berlin, G. Reimer, 1819, 30; C.F. Kleinert (ed.), *Allgemeines Repertorium der gesammten deutschen medizinisch-chirurgischen Journalistik,* vol. 4, no. 9, 1830, 104; A. Henke, *Lehrbuch der gerichtlichen Medizin. Zum Behufe akademischer Vorlesungen und zum Gebrauch für gerichtliche Ärzte und Rechtsgelehrte,* Berlin, Ferdinand Dümmler, 1832, 107.

physical examination, and the second part of his text is based on his observations of the woman's body.[134]

In the first part of the case history, by contrast, Ruggieri gave a detailed account of the woman's childhood, based on the discussions he had with her family. Ruggieri reported on the girl's strange behaviour towards animals: while she
used to hate all kinds of birds, she showed herself extremely fond of dogs.[135]
In order to deliver a medical explanation for the woman's physical 'monstrosity', Ruggieri consequently discussed different hypotheses, among them the
popular medical explanation of the influence of maternal imagination on the
foetus,[136] and the popular idea that the girl's mother had possibly had sexual
intercourse with an animal.[137] Admitting that current medical science lacked
the knowledge to properly explain such phenomena, Ruggieri concluded that
some disease already suffered in the uterus had caused the physical defect.[138]
At the end of his case history, Ruggieri maintained that the marriage had to be
annulled because of the woman's monstrosity. He justified his decision with a
social and a medical argument: the disgust of the husband would make sexual
intercourse between the couple impossible; and because of the risk of degra-
dation, the children of the couple would probably inherit the physical defect
of the mother.[139]

All three *storie* by Ruggieri thus dealt with problems that went far beyond
the traditional competences of a surgeon as described at the beginning of this
chapter. As none of the three cases required complicated surgical procedures,
Ruggieri could not shine with surgical-anatomical knowledge and techniques,
but had to prove his abilities in other areas. This was exactly the great potential of the three cases: they gave Ruggieri the chance to demonstrate his all-
embracing expertise as a medical specialist who had a say in both internal and
external diseases as well as in social, moral and legal matters. In brief, they gave
him the chance to present himself as a 'guardian angel' triumphing over societal subversion, as he himself had described the ideal physician.[140]

---

134   Ruggieri, *Storia ragionata di una donna*, 21.
135   Ibid., 4ff.
136   The explanation of bodily anomalies as caused by pathological imagination was a fre-
        quent feature in enlightenment discourse, see for this theme L. Daston and K. Park, *Won-
        ders and the Order of Nature 1150–1750*, New York, Zone Books, 1998, 339, and L. Daston,
        Wunder, Beweise und Tatsachen. Zur Geschichte der Rationalität, Frankfurt, Fischer, 2011,
        99–126.
137   Ruggieri, *Storia ragionata di una donna*, 39.
138   Ibid., 48.
139   Ibid., 35.
140   Ruggieri, *Dei doveri di chi studia e di chi esercita la medicina*, 31.

The particularities of the three *storie* become even clearer if we compare them briefly to some of the surgical case histories, which Ruggieri published in various journals of practical medicine. Here, his professional background in surgery and anatomy came to the fore. In 1814 he published a case history (*osservazione*) of ten pages in Valeriano Luigi Brera's *Giornale di medicina pratica*, in which he reported on the treatment of a patient who suffered from a urinary stone and died in consequence of Ruggieri's operation.[141] A 67-year old man felt such big pain over several months while urinating that he finally came to Ruggieri to ask for an operation.[142] Ruggieri warned his patient against the great risks of such an operation, and even encouraged him to consult other physicians before.[143] But the man insisted on being operated by Ruggieri and also asked for a dissection of his body in case he died during the operation.[144] The patient did in fact died, and Ruggieri conducted a post-mortem with two colleagues.

Ruggieri published another surgical case history in 1818 in the *Nuovi commentarj di medicina e di chirurgia*, a follow-up to Brera's journal, which was co-edited by Ruggieri and Floriano Cladani and launched in Padua from 1818 onwards.[145] This *Osservazione medico-chirurgica* was an account of the treatment of a young carpenter, who suffered from pains in the movement of his left arm. According to Ruggieri's report, prior treatments by other physicians had not been successful. After having discovered that the disease was caused by a dysfunction of the nerves, Ruggieri successfully carried out an operation of the arm.[146] Thanks to his treatment, the patient recovered completely.[147]

As these two examples show, Ruggieri's surgical case histories display his self-understanding as a surgeon and medical practitioner who mastered the manual art of surgery in all its refinements. While the first case history allowed Ruggieri to justify both the fatal result of his operation and the anatomical

---

141   C. Ruggieri, *Aneurisma vastissimo dell'aorta, causa di morte in un operato di pietra. Osservazione del Signor Dottore Cesare Ruggieri professore di chirurgia in Venezia*, Padua, Nella Tipografia del Seminario, 1814, 5–15.

142   Ibid., 8.

143   Ibid., 9.

144   Ibid., 10.

145   C. Ruggieri, 'Dolore spasmodico riccorrente alla parte interna dell'anti-braccio sinistro, che apportò la piegatura della mano sull'anti-braccio medesimo con contrazione di tutte le dita; osservazione medico-chirurgica', *Nuovi commentarj di medicina e di chirurgia pubblicati dai Signori Valeriano Luigi Brera Cesareo-Regio Consigliere, Cesare Ruggieri, e Floriano Caldani professori di medicina e chirurgia nell'imperiale regia università di Padova etc.*, vol. 1, no. 3, 1818, 97–104.

146   Ibid., 101.

147   Ibid., 103f.

dissection to his colleagues and his patient's relatives,[148] the account of a successful operation helped Ruggieri to demonstrate his surgical expertise to his colleagues. Both the demonstration of efficacy and the claim for the validity of a judgement are two purposes that surgeons and physicians had traditionally pursued with the publication of case histories, as Charlotte Furth has argued.[149]

Ruggieri's strong identity as a surgeon is further demonstrated by the fact that he even sought to publish an illustrated collection of surgical cases. At Ruggieri's funeral, his Paduan colleague Floriano Caldani remarked in his speech that,

> [...] for quite a while, he [Ruggieri] had the great idea to publish a truthful history of the most extraordinary diseases he had cured. This work, as well as the illustrations representing some unusual monstrous tumours of the external body, or some disturbances of an inner limb, was almost finished. It described the physical condition of many sick persons, of the development of their disease, the successful or unsuccessful result of the cure. [...] Undoubtedly, this significant work would have spread the glory of our school amongst the nations; but because the decrease of his physical forces did not permit him to give it the elaboration he wanted, he feared to face the same fatal sentence with which Virgil judged his inimitable poem.[150]

Tellingly, Caldani alludes to a comment of the Church Father St. Augustine, on Virgil's desire to burn his *Aeneid*. According to Augustine's interpretation, Virgil sought to burn his *Aeneid* before he died because he was not satisfied

---

148   Ibid., 11.

149   C. Furth, 'Introduction. Thinking with Cases', in C. Furth, J.T. Zeitlin, and P. Hsiung (eds.), *Thinking with Cases. Specialist Knowledge in Chinese Cultural History*, Honolulu, University of Hawaii Press, 2007, 1–27, 2.

150   Caldani, *Discorso funebre*, 15f.: '[...] la grande idea da qualche tempo concepì di pubblicare colle stampe la verace storia delle più singolari malattie da lui curate. Pronta è in gran parte quell'opera, e pronto il disegno di alcune insolite mostruose escrescenze esteriori, o del guasto interno di qualche membro; descrisse lo stato di molt'infermi, l'avanzamento di lor malattia, e l'esito felice od infausto che n'ebbe la cura; perocchè sincero il Ruggieri, e conoscitore dell'arte sua, ben sapea che nella medicina non val mentire, che riverenza e gratitudine merita l'ingenuità del maestro, e che può lo studioso approfittare persino dell'infelice riuscita d'una cura. Quell'insigne lavoro accrescer dovea certamente tra le nazioni lo splendore della nostra scuola; ma perchè l'affievolimento delle sue forze non gli permise dargli il compimento che divisava, odo essere uscita contr'esso la fatale sentenza, cui Virgilio condannò il suo inimitabil poema'.

with it, but friends stopped him from doing so.[151] Caldani's reference thus suggests that Ruggieri had prepared a collection of surgical case histories, but then destroyed it, or at least refused to publish it.[152] Most likely, this work was the *Nuovo trattato sui tumori di singulare natura corredato di pratiche osservazioni, e varie tavole in rame*, a manuscript listed in Ruggieri's autograph but untraceable in Italian libraries and archives.[153]

Hence, while the surgical case histories allowed Ruggieri to promote himself as a master of his profession within the local and national community of surgeons, he used the elaborate three *storie* as a platform to present himself to an international medical audience as a new 'scientific' surgeon, a medical specialist whose expertise went beyond surgery, and whose medical advice was requested by patients as well as by state authorities. While the surgical cases reported primarily on specific diseases and surgical interventions and treatments, his three *storie* told stories about individual patients with real characters and biographies. As we have seen, Ruggieri described his patients in their respective social environment, showing empathy and commitment to their needs. But the three *storie* not only reported on individual patients, they also spoke about a successful Venetian Professor of Surgery who knew how to handle all kinds of delicate medical and moral problems. They proved that Ruggieri was not only a specialised medical practitioner but also a good reasoner and a gifted writer of case histories.[154] Publishing the three *storie* as book-like publications rather than articles, Ruggieri seems to have been quite aware of their compelling themes and their potential on the international bookmarket. Because all three *storie* implicitly conveyed major or minor social scandals and therefore provoked social judgement, he probably foresaw that they would not only receive attention in international medical debates but also arouse the interest of a broader lay readership.

---

151   See for this issue A.M. Bowie, 'The Death of Priam: Allegory and History in the *Aenedid*', *Classical Quarterly*, vol. 40, no. 2, 1990, 470–481, 474.

152   Caldani, *Discorso funebre*, 16: 'Ma se dall'incendio fu risparmiata la narrazione vaghissima di tanti pericoli e di tante rovine, potrem noi credere che, per secondare la modestia del nostro Ruggieri, riguardo alcuno usar non si voglia alla vita ed alla salute degli uomini? Ah no: *Frangatur potius legum veneranda potestas,/Quam tot congestos noctesque diesque labores/Hauserit una dies*.' For an English translation of these Latin verses see G. Puttenham et al. (eds.), *The Art of English Poesy*, Ithaca, Cornell University Press, 2007, 13: 'The great power of the laws, which is to be venerated, should be broken rather than one day should have consumed what the poets' labors built up over so many days and nights'.

153   See the *Autograph of Cesare Ruggieri*, No. 9 in the list.

154   On the importance of writing for the professionalisation of nineteenth-century physicians see L. Gafner, *Schreibarbeit. Die alltägliche Wissenspraxis eines Bieler Arztes im 19. Jahrhundert*, Tübingen: Mohr Siebeck, 2016.

5   The Art of Medical Observation: Between the Individual and the
       Collective

In all of his case histories, Ruggieri emphasised the epistemic practice of 'observing' in order to underline his self-understanding as a medical practitioner
whose primary source of both knowledge and reputation was his first-hand
experience. For Ruggieri, the art of medical observation was the most important programme for directing medicine towards a more empirically grounded
and thus more certain science. He directly reflected on his individual 'doctrine
of observation' in a lecture he gave in Padua on the occasion of his appointment to a professorship for Clinical Surgery in 1822, entitled *Dei doveri di chi
studia e di chi esercita la medicina.*[155] Addressing his students, he argued that
no one could become a good physician without learning the right techniques
of clinical observation. The observation of the visible facts had to be the starting point for any cognitive process in the medical sciences: 'One therefore has
to start with the observation of the facts, and the theoretical explanation of
these facts as well as their systematic coordination have to be made afterwards
to constitute the science'.[156] Emphasising the primacy of empirical observation over theory, Ruggieri proclaimed that 'The simple doctrine of observation
is clear, unchangeable, evident, it convinces everybody, and it alone rules in
contrast to the numerous, diverse, changeable, abstract and difficult theories
and opinions [...]'.[157]

    Already in his inaugural speech from 1803 Ruggieri had asked the rhetorical
question 'who does not recognise that all the theories would have remained
undeveloped, and of very little help, if not through repeated observation at the
bedside of the sick, our art had become stronger and stronger, so that it is no
longer based on abstract ideas, but can rely on the trustworthy ground of experience and reach a higher grade of certainty?'[158] Notwithstanding this emphasis on experience, in his Paduan lecture Ruggieri emphasised the importance

155   Ruggieri, *Dei doveri di chi studia e di chi esercita la medicina.*
156   Ibid., 19: 'Bisogna dunque cominciare dall'osservazione dei fatti, e la spiegazione teorica
      di questi fatti, e la loro coordinazione sistematica devono venir in seguito per costituire la
      scienza'.
157   Ibid., 26: '[...] la dottrina semplice dell'osservazione è chiara, immutabile, evidente,
      che convince tutti, e sola regge al confronto delle molteplici, diverse, mutabili, astratte,
      non che difficili teorie ed opinioni, sulle quali talvolta un raggio appena rifulge dei loro
      inventori'.
158   Ruggieri, *Prolusione intorno ai progressi ed avvanzamenti della chirurgia*, XXXIIIf.: '[...] e
      chi non vede che le teorie tutte sarebbero ben addietro rimaste, e ben poco giovevoli
      all'intento, se colla sedula e moltiplicata osservazione al letto degli ammalati l'arte non
      fosse venuta via via fortificandosi ed aggrandendosi a segno che non più camminando

of previous knowledge and theoretical reasoning for the ability to observe well, arguing that

> One has to be clear about that *to observe* is by no means a synonym for *looking at something*, and a physician who deserves to be called an observer first has to be instructed in as many analogous facts as possible. This is why deep study and reading is necessary. Then, the disease has to be observed among others, or at least with regard to the principal relations or differences that this disease can have with other disorders of the human body. This is why good reasoning powers and a good faculty of judgement are necessary. Whenever possible, the inner disease has to be observed by looking at the analogous lesions of the external human body, which, because they are subject to the senses, reveal the facts. This proves the indispensible necessity of surgical expert knowledge. Finally, one has to consider as often as possible experimental and inductive philosophy in order to discern the true type of action of the medical substances, and also, in order to determine the relation between them and the specific type of the pathological alterations constituting the disease. Only a man who is already familiar with the principal parts of the natural science is able to do this.[159]

This passage reveals the reciprocity between practice and theory in the medical idea and practice of observation. In order to understand the specificities of the disease under examination, individual observations needed to be related to numerous analogous observations. To this end, the physician had to draw

---

sopra le idée astratte, ma sopra i saldi sostegni dell'esperienza potè francamente poggiare al più alto grado di sicurezza?'

159 Ruggieri, *Dei doveri di chi studia e di chi esercita la medicina*, 28f.: 'E qui deve avvertirsi, che l'osservare non è in verun conto sinonimo di vedere, e che il medico degno del titolo d'osservatore, deve esser primieramente istruito del maggior numero possibile di fatti analoghi a quelli, ch'egli ha sott'occhio, donde la necessità di un assiduo studio e della lettura; poi considerare la malattia osservata sotto tutte, o almeno le principali relazioni o differenze, ch'essa può avere cogli altri disordini del corpo umano, donde la necessità d'un buon raziocinio e d'un giusto discernimento; quindi paragonare, ogni qualvolta ciò possa farsi, l'interna malattia osservata colle lesioni analoghe esteriori del corpo umano, le quali essendo soggette ai sensi, forniscono direttamente molti interessantissimi lumi, lo che prova l'assoluta indispensabile necessità delle cognizioni chirurgiche; finalmente servirsi il più spesso possibile della sperimentale ed induttiva filosofia, onde arrivare a discernere il vero tipo d'azione delle sostanze medicinali, non che a determinare il rapporto, che v'ha tra esso ed il tipo specifico dell'alterazione morbosa costituente la malattia, lo che non può farsi se non da chi è già versato nelle principali parti della scienza della natura'.

from previous knowledge gained by both experience and doctrine. This experience, in turn, could only be made through the repeated practice of individual observations. With this two-fold approach, Ruggieri was in line with medical authors since the seventeenth century who had likewise argued for the right balance between direct observation and theory – an approach that Pomata describes as 'Hippocratic-Galenic rational empiricism'.[160] Around 1800, we find similar claims for a 'combination of notions deriving from rational theory with those deriving from rational practice' in many contemporary reflections on the art of medical observation.[161]

However, the art of medical observation not only embraced cognitive capacities of physicians, it also meant the ability to document, to write down and to publish the observations in an appropriate way. Ruggieri explicitly reflects on this transformation of medical observations into narrative case histories in one of his *storie*. In the foreword to the *Storia di una blennorea*,[162] he refers to the ancient historian Thucydides as a model of impartial writing in order to compare the method of physicians with that of historians.[163] Ruggieri argues that 'it is not without reason that Mr Rousseau calls Thucydides the true model of a historian, because Thucydides always tells the facts without judging, thereby enabling the reader to make his own judgements. In fact, our spirit in writing case histories (*osservazioni*) must be free of any prejudice, and of any other useless passion, if we seek to reveal the truth properly'.[164] Referring to an important book on 'experience in the medical science',[165] published in

---

160   Pomata, *Praxis Historialis*, 136.

161   See for instance the entry 'osservazione' in Ruggieri's translation of the *Encyclopédie mé-thodique*: C. Ruggieri, *Dizionario enciclopedico di chirurgia. Tradotto dal francese in italiano ed accresciuto di aggiunte e note,* vol. 3, Padua, Nella Stamperia del Seminario presso Tommaso Bettinelli, 1806, 402: 'La natura deve parlar sola nelle Osservazioni, ma siccome il suo linguaggio anche allorquando se lo trascrive fedelmente, è quasi sempre involuto ed ambiguo, e spesso anche ingannatore, bisogna per interpretarlo far insieme concorrere le nozioni depurate di una teoria giudiziosa, con quelle di una pratica ragionata'.

162   Ruggieri, *Storia di una blennorea*, v.

163   This comparison was a commonplace in humanist medical writings, see Pomata, *Praxis Historialis,* 107.

164   Ruggieri, *Storia di una blennorea*, v: 'Non senza ragione il sig. ROUSSEAU chiamò TUCI-DIDE il vero modello degli Storici, perchè TUCIDIDE non fece che raccontare i fatti senza giudicarne, che possono mettere il lettore in istato di darne giudizio. Difatti il nostro spirito nello scrivere osservazioni deve essere sgombro d'ogni pregiudizio, e da qualunque altra inutile passione, se vuole disporsi bene a vedere la verità [...]'. Ruggieri refers here to Jean-Jaques Rousseau's book *Emile, où, de l'éducation,* Paris, Garnier Frères, 1961. The respective passage is in the fourth book.

165   J.G. Zimmermann, *Von der Erfahrung in der Arzneykunst. Neue Auflage,* Zurich, Orell, 1777. On Zimmermann see M. Dinges, 'Zimmermann, Johann Georg', in W.E. Gerabek

1777 by the Swiss physician Johann Georg Zimmermann (1728–1795), Ruggieri warns that as soon as prejudices are involved, 'one only sees what one wants to see'.[166] His ideal of observing nature and of writing impartial case histories as announced in the *Storia di una blennorea* was therefore as follows:

> The histories of diseases must be true, they must be written accurately, they must be simple and free of any hypothesis, containing only the pure and isolated description of the case (*fatto*). Nature wants to be painted as it is; and we should not add ornaments that disfigure it.[167]

Ruggieri's ideal of observation was not unusual. Rather, it has to be seen in the context of a broader endeavour to promote medicine as an empirical practical science, a programme which many European physicians pursued at that time. Philip Rieder has described this endeavour as characterised by a strong reliance on medical knowledge that derived from the observation of particular cases, which went together with a general mistrust of abstract medical systems.[168] Reflecting the emergence of a professional identity, medical societies were one of the many places in which such a practical medicine was promoted.[169] For this reason, it is worth considering that Ruggieri was a member in the Venetian medical society *Società Veneta di Medicina*. His participation in that circle shows that different visions of 'practical medicine' and the role of medical case histories in it co-existed in the early nineteenth century. In the *Società Veneta di Medicina*, Ruggieri's individual use of extraordinary cases to make a name for himself conflicted with the goal of a collective empiricism as pursued by the Venetian society, as we will see in the following.

The *Società Veneta di Medicina* had been founded during the time of the Venetian Republic, as an answer to a perceived crisis in Venetian medicine. During the political upheaval after the fall of the Venetian Republic, the existence

---

et al. (eds.), *Enzyklopädie Medizingeschichte*, Berlin and New York, Walter de Gruyter, 2005, 1530.

166   Ruggieri, *Storia di una blennorea*, V: '[...] e non basta nemmeno che senza parzialità, senza resistenze ed inciampi la rintracci, ma è altresì necessario che altro non cerchi, nè vagheggi che essa, mentre per quanto spirito di osservazione si possieda, dice sensatissimamente il celebre ZIMMERMANN, subito che vi si introducono gl'inciampi dei pregiudizj, quello solamente si vede, che si ha voglia di vedere [...]'.

167   Ibid.: '[...] Le istorie dunque delle malattie devono esser vere, devono esser scritte accuratamente, esser semplici e libere d'ogni ipotesi, contenendo soltanto la pura ed isolata relazione del fatto. La natura vuol esser depinta come si trova, nè occorre imprestarle ornamenti che poi la sfigurino'.

168   Rieder, *La médecine pratique*, 4.

169   Ibid., 8.

of the organisation was threatened several times. In 1810, it merged with two
literary societies to form the *Ateneo Veneto*, an important scholarly institution
that, in the course of the nineteenth century, became the centre of intellectual
debates in Venice.[170] While Ruggieri was not among the founding members
of the *Società di Medicina*,[171] he must have joined the unofficial meetings in
1806,[172] two years before the Minister of Internal Affairs of the French *Regno
d'Italia* officially re-founded the Society in 1808.[173] By then, it included 24 physicians practising in Venice, most of them members of the former *Collegio dei
Medici*.[174] The printed introductory speech of the first session of the re-founded
Società di Medicina mentions Ruggieri as Vice-Secretary, and describes him as
a man of broad knowledge with extraordinary skills in the surgical science.[175]

---

170   See Vanzan Marchini, *La politica sanitaria*, 160–172 and Pelizza, *Da 'alberghi informi di
      ammalati'*. So far, no profound research has been done on the *Società di Medicina*. A lot of
      archival material was destroyed during the political upheavals at the end of the Venetian
      Republic. The remaining material is today conserved in the archive of the Ateneo Veneto
      in Campo San Fantin. On the history of the building see P. Zampetti, *Guida alle opere
      d'arte della scuola di S. Fantin*, Venice, Ateneo Veneto, 1973. See also M. Gottardi (ed.),
      Venezia suddita (1798–1866), Venice, Marsilio, 1999, esp. the chapter by B. Rosada, 'Let-
      teratura e vita culturale a Venezia nella prima metà dell'ottocento', 107–126. The domicile
      of the *Ateneo Veneto* was (and still is) situated next to the *Teatro La Fenice*, in the former
      Scuola di S. Gerolamo on Campo San Fantin. It had very representative rooms, and the
      academy owned a precious library of medical books, see D. Raines (ed.), *Anatomia di una
      biblioteca: cinquanta volumi di medicina dalla collezione storica dell'ateneo veneto*, Venice,
      Ateneo Veneto, 2007. On the initial change of the residencies of the Società di Medicina
      see ibid., 18 and the files in ATV, Società Veneta di Medicina, b. 1, fasc. 4 (=anni 1792 a 1810,
      atti riguardanti la sede della società e a sua chiesa).
171   His name neither appears in the files of ATV, Società Veneta di Medicina, b. 1, fasc. 1 (=anni
      1789–1810, Statuti e regolamenti) nor in the files regarding the members, see ATV, Società
      Veneta di Medicina, b. 8.1 (=anni 1808–1862, Elenchi dei soci, prospetti e relazioni).
172   In a publication of 1806, Ruggieri is mentioned as a member, together with his brother
      Gaetano Alfonso Ruggieri: G. Moschini, *Della letteratura veneziana del secolo XVIII fino ai
      giorni nostri*, vol. 3, Venice, Dalla Stamperia Palese, 1806, 262.
173   P. Pezzi, *Discorso pronunciato dal vice-presidente Pezzi alla società di medicina di Vene-
      zia nella prima sessione di settembre dell'anno 1807 diciottesimo della sua istituzione prima
      della sua riforma*, Venice, Per Giuseppe Picotti, Stampatore della suddettta Società, 1808,
      25–48.
174   Giormani, *Contrasti tra l'università di Padova*, 67.
175   Pezzi, *Discorso pronunciato*, 38: '[...] colti in ogni ramo dell'umano sapere, ma eruditis-
      simo uno ed abilissimo nella scienza Chirurgica'. From the the printed papers of the first
      session results that Ruggieri belonged to the first class of the natural sciences that was
      medicine. Here, he is mentioned as professor and 'Elettore nel Collegio dei Dotti', see
      Società Scientifiche e Letterarie formanti l'ateneo Veneto (ed.), *Relazioni accademiche
      delle società scientifiche e letterarie formanti l'ATENEO VENETO. Prima pubblica sessione 21
      novembre 1812*, Venice, Nella Tipografia Picotti, 1812, 8.

The secretary was his brother Gaetano, who was responsible for the compilation and publication of all the academic lectures given in the *Ateneo*.[176]
The explicit model of the *Società Veneta di Medicina* was the *Société de Médecine* of Paris, the successor of the famous *Société Royale de Médecine* that
had been dissolved in 1793 during the French Revolution.[177] The principal concern of that Parisian society had been the collection of medical observations
from the whole country, regarding environmental and climatological factors
in relation to disease. The ultimate purpose of these collective observations
was to gain a general picture of the country's health condition, that is a medical topography, in order to effectively combat epidemics.[178] Under the guidance of its first secretary Francesco Aglietti, whom I have already introduced

176   Gaetano Ruggieri was temporarily editor of the *Sessioni pubbliche dell'ateneo veneto*, Ven-
      ice, Vitarelli, 1812–1817 and the *Esercitazioni scientifiche e letterarie dell'ateneo di Venezia*,
      Venice, Presso G. Picotti, 1827–1829. He also published an essay on the history of the *At-
      eneo Veneto*: G. Ruggieri, 'Ricordi storici sull'ateneo di Venezia, compilati dal Dott. Gaeta-
      no A. Ruggieri, membro ordinario, e vice-presidente', in G. Ruggieri (ed.), *Esercitazioni
      scientifiche e letterarie dell'ateneo di Venezia*, vol. 1, Venice, Presso G. Picotti, 1827, 2–16 and
      contributed to the debate on pellagra, see G. Ruggeri [sic!], *Riflessioni intorno ad una me-
      moria del p. trivigiano Giambattista Marzari, intitolata della pellagra e della maniera di
      estirparla in Italia*, Padua, Nella tipografia del Seminario, 1815.
177   ATV, Società Veneta di Medicina, b. 1, fasc. 1 (=anni 1789–1810, Statuti e regolamenti), *Piano
      per la istituzione di una società di medicina pratica esteso per commissione della medesi-
      ma dal Sign. Dott. Aglietti, letto il dì 3-di settembre del 1789, esaminato ed approvato in tre
      susseguenti sessionio, e sottoscritto dai membri componenti la Società medesima il dì primo
      ottobre*, 3: 'Nell'eseguimento della quale impresa io vi avverto a Signori che seguirò passo
      a passo e ricopierò luogo a luogo le savie istruzioni già per un simile oggetto pubblicate
      dalla illustre Società Medica di Parigi fino dalla prima epoca della sua fondazione'. On the
      Société Royale see R. Mandressi, 'Le passé, l'enseignement, la science: Félix Vicq d'Azyr
      et l'histoire de la médecine au XVIIIe siècle', *Medicina nei secoli. Arte e scienza*, vol. 20,
      no. 1, 2008, 183–212. The Society also published his own journal from 1796 onwards: So-
      ciété Royale (ed.), *Recueil périodique de la société de médecine de Paris*, Paris, Croullebois
      & Barrois, 1797–1802; Société Royale (ed.), *Journal général de médecine, de chirurgie et de
      pharmacie, françaises et étrangères; ou recueil périodique de la société de médecine de Paris*,
      Paris, Croullebois, T. Barrois jeune, 1802–1830.
178   Such projects were inspired by Thomas Sydenham's programme of studying the natural
      history of populations. Sydenham's primary concern was to study epidemic diseases, and
      he questioned the use of individual cases in medicine, see T. Sydenham, *Medical Observa-
      tions Concerning the History and the Cure of Acute Diseases. Translated from the Latin Edi-
      tion of Dr. Greenhill with a Life of the Author by R.G. Latham*, London, Sydenham Society,
      1848; see in particular vol. 1, 'Preface to the Third Edition', 17f. On the making of general
      observations see J.A. Mendelsohn, 'The World on a Page. Making a General Observation
      in the Eighteenth Century', in L. Daston and E. Lunbeck (eds.), *Histories of Scientific Ob-
      servation*, Chicago, University of Chicago Press, 2001, 396–420. On collective empiricism
      see also Gillispie, *Science and Polity in France*, 226–244.

as Ruggieri's partner in the Venetian Clinical School, the Venetian *Società di Medicina* sought to imitate this French model of collective empiricism.

Aglietti was an erudite physician, anatomist and medical writer who played a pivotal role in Venetian medical debates around 1800.[179] In 1789 he drafted an 'outline for the formation of a society for practical medicine', in which he programmatically called for a *collective* endeavour of observing nature:

> All sciences that have as their object the observation of nature, and that can only improve by means of observation, need to be cultivated collectively. Nature is so large and magnificent in its doctrines; she has come to vary in many aspects and at the same time she reunifies in so many relations that it is absolutely impossible that one single man, isolated and restricted in the narrow limitations of his own activity, could ever make a step towards the acquisition of these indefinable series of truth that can actually lead to the discovery of any of the multiple operations of the great mother [nature].[180]

In this spirit of collective inquiry, the Venetian society sought to bring physicians together in order to compose 'an exact history of the diseases present in the country, considered in their various relations to climate, temper, and the

---

179   Under Austrian rule, Francesco Aglietti (1757–1836) became the personal physician of the Emperor Francis I, see Vanzan Marchini, *La memoria della salute*, 236. See also C. Maccagni, 'Francesco Aglietti e il suo tempo', in Istituto Veneto di Scienze Lettere ed Arti (ed.), *Le scienze mediche nel veneto dell'ottocento*, Venice, Istituto Veneto di Scienze Lettere ed Arti, 1990, 155–169. There is also a contemporary biography on Aglietti: Zannini, *Biografia di Francesco Aglietti*. Archival documents regarding Aglietti (correspondence, certificates) are conserved in ATV, Società Veneta di Medicina, b. 1, fasc. 1 (=anni 1789–1810, Statuti e regolamenti).

180   Aglietti, *Piano per la istituzione di una società di medicina pratica*, 1: 'Tutte le Scienze, le quali hanno per oggetto la contemplazione della natura, e le quali non possono perfezionarsi che per mezzo dell'osservazione abbisognano di essere coltivate in commune. La Natura è cosi grande e magnifica nè suoi magisterj, a ella saputo diversificarsi sotto tanti aspetti e riunirsi nel medesimo tempo con tanti si varj rapporti ch'egli è assolutamente impossibile che l'uomo isolato e ristretto negli angusti confini della propria attività possa mai fare alcun passo verso l'aquisto di quella serie indefinibile di verità, che menano adirittura allo scoprimento di qualcheduna fra le moltiplici operazioni della gran madre'. Aglietti likewise expressed his admiration of the collective empiricism of the Parisian society in a journal he edited in the 1780s, in which he occasionally published contributions written by some of its members, see F. Aglietti (ed.), *Giornale per servire alla storia ragionata della medicina di questo secolo*, Venice, Nella Stamperia Pasquali, 1783–1793. On this journal see A. Castiglioni, *Gli albori del giornalismo medico italiano*, Trieste, Tipografia del Lloyd triestino, 1923, 22f.

way of life of the inhabitants, as well as to natural incidents and the effects of the seasons'.[181] In order to achieve such a general history of current diseases, the single observations written by the different members needed to be collected and united in a central place.[182] This general medical history as proposed by Aglietti included three main subjects: a 'medical topography' of the city, meteorological observations, and a description of all the current diseases, categorised as sporadic, endemic, and epidemic.[183] According to a contemporary observer, the overall aim of the Society was the improvement of the medical provision in the city of Venice – in modern terms, it pursued public health goals.[184]

The writing of medical observations was one of the most important duties of the members. Aglietti wrote in his outline that

> [...] it is necessary that every physician keeps an exact record of all the cases that he observes, and writes down with the greatest accuracy all the visible circumstances of the given case, whether they are effects or natural consequences of the disease, but also those that can be considered products or effects of remedies, and of all the coincidences that can occur. The compilation of such a journal is not very difficult; the physicians only has to get rid of any kind of preconception and carry it out with the sincerity that a true adherent and servant of nature must have.[185]

---

181   Aglietti, *Piano per la istituzione di una società di medicina pratica*, 1: '[...] una Storia esatta delle malattie dominanti in un dato paese, considerate sotto i varj rapporti del clima, del temperamento, e della maniera di vivere degli abitanti, e delle vicende naturali e avventizie delle stagioni [...]'.

182   Ibid.

183   Ibid., 3: 'La Storia medicinate di una Città o Provincia deve soddisfare a tre oggetti essenzialissimi: I. Ricerche ed osservazioni sulla costituzione fisica e morale, ossia Topografia medica della Città; II. Osservazioni Meteorologiche; III. Descrizione esatta e complessa delle malattie insorgenti considerate sotto i tre conosciuti rapporti di Sporadiche, Endemiche, ed Epidemiche'. The interest in medical topography was a more general trend, see A. Valatelli, *Della topografia fisico-medica di Venezia. Dissertazione*, Venice, s.n., 1803.

184   See Moschini, *Della letteratura veneziana*, 225.

185   Aglietti, *Piano per la istituzione di una società di medicina pratica*, 3: '[...] ed a tal uopo é necessario che ogni Medico tenga un giornale esatto di tutti li casi che a mano a mano gli si anderan presentando, notando con ogni più scrupolosa diligenza tutte le più minute circostanze percettibili nel dato caso, tanto quelle sono effetti o successioni naturali della malattia, come quelle che si potran risguardare come prodotti o consequenze de' rimedj, e di tutte le accidentalità, che mai potessero per avventura combinarsi. La compilazione di un simile Giornale non è poi un impresa gran fatto difficile, e basta che il Medico vi si conduca spoglio da ogni spirito di sistema, e con quella sincerità che si conviene a un fedele seguace e ministro della natura'.

Referring to Hippocrates as the best model for the recording of medical observations, Aglietti specified the way in which the members were to write their
case records. They had

> I. To record everything that may have an influence on the disease under
> examination, however remote it may seem, such as the season, the sky,
> and the current diseases. II. To mention the cause of the disease, if there
> is an obvious one, but paying attention not to declare it as the truth if
> there is any uncertainty. III. To explain with great accuracy the temper,
> the sex, and the previous condition of the sick. IV. To pay special attention
> to the course of the disease, recording the excesses, the aggravations, the
> intermissions, the critical moments, the relapses.[186]

As prescribed in the *Regolamento per la società di medicina*, the Society's printed rules published in 1808,[187] every member had to present his case record to
the Society once a month.[188] They contained a series of cases and were meant
to contribute to a medical topography of Venice. As sociologist Wolf Lepenies
has remarked with view to the Parisian *Société Royale de Médecine*, the Venetian Society's model, while 'the narration of singular monstrous cases was the
duty of a single scholar and satisfied his curiosity, the observation of epidemics required to be done by groups of scholars, because they occurred at distant
places'.[189] Notwithstanding this focus on collective inquiry, the members were
also obliged to regularly present individual observations on practical medicine

---

186   Ibid.: 'I. Di notare tutto quello che può influire sulla data malattia, quantunque straniero
       ad essa, come la stagione, lo stato del Cielo, e le malattie regnanti. II. Di far menzione
       della causa, quando però ve ne' abbia una di apparente, avvertendo bene di sfuggire at-
       tentamente il pericolo di proporne come vera qualcheduna di incerta. III. Di esporre con
       ogni diligenza il temperamento, l'età, il sesso, e lo stato anteriore degli infermi. IV. Di pre-
       stare una speziale attenzione all'invasione della malattia, notarne esattamente gli accessi,
       le esacerbazioni, le intermissioni, li movimenti critici, le recidive'.
187   In the files of the ATV, there are different manuscript drafts of this text: ATV, Società Ve-
       neta di Medicina, b. 1, fasc. 1 (=anni 1789–1810, Statuti e regolamenti), *Regolamento della
       pubblica società di medicina di Venezia*. See for the published version of this text: Società
       di Medicina di Venezia, *Regolamento della pubblica società di medicina di Venezia*, Venice,
       Per Giuseppe Picotti, Stampatore della suddettta Società, 1808.
188   ATV, *Regolamento della pubblica società di medicina di Venezia*: 'Occupazioni e doveri de'
       Socj [...]'.
189   W. Lepenies, *Das Ende der Naturgeschichte. Wandel kultureller Selbstverständlichkeiten
       in den Wissenschaften des 18. und 19. Jahrhunderts*, Frankfurt, Carl Hanser, 1978, 91: '[...]
       während die neugierbefriedigende Erzählung monströser Krankheitsfälle die Sache
       Einzelner war, konnte die Beobachtung voneinander entfernt auftretender Epidemien
       nur durch Gruppen erfolgen'.

(*osservazioni di medicina pratica*), called *memorie particolari* or *memorie di do-veri*. Afterwards, the secretary collected these individual case histories for censorship (*le necessarie censure*).[190] The authors had to write their case histories in Italian, French or Latin, and they were not allowed to publish any papers delivered in the Society without prior permission of the secretary.[191] From 1810 onwards, the *Ateneo Veneto* continued with a similar procedure. In every session, one member had to give a lecture on a topic of his particular interest. In the case of physicians, the papers usually reported on individual medical cases they had observed in their medical practice.[192] In the subsequent session, the members present would approve the paper on the basis of the minutes.[193]

Ruggieri had some problems with these rules. As an ordinary member, he regularly participated in the assemblies of the *Società di Medicina*.[194] While there is no evidence that Ruggieri presented Lovat's case to the Society, he did present his other two *storie*. In the *Storia di una blennorea,* published in 1809, he wrote: 'I think I have to inform the reader that so far, the Society has not yet pronounced a judgement of this case, this means that I am not disrespecting the article 60 of the Society's rules prohibiting publishing anything that has been read to the society and that has not yet been approved of by the secretary'.[195] Clearly, this was a rather liberal interpretation of the rules – it seems that Ruggieri simply did not want to wait with the publication of his case history until the judgement of his colleagues. Was he afraid that his colleagues would not authorise the publication of the *Storia di una blennorea* because it dealt with the delicate subject of bestiality? In any case, Ruggieri chose to publish his case history independently rather than in one of the Societies' journals.

---

190   ATV, *Regolamento della pubblica società di medicina di Venezia*. In the published rules, these lectures were later called *memorie di dovere*, see Società di Medicina di Venezia, *Regolamento della pubblica società di medicina di Venezia*, 8.

191   Ibid., 20f.

192   See a manuscript of the *Regolamento dell'ateneo veneto* in BMC, Cod. Cicogna, 2999, fasc. 12: 'Titolo IX. Dei Membri Ordinarj. 37. I Membri Ordinarj risiedono nella Città di Venezia [...]'.

193   See the minutes of the sessions in ATV, Adunanze/processi verbali, b. 13 (=anni 1812–1826, Corpo academico). A register of these sessions can be requested by the personell of the ATV. See also the list of external members and correspondents, mirroring the structure of the institution, in Società Scientifiche e Letterarie formanti l'ateneo Veneto (ed.), *Relazioni accademiche delle società scientifiche*, 75–97.

194   His name appears in some minutes of sessions during the year 1811, for instance: ATV, Società Veneta di Medicina, b. 1, fasc. 2 (= anni 1790–1811, Relazioni sull'attività della società e verbali delle sedute; Rese di conti, cariche onorarie), *Processo verbale della sezione tenuta dalla pubblica società di medicina il dì 14 dicembre 1811.*

195   Ruggieri, *Storia di una blennorea*. In the edition of 1814, this preface was not reprinted.

Some years later, Ruggieri presented the *Storia ragionata di una donna* to the Society, again provoking a conflict.[196] Although he intended to publish the case, he refused to leave a copy of his lecture in the archive of the *Ateneo Veneto*.[197] He even denied the secretary a chance to take a closer look at his manuscript.[198] Ruggieri's obstinate behaviour caused a stir in the Society. The secretary called on the president of the *Ateneo Veneto* in order to inquire if such behaviour was acceptable: 'Is this in accordance with the dignity of the *Ateneo Veneto*, and with the spirit of the rules that we have approved with the greatest consent, stating that none of the ordinary members gives any presentation against which the audience of the *Ateneo* has no right of veto, or which is not properly registered in the files of the *Ateneo*?'[199]

These conflicts surrounding the presentation of Ruggieri's two *storie* in front of the *Società di Medicina* suggest two conclusions. Firstly, they show that Ruggieri wanted to take the publication of his case histories into his own hands. Most likely, he mistrusted the Society's examination procedures because he feared that his case histories, because of their delicate subjects, would not be published at all but instead buried in the Society's archive. Also, he might have hoped that publishing his case histories independently in the form of booklets would be more rewarding for his own reputation, as the *Storia della crocifissione* had proved. Secondly, rather than merely representing a curious anecdote of Ruggieri's amour-propre, these conflicts point to two conflicting conceptions of case writing at the time. In the *Società di Medicina*, the serial and collective recording of medical cases served the making of so-called general observations, which in turn were used to construct a medical topography

---

196 In the files from the year 1814, we find the minutes of a session in which Ruggieri gave a lecture entitled 'Relazione ragionata del tricazoodes osservato in una donna' ATV, Adunanze/processi verbali, b. 13 (=anni 1812–1826, Corpo academico), Processo verbale della 17a sessione dell'ateneo veneto tenuta lì 22 dicembre 1814. The title confirms that this was the same case history Ruggieri published independently in 1815 under the title *Storia ragionata di una donna avente gran parte del corpo coperta di pelle:* the term *tricazoodes* is the same term Ruggieri uses in his published text to describe the pelt of the woman.

197 Ruggieri participated in most of the assemblies between 1812 and 1815, but in the files containing the papers of the members no papers authored by him can be found, see ATV, Ateneo Veneto, b. 28 (=anni 1812–1817, Attività letteraria e scientifica, memorie e studi) and b. 13 (=anni 1812–1826, Corpo accademico, adunanze, relazioni annuali).

198 See the complaints in the respective minutes: ATV, Adunanze/processi verbali, b. 13 (=anni 1812–1826, Corpo academico), *Processo verbale della 17a sessione dell'ateneo veneto tenuta lì 22 dicembre 1814.*

199 Ibid.: 'Convien egli dal decoro dell'Ateneo, ed'allo spirito del Regolarmento che di massimo consenso abbiamo approvato che venga fatta da qualunque siasi fra i soci ordinarj alcuna lettura sulla quale l'Ateneo uditore non debba [illegible; probably pronunciare, M.B.] il suo veto, o della quale non debba tenersi ragionato ricordo nei registri dell'Ateneo?'

of the Venetian state for the purpose of public health. In contrast, Ruggieri relied on the early modern tradition of writing remarkable case histories, which had a totally different epistemic purpose, as they focused on the idiosyncrasies of individual patients and their ailments rather than on epidemic diseases. As we have seen, there was space for such individual case histories in the Venetian society. Yet, rules were to be followed, collaboration was required and a rigid system of censorship was applied.[200] This normative framework conflicted with Ruggieri's individual professional interests. In contrast to the collective enterprise of the Society, he regarded medical case histories to be the property of their author. That Ruggieri published his three *storie* in book-like publications in several editions and followed their success beyond Venice with great interest, confirms his self-confidence as an independent medical writer.

Despite these tensions, being a member of the *Ateneo Veneto* had professional advantages for Ruggieri. As the Society had many correspondents in different European cities, Ruggieri had access to a broad international network.[201] Among the corresponding members were physicians from Florence and Pisa but also from Edinburgh, Berlin, Göttingen, Leiden, London, Munich, Paris, Vienna, Petersburg and Copenhagen.[202] Some of the external members would later show great interest in Ruggieri's *Storia della crocifissione*. This proves that the dissemination of Ruggieri's *storie* profited from the *Ateneo*'s international network.

Focusing on Ruggieri's role as a Professor of Surgery and on his publications, this chapter has shown how a medical author's choice to publish in a certain epistemic genre depended on a variety of factors. First of all, Ruggieri *wrote down* case histories in the *observationes* genre because this was the textual form traditionally used to communicate knowledge gained from medical practice. Although Ruggieri was eager to present himself as a 'scientific' surgeon, his self-understanding was ultimately that of a practitioner. He was convinced that medicine had to be based on empirical knowledge gained through observation in order to become a more certain science. Secondly, *printing* and *publishing* his case histories in the way and form he wanted was very important

---

200 A detailed description of this system can be found in a foreword to a case history conserved in ATV, Società di Medicina, b. 2, fasc. V a (=anni 1790–1810, Lavori accademici), fasc. 14.

201 The publications of the *Ateneo Veneto* give an interesting insight into the international dimension of the medical culture of nineteenth-century Venice, see the bibliography of the works published by the Ateneo Veneto, *L'ateneo veneto nel suo primo centenario 1812–1912*, Venice, Ateneo Veneto, 1912.

202 Società Scientifiche e Letterarie formanti l'Ateneo Veneto (ed.), *Relazioni accademiche delle società scientifiche*, 79 and 93–97.

for Ruggieri. He wanted to see his name in print, and he strove for the attention of an international readership. His eagerness in getting his case histories published is itself revealing, as it points to a broader development in medical publishing, namely the growing new need to publish in print which was an effect of the print revolutions of the eighteenth century. As George Rousseau and Roy Porter have argued, during the long eighteenth century, publication had become the cornerstone for the developing professional identity of physicians.[203] Publishing was vital for the professionalisation of medicine because the making and dissemination of reliable knowledge, and therefore medical progress, had come to depend on it. As Rousseau has suggested, only printed discoveries were discoveries, and news was only news if printed.[204] In order to become a real science, medical knowledge had to go public, and print was the best and only 'legitimate proof of professionalization'.[205] Ruggieri's case histories, in particular the erudite *storie*, therefore helped him to construct his identity as an academic surgeon who, by way of publishing, contributed to the making of surgery as a new medical specialty. That Ruggieri was so keen to get his name into print by publishing elaborated case histories was therefore not only an individual penchant of a vain professor, but signalled a new professional consciousness that heavily relied on publishing in print.

---

203   G.S. Rousseau, '"Stung into Action...": Medicine, Professionalism, and the News', in J. Raymond (ed.), *News, Newspapers, and Society in Early Modern Britain*, London, Frank Cass and Company, 1999, 176–205; R. Porter, 'The Rise of Medical Journalism in Britain to 1800', in W.F. Bynum, S. Lock, and R. Porter (eds.), *Medical Journals and Medical Knowledge. Historical Essays*, London, Routledge, 1992, 6–28.
204   Rousseau, *'Stung into Action...'*, 186.
205   Ibid., 194.

CHAPTER 3

Making the Case Travel: Translation, Media, Reading

In 1807 a German translation of Ruggieri's *Storia della crocifissione* appeared on the German book market.[1] In the foreword dating from 30 May, the translator explained that,

> I received this story on the seventeenth of May from Venice, together with a letter dating from the second of May, which, among other things, contained the note that the story had been released only a few days ago, printed in quarto; he (the sender) would not need to confirm the authenticity of this unheard story of crucifixion – for the fast and generous communication of it I herewith thank the sender publicly – : for all the inhabitants of Venice, like for himself, the fact would still be fresh in the memory.[2]

The author of the translation was Julius Heinrich Gottlieb Schlegel (1772–1839), a German physician who had served as the official physician of the town of Ilmenau in Saxony since 1796 and became known for his 1803 book on practical medicine and public health, entitled *Materialien für die Staatsarzneiwissenschaft und praktische Heilkunde*.[3] It is clear from the preface that Schlegel had received the French version of the *Storia della crocifissione*, which had been

---

1 C. Ruggieri, *Geschichte der durch Mathieu Lovat zu Venedig im Jahr 1805 an sich selbst vollzogenen Kreuzigung. Bekannt gemacht von Cesar Ruggieri [...] Aus dem Französischen übersetzt und mit Anmerkungen versehen von Julius Heinrich Gottlieb Schlegel [...]*, Rudolstadt, Klüger, 1807.

2 Ibid., 5: 'Gegenwärtige Geschichte erhielt ich am 17ten May 1807 aus Venedig, begleitet von einem den 2ten May datierten Briefe, der unter andern die Bemerkung enthielt, daß sie erst vor einigen Tagen, in 4. Gedruckt, ausgegeben worden sey; er (der Einsender) habe nicht nöthig mir die Echtheit dieser unerhörten Geschichte der Kreuzigung – für deren schnelle, gütige Mittheilung ich demselben öffentlich hierdurch meinen verbindlichen Dank abstatte – zu bezeugen: allen Einwohnern Venedigs, so wie ihm selbst, sei das Faktum noch in frischem Andenken'.

3 J.H.G. Schlegel, *Materialien für die Staatsarzneiwissenschaft und praktische Heilkunde*, Jena, Goepferdt, 1800–1803. Schlegel was the 'Herzogl. Sachs.-Weimar. Amts-und Stadt-Physikus zu Ilmenau', see J. Pagel, 'Schlegel, Julius Heinrich Gottlieb', in Historische Kommission bei der Bayerischen Akademie der Wissenschaften (ed.), *Allgemeine Deutsche Biographie*, vol. 31, Munich, Duncker & Humblot, 1890, 389. In 1810, he was appointed to the post of a court physician of Saxony ('Sachsen-Weimarischen und Meiningischen Hofmedicus'), and in 1811 he became a court counsellor ('fürstlich Schwarzburg-Sondershausenschen Hofrath').

printed in quarto in Venice in 1806. Ruggieri had sent the booklet to him in a letter, and it took Schlegel only a few days to translate the French text and to publish a German translation with a commentary. The *Geschichte der durch Mathieu Lovat zu Venedig im Jahr 1805 an sich selbst vollzogenen Kreuzigung* appeared in the same format as the French original and included a high quality reproduction of the two original illustrations (see illustration 5). From 1807, it was distributed by a bookshop in the German town of Rudolstadt, and was printed in a second edition in 1821.[4]

Schlegel's translation, to which we will turn in greater detail below, shows the crucial role of translations in the dissemination of Ruggieri's case history beyond Venice. The precondition for the effective circulation of Lovat's case in different European countries was the production of a German and an English translation, in addition to Ruggieri's own French edition. Together, the three translations communicated Lovat's case to an international readership and thus triggered the Europe-wide reactions to it. To a large extent, the translations determined where, when and how Ruggieri's case history was received in the different countries.

The other determining factor in the dissemination of the *Storia della crocifissione* in the nineteenth century was the existence of an ever-growing media landscape, which had emerged in Europe as an effect of the print revolutions during the early modern period.[5] Historians of the book, publishing and reading have shown how the nineteenth century saw the rise and pluralisation of new media, which helped bring about the development of a much wider reading public.[6] Addressing the increasing literacy and education of the public, different sorts of publications had established their own genres and audiences by the early nineteenth century. Besides the book, these included various periodical publications such as newspapers and magazines, which had developed with distinct national specificities since the seventeenth century and provided

---

4   C. Ruggieri, *Mathieu Lovat's Selbstkreuzigung zu Venedig im J. 1805. A. d. F. von dem Hofrath und Ritter Julius Heinrich Gottlieb Schlegel. Unveränderte, wohlfeile Ausgabe*, Meiningen, In der Reyßnerschen Hofbuchhandlung, 1821.

5   E.L. Eisenstein, *The Printing Press as an Agent of Change: Communications and Cultural Transformations in Early-Modern Europe*, Cambridge, UK, Cambridge University Press, 1994; M. Giesecke, *Der Buchdruck in der frühen Neuzeit. Eine historische Fallstudie über die Durchsetzung neuer Information- und Kommunikationstechnologien*, Frankfurt, Suhrkamp, 1991; J. Raymond and N. Moxham, 'New Networks in Early Modern Europe', in J. Raymond and N. Moxham (eds.), *News Networks in Early Modern Europe*, Leiden and Boston, Brill, 2016, 1–18.

6   See for instance M. Lyons, *Reading Culture and Writing Practice in Nineteenth-Century France*, Toronto, University of Toronto Press, 2008; M. Lyons, *Readers and Society in Nineteenth-Century France. Workers, Women, Peasants*, Basingstoke, Palgrave, 2001; H. Martin and R. Chartier (eds.), *Le temps des éditeurs. Du romantisme à la belle époque*, Paris, Promodis, 1985.

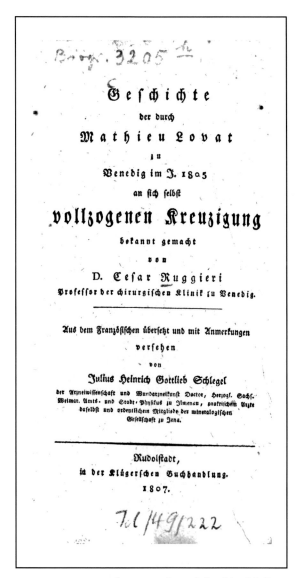

ILLUSTRATION 5   Julius Heinrich Gottlieb Schlegel (ed.),
                  Geschichte der durch Mathieu Lovat zu
                  Venedig im Jahr 1805 an sich selbst
                  vollzogenen Kreuzigung, 1807.

quick information, education and entertainment for a broader readership.[7]
New reading practices developed as a response to the growing trade in

7   See E. Fischer, 'Buchmarkt', *Europäische Geschichte Online*, [website], 2010, http://ieg-ego.eu/
     de/threads/hintergruende/buchmarkt/ernst-fischer-buchmarkt, (accessed 12 July 2017).

publishing, with a shift from intensive to extensive reading habits, leading to a demand for new forms of publications.[8] In particular periodicals, both specialist and generalist, allowed for the emergence of discursive spaces in which the reading public gradually developed secular worldviews and political opinions.[9] In this sense, publishing constructed new public spheres, creating the cultural and technical preconditions for the circulation of Lovat's case.[10]

As part of this emerging media landscape, medical journalism and a specialised medical press played an important role in the Europe-wide dissemination of the case.[11] As historian George Rousseau has emphasised, publishing in print had become an important means for physicians to assert progress and professionalisation, prompting questions about the elite or public character of medical knowledge. In the course of the eighteenth century, a causal relation had emerged in medicine between the act of publishing and professional consciousness:

> If a developing profession – for example, medicine – wished to gather status, it *had* to publish. Otherwise, it would remain a private rather than public enterprise, an activity for private persons writing unpublished letters to each other no matter how dire the need for medical diagnosis and cure. The historical issue for medical news may then be not so much its publication as its professionalisation in the eighteenth century, with print culture as living proof that it was indeed professionalising.[12]

Hence medical news, and also that transmitted in the form of case histories such as Lovat's case, gained in importance in part through the act of publishing.[13]

This chapter briefly considers the impact these broader developments had on the travelling of Lovat's case in the different countries and through different

---

8   Ibid., 25.

9   See H. Böning, 'Weltaneignung durch ein neues Publikum. Zeitungen und Zeitschriften als Medientypen der Moderne', *Historische Zeitschrift. Beihefte*, vol. 41, 2010, 105–134, 133.

10   Jouhaud and Viala, *De la publication entre renaissance et lumières*, 10.

11   On medical journalism see Porter, *The Rise of Medical Journalism in Britain to 1800*, and W.F. Bynum and J.C. Wilson, 'Periodical Knowledge: Medical Journal and Their Editors in Nineteenth-Century Britain', in W.F. Bynum, S. Lock, and R. Porter (eds.), *Medical Journals and Medical Knowledge. Historical Essays*, London, Routledge, 1992, 29–48.

12   Rousseau, 'Stung into Action...', 180.

13   On the relation between medicine and print see also J.J. Connor, 'Introduction. Book Culture and Medicine', *Canadian Bulletin of Medical History*, vol. 12, no. 2, 1995, 203–214 and, with a broader focus on science, R.D. Apple, G.J. Downe, and S.L. Vaughn (eds.), *Science in Print: Essays on the History of Science and the Culture of Print*, Madison, University of Wisconsin Press, 2012.

genres. It does so by taking a close look at the physical appearance of the three translations in their respective local contexts, and by examining the reasons for the early discussion and transnational dissemination of Lovat's case in French, German and English periodicals. While the later chapters focus on how different 'interpretive communities' read, understood and rewrote Lovat's case in terms of its meaning and interpretation, this chapter considers the simple fact that, to a certain extent, the medium always shapes the message: not only does the form of a text itself determines its meaning, the publication in which a text appears also affects its form and content. As we shall see, it made a difference if Lovat's case was published in a magazine directed at a broader lay readership, or if it was included in a textbook for specialists. Various publications discussed Lovat's case, and the purposes of these publications varied. It is important to consider these different purposes of the vehicles of Lovat's case because they reveal not only why and how authors or editors republished Lovat's case, but also what readers might have expected when reading it. From the perspective of the history of printing, therefore, Lovat's case demonstrates the effects which the nineteenth-century growth in the number of publications had on the circulation of case histories.

1   The French Translation (1806)

As mentioned in the previous chapter, the French edition of Ruggieri's case history, entitled *Histoire du crucifiement éxécuté sur sa propre personne par Mathieu Lovat, communiqué au public dans une lettre de César Ruggieri docteur en medecine et professeur de chirurgie clynique à Venise. A un medecin son ami* had been printed by Ruggieri himself.[14] Schlegel's foreword to his German translation suggests that the French booklet was published in Venice only in 1807, while Ruggieri had written the text in 1806 and had also published his Italian *Storia della crocifissione* in Carlo Amoretti's miscellanea in the same year.[15] Was Ruggieri thus the first translator of his own case history? Simone Bandirali, who edited the 1814 edition of the *Storia della crocifissione*, presumes that the Italian version published by Amoretti was the very first draft of Ruggieri's case history.[16] She argued that in order to produce the French version, Ruggieri translated this first Italian edition.[17] Bandirali presumed that with several

---

14   Ruggieri, *Histoire du crucifiement éxécuté sur sa propre personne par Mathieu Lovat.*
15   Ruggieri, *Geschichte der durch Mathieu Lovat zu Venedig im Jahr 1805 an sich selbst vollzogenen Kreuzigung*, 5f.
16   Bandirali, *Storia della crocifissione*, 30–42.
17   See the bibliographical notes ibid., 8.

additional annotations, Ruggieri sought to give the French edition a more academic style because he intended to address it directly to the circle of the first
French psychiatrists (*aliénistes*).[18]

Indeed, Ruggieri intended to reach an international readership, and the existence of the French pamphlet led to the circulation of Lovat's case not only
in France, but also in Germany and Britain. However, there is no evidence that
the French text actually had a specific French readership in mind right from
the beginning: as Schlegel's foreword confirms, the French booklet first arrived
in Germany, and only a few years later in Paris. Hence, rather than addressing a specific French colleague, Ruggieri presumably chose French as a *langue
universelle* to communicate his case to the international medical community.
Also, the political circumstances might have influenced Ruggieri's linguistic
choice: In 1806, Venice fell under Napoleonic rule. As a consequence, corresponding in French had much to recommend it. That the French edition is
more elaborate than the first Italian version is probably due to the fact that
Ruggieri sought to edit the case in the form of a booklet: the different format
required a certain length and some more elaboration. The French edition thus
confirms what Isabelle Pantin has stated considering the functions of scientific
translations in the early modern period:

> [t]he translation of a modern work could serve different purposes. Its
> original language – either Latin or vernacular – was chosen according to
> the requirements of the context. As a rule, the decision to translate it did
> not mean that this context had changed, but that the role assigned to the
> work and the way in which its reception was envisaged, were altered. Two
> principal factors came into play: the new public and the prestige associ-
> ated with a change in the status of the work.[19]

Not only the addressee but also the status of the French booklet appears ambiguous: as mentioned before, the typographic details are lacking, which means
that Ruggieri had it printed at his own expense and that it was not officially
distributed by a Venetian printer. Schlegel's translation confirms that the
French edition soon circulated via informal ways such as letters or private

---

18   See ibid., 6.
19   I. Pantin, 'The Role of Translations in European Scientific Exchanges in the Sixteenth and
      Seventeenth centuries', in P. Burke and R. Po-Chia Hsia (eds.), *Cultural Translation in Early
      Modern Europe*, Cambridge, UK, Cambridge University Press, 2007, 163–179, 167. On the
      role of translations see also S. Stockhorst (ed.), *Cultural Transfer through Translation. The
      Circulation of Enlightened Thought in Enlightened Europe by means of Translation*, Amster-
      dam and New York, Rodopi, 2010.

hand-to-hand distribution. It thus seems that Ruggieri used the French edition as kind of a backup: he probably feared that his case history, if published exclusively in Carlo Amoretti's collection, would receive only a little attention by an Italian readership, but never reach foreign colleagues. As it turned out, Ruggieri was right to have this concern: Carlo Amoretti's first edition of the *Storia della crocifissione* was met with almost complete disregard. Throughout the nineteenth century, no detailed commentary on Lovat's case was made on the basis of this first Italian edition. If Amoretti's edition was mentioned at all, it was in the context of general reviews of Amoretti's editorial project.[20] By producing an autonomous publication in French, Ruggieri probably hoped that it would not only reach an international readership and was therefore a better means to enhance the reputation of its author, but it would also stress the singularity of Lovat's case much more than an article in a collective volume. As the career of Lovat's case described in the following chapters shows, his strategy bore fruit.

Beyond the specific purpose of Ruggieri's French translation, the fact that he considered it important to publish his case history in more than one language also reflects a much broader historical development, namely the rise of national languages during the eighteenth century that replaced Latin as the language of the academic elite.[21] By the early nineteenth century, the European scientific community relied on national languages for correspondence, in particular on French, and published texts were read either in their original languages or as translations.[22] As an effect, the demand for foreign publications and translators increased and plural ways of distribution, both official and private, emerged. Scientific networks played an important role in the communication of new publications, and travelling scholars frequently functioned as book suppliers and important agents in their distribution.[23] These circumstances explain why Ruggieri considered it promising to have a special edition printed in French, which he could distribute via his personal network

---

20   For instance, this is the case in a German journal on natural sciences: A.F. Gehlen (ed.), *Journal für die Chemie, Physik und Mineralogie*, vol. 4, Berlin, Realschulbuchhandlung, 1807, 51.

21   Fischer, *Buchmarkt*, 21. On vernacular translations in the realm of medicine see A. Carlino and M. Jeanneret (eds.), *Vulgariser la médecine. Du style médical en France et en Italie*, Geneva, Droz, 2009.

22   Fischer, *Buchmarkt*, 21.

23   Ibid., 22. See also M. Werner, 'Les libraires comme intermédiaires culturels: remarques à propos du rôle des libraires allemands en France au xixe siècle', in F. Barbier, S. Juratic, and D. Varry (eds.), *L'Europe et le livre. Réseaux et pratiques du négoce du librairie XVIe–XIXe siècles*, Paris, Klinksieck, 1996, 527–542.

and according to his individual needs. Not only did he send the French pamphlet via mail to specific addressees, like Schlegel, but he also took it with him
when he travelled. In 1811, that is four years after he had the French edition
printed, he brought it with him when he visited Paris in order to personally
hand it over to a medical colleague. Ruggieri's publishing strategy thus confirms historian Peter Burke's argument that '[l]ike other forms of speech and
writing, translating is a kind of action'.[24]

2   The German Translation (1807)

Schlegel was not only interested in translating Ruggieri's case history because
of various specific medical topics it referred to, but also because it allowed him
to get his own name into print and to communicate with other physicians. He
dedicated his translation to the German physician Johann Christian Friedrich,
who was a court councillor and the private physician of the prince of Lippe
in Detmold, as well as to David van Gesscher, Lecturer in Theoretical Surgery
in Amsterdam.[25] Still in 1807, Schlegel produced a Dutch translation of Ruggieri's case history, on the basis of his own German text.[26] Schlegel was generally
known to be a great correspondent and regularly exchanged letters not only
with medical colleagues but also with well known German writers, including
Goethe.[27] But what were Schlegel's professional ambitions as a physician, and
what exactly did he seek to achieve with the two translations of Lovat's case?

Schlegel's *Geschichte der durch Mathieu Lovat zu Venedig im Jahr 1805 an sich
selbst vollzogenen Kreuzigung* provided a direct translation of Ruggieri's French
text. However, Schlegel added several footnotes in which he commented in

---

24   P. Burke, 'Cultures of Translations in Early Modern Europe', in P. Burke and R. Po-Chia
      Hsia (eds.), *Cultural Translation in Early Modern Europe*, Cambridge, UK, Cambridge Uni-
      versity Press, 2007, 7–38.

25   Ruggieri, *Geschichte der durch Mathieu Lovat zu Venedig im Jahr 1805 an sich selbst vollzo-
      genen Kreuzigung*, 3f.

26   C. Ruggieri, *De kruissiging van Matthieu Lovat, aan zich zelven volbragt te Venetie, in den
      jaare 1805, medegedeeld door Cesare Ruggieri; volgens de hoogduitsche overzetting, naar het
      fransch, met de aanmerkingen van J.H.G. Schlegel, en ook van den nederduitschen vertaaler*,
      Amsterdam, Esveldt-Holtrop, 1807. This suggests that Lovat's case was also discussed by a
      Dutch readership, something that I do not examine in this book.

27   Between 1796 and 1804, Schlegel addressed some letters to Goethe regarding the publica-
      tion of his books, see the online database Klassik Stiftung Weimar (ed.), *Briefe an Goethe.
      Gesamtausgabe in Regestform*, http://ora-web.swkk.de/swk-db/goeregest/index.html,
      (accessed 7 July 2017). The numbers of the respective regests are 2/509, 2/1070, 2/1126,
      3/57, 3/760, 3/1256, 4/949, and 4/1457.

detail on those aspects of Lovat's case in which he believed himself to have expertise. These annotations recall the wide spectrum of medical problems addressed in Ruggieri's *Histoire du crucifiement* and reveal which aspects of it Schlegel considered to be particularly relevant either to himself or to the German medical readership. In contrast to most of the future authors who would simply ignore Ruggieri's remarks on the local disease pellagra when reproducing Lovat's case, Schlegel conveyed this diagnosis by referring to his publication *Briefe einiger Ärzte in Italien über das Pellagra* (Letters of Italian physicians concerning Pellagra).[28] Like Ruggieri, Schlegel was a traveller and a translator. In the 1790s, he had travelled through Southern Germany and Northern Italy.[29] He described the medical experiences he had during his journey in a book published in 1807.[30] In the same year he also edited his *Briefe einiger Ärzte in Italien über das Pellagra*. This work, one of the first German publications on pellagra, documents his encounter with the new disease in Italy.[31] One reason for Schlegel's special interest in Lovat's case was thus his familiarity with the Italian medical context and his previous knowledge about pellagra.

Referring to many other medical cases, Schlegel also comments on various other aspects of Lovat's health condition and behaviour as described by Ruggieri. For Schlegel, the fact that Lovat was a shoemaker by profession explained some of his health problems. Starting from Ruggieri's hypothesis that Lovat's health changed for the worse due to the specific working conditions of a shoemaker, Schlegel argues that every trade brings about a specific temper and physical condition, the so-called 'Zunft-Temperament', and this is particularly true for shoemakers. A shoemaker's bad posture would affect his back, and his seated position would affect his gastric organs, hinder the digestion and bring about different kinds of diseases. Like the scholar, he would consequently suffer from 'hypochondria'. To confirm his argument, Schlegel cites German and

---

28 Ruggieri, *Geschichte der durch Mathieu Lovat zu Venedig im Jahr 1805 an sich selbst vollzogenen Kreuzigung*, 7.

29 According to a contemporary biographer, Schlegel's original plan was to stay in the Italian city of Pavia for a while to broaden his medical knowledge with the famous German physician Johann Peter Frank, who held a chair as Professor there. However, as Frank was appointed to a professorship at the General Hospital in Vienna, Schlegel followed him to Vienna, see B.F. Voigt, *Neuer Nekrolog der Deutschen*, vol. 18, no. 1, Weimar, Bernh. Friedr. Voigt, 1842, 9.

30 J.H.G. Schlegel, *Reise durch das mittägliche Deutschland und einen Theil von Italien. Mit Kupfern*, Gießen and Wetzlar, Tasche und Müller, 1807.

31 J.H.G. Schlegel (ed.), *Briefe einiger Ärzte in Italien über das Pellagra. Aus dem Italienischen übersetzt und mit beygefügter Literatur*, Jena, Joh. Christ. Gottfr. Göpferdt, 1807. The book contains an outline of existent Italian publications on *pellagra* as well as some letters of Italian physician concerning the disease, translated and commented by Schlegel.

Italian authors who had previously written on the topic,[32] and he relates the case of an English shoemaker who had been incurably sick for twenty years until he invented a machine allowing him to stand upright while working, which cured him.[33] In this way, Schlegel used Lovat's case to pursue an important eighteenth-century medical debate on workers' diseases.[34]

With regard to Lovat's self-mutilation, Schlegel briefly cites the parallel case of a 75-year-old English man who had cut off his genitals during an 'attack of melancholy', and was completely cured after seven weeks.[35] As to Ruggieri's elaborate description of Lovat's self-crucifixion, Schlegel refers to his own book, the *Materialien für die Staatsarzneiwissenschaft*, in which he had reported similar cases of suicide attempts that all showed the same 'truth': '[...] that men driven by heroic passions concentrate all their conscious energy on one single point, so that their freedom of will does not lay in their decision for a certain action, but only in the choice of the means applied'.[36] Another point Schlegel comments on is that Lovat refused to eat while he was hospitalised at San Servolo. He remarks that during illness, voluntary fasting, even over several weeks, would be more frequent than it would be in a healthy state. Here again, Schlegel refers to a specific case he had published elsewhere, which argued that men could live ten days without eating.[37]

Some of Schlegel's comments highlight his interest in contributing to the emerging specialist debate on mental diseases, an interest which is also displayed in the many individual case histories Schlegel himself published

---

32   Schlegel refers to: G. Adelmann, *Über die Krankheiten der Künstler und Handwerker nach den Tabellen für kranke Gesellen der Künstler und Handwerker in Würzburg von den Jahren 1786 bis 1802 nebst einigen allgemeinen Bemerkungen*, Würzburg, Bey den Gebrüdern Stahel, 1803. More important in the Italian discourse was probably the older study by B. Ramazzini, *De morbis artificum diatriba*, Mutinae, Typis Antonii Capponi, impressoris episcopalis, 1700.

33   See the note on 9f. The story had been published in Germany shortly before: H. Fettleworth, *Neue Erfindung für S., Schuhe u. Stiefeln mittelst einer Maschine stehend zu verfertigen*, Leipzig, s.n., 1805. The title is cited in several contemporary medical publications but cannot be verified in today's library catalogues.

34   Most influential in the Italian context was Ramazzini, *De morbis artificum diatribe*. At the beginning of the nineteenth century, medical writers still published on the topic, see for instance Adelmann, *Über die Krankheiten der Künstler und Handwerker*.

35   Ibid., 8.

36   Schlegel, *Geschichte der durch Mathieu Lovat zu Venedig im Jahr 1805 an sich selbst vollzogenen Kreuzigung*, 15: '[...] daß Menschen, von heroischen Leidenschaften gefesselt, alle Besinnungskraft auf einen Punkt concentrieren, daß sich ihre Freiheit nicht bei der Fassung des Hauptentschlusses, sondern nur bei der Wahl der Mittel dazu zeigen könnte'.

37   Ibid., 27f. The book he refers to is: D. Collenbusch, *Der Rathgeber für alle Stände, in Angelegenheiten, welche die Gesundheit, den Vermögenserwerbstand und den Lebensgenuß betreffen*, Schneeberg, In der neuen Verlagshandlung, 1802.

on the topic.[38] Accordingly, his longest comment concerns Lovat's excessive sunbathing – a behaviour that Ruggieri had identified as typical for a particular kind of mania.[39] For Schlegel, however, 'this does not indicate a special kind of mania, but rather the most certain sign of dull madness, called *Melancholia lattonita*, in which the inactivity of the nervous system has reached its highest degree; and the affected usually stays immobile like a column, stands or sits at one point, does not desire for food or drinks, or, if he is forced to, devours it without reason'.[40] To explain Lovat's striking insensitivity towards the sun, Schlegel refers to a book by Thomas Barnes, arguing that religious convictions strongly affect a person's sensitivity.[41] He stresses that in a condition of madness, the sensitivity of the nerves is sometimes completely interrupted, so that the insane becomes unaware of his feelings of hunger, cold or heat. In the rest of the comment, Schlegel discusses the ambivalent effects that sunlight that can have on the diseased mind.[42] As an example of a negative effect, he refers to Vicenzo Chiarugi's book on *pazzia* in which the Florentine physician described the increase of madness among peasants during harvest time.[43] As a positive example, he describes a 'therapeutic' practice of Benedictine monks in a convent in Upper Carinthia in Austria that he himself had observed during his travels.[44] In order to cure 'obsessed and raving mad, deaf and dumb, blind people and those affected by headaches', these monks allegedly used big crystal balls which, according to a legend, they had received from Saint Mary in 1300. The mentally affected were put in the sunlight in front of the church where a priest spotlighted them by holding the balls into the light. According

---

38   The list of Schlegel's works contains many reports on patients suffering from mental disturbances, see A. Callisen, *Medicinisches Schriftsteller-Lexikon der jetzt lebenden Aerzte, Wundärzte, Geburtshelfer, Apotheker, und Naturforscher aller gebildeten Völker*, vol. 17, Copenhagen, Reitzl, 1833, 158–166.

39   Ruggieri, *Geschichte der durch Mathieu Lovat zu Venedig im Jahr 1805 an sich selbst vollzogenen Kreuzigung*, 29f.

40   Ibid., 29: 'Dieß verrieth wohl weniger eine besondere Art einer Manie, als vielmehr das sicherste Kennzeichen des dumpfen Wahnsinns, der Melancholia lattonita, in welchem die Unthätigkeit des Nervensystems den nöchsten Grad erreicht hat, der Kranke gewöhnlich, wie eine Bildsäule, unbeweglich ist, auf einer Stelle steht, oder sitzt, weder Speise, noch Trank begehrt, oder diese, wenn man sie ihm bringt, ohne Besonnenheit verschlingt'.

41   The book he refers to is T. Barnes, *Memoirs of the Literary and Philosophical Society of Manchester*, vol. 2, Manchester, T. Cadell, 1785.

42   Schlegel refers here to a debate which later became known as helio-therapy, see T. Woloshyn, 'Le pays du soleil: The Art of Heliotherapy on the Côte d'Azur', *Social History of Medicine*, vol. 26, no. 1, 2013, 74–93.

43   See V. Chiarugi, *Della pazzia in genere, e in specie: trattato medico-analitico: con una centuria di osservazioni*, Florence, Presso Luigi Carlieri, 1793–1794.

44   Schlegel refers to his above mentioned book *Reise durch das mittägliche Deutschland*.

to the monks' account, the patients were all cured except from those who were 'adherents to Bacchus and Venus'.[45] Probably, Schlegel referred here to patients who were alcoholics or sex-crazed.

Finally, Schlegel comments on the two diagnostic categories Ruggieri suggested at the end of his case history, namely that Lovat's madness should be defined as 'delirium melancholicum' and 'mania cum studio'. Schlegel concludes that, 'When the fools are not mad but in one point, Erhard calls this *Moria melancholica*. For men, the point that the folly is generally about is more pride than love'.[46] By emphasising 'pride', Schlegel refers to the contemporary notion of enthusiasm in which pride, as we will see below, was considered a typical trait of people exhibiting an extreme religious zeal.

Considered together, Schlegel's long and sometimes cryptic comments show how he used his translation to engage scientifically with Ruggieri, as a way to respond to Ruggieri's medical explanations and diagnoses. At the same time, his annotations allowed him to display his specialist knowledge and expertise in the context of various medical problems. In particular, the citation of comparable case histories allowed Schlegel to demonstrate his own knowledge about various topics as well as his membership of the medical community. Like Ruggieri, Schlegel elaborated especially on those aspects of Lovat's case that were to become major topics for the early psychiatrists: suicide, religion and madness. And like Ruggieri, he did not connect Lovat's insensibility or his mental derangement to the fact that Lovat was a victim of pellagra – a connection which was not yet established at the time. Clearly Schlegel used the publication of his translation for the purpose of professional self-advertisement: he considered the promotion of his translation of Lovat's case as a chance to gain the attention of medical colleagues.

As we shall see in the following chapters, Schlegel's German translation was advertised in several review journals and triggered the further spread of Lovat's case in many scientific and popular debates in Germany. It is therefore surprising that in 1842, a biographer of Schlegel retrospectively commented on Schlegel's publishing efforts with a certain derision:

> In the year 1807, which was so bad for the booktrade [...] a small brochure was published in Rudolstadt [...] This small brochure, of which the

---

45   Ruggieri, *Geschichte der durch Mathieu Lovat zu Venedig im Jahr 1805 an sich selbst vollzogenen Kreuzigung*, 30f.

46   Ibid., 32: 'Die Art Narrheit, wo die Narren nur in einem Punkt verrückt sind, nennt Erhard Moria melancholica. Bei Männern ist der Punkt, um den sich die Narrheit größtentheils dreht, mehr Stolz, als Liebe'.

content was indeed of the highest psychological interest, but which as a whole was rather an ephemera, was edited by Schlegel at his own expense. As it did not sell, he caused himself and his friends a lot of useless

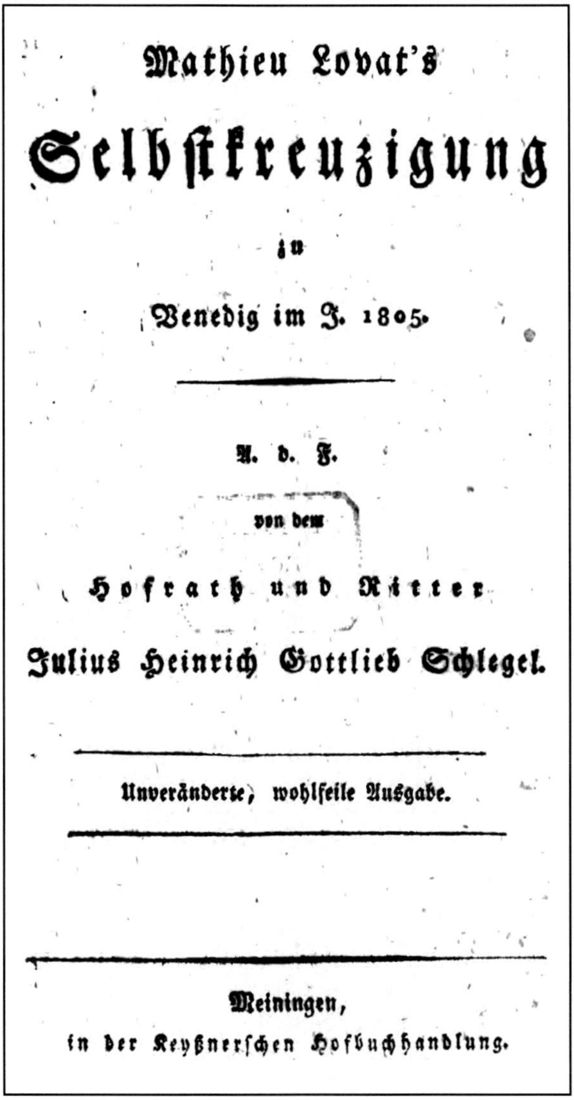

Mathieu Lovat's

Selbstkreuzigung

in

Venedig im J. 1805.

A. d. F.

von dem

Hofrath und Ritter

Julius Heinrich Gottlieb Schlegel.

Unveränderte, wohlfeile Ausgabe.

Meiningen,
in der Keyßnerschen Hofbuchhandlung.

ILLUSTRATION 6   Julius Heinrich Gottlieb Schlegel (ed.),
                   *Mathieu Lovat's Selbstkreuzigung zu Venedig
                   im J. 1805*, 1821.

trouble; sold it on commission but did not market it in the end; so that it provoked some good jokes.⁴⁷

This comment gives us a rare insight into how those readers might have responded to Lovat's case who never bothered reproducing or citing it: while many physicians – like Schlegel – considered it interesting and important and therefore reproduced it, others laughed at the efforts to distribute such an 'ephemera'. Nevertheless, in 1821 Schlegel even launched a second edition of his translation, under a slightly different title with another printer (see illustration 6).⁴⁸

Yet, some reviews in literary journals were not supportive and recalled that Schlegel's first edition 'had not found many lovers'.⁴⁹ This shows that within the growing German publishing business, publications were rated not only with regard to their contents, but also with regard to their economic value. However, more important than the number of copies published and sold was the fact that the narrative of Lovat's self-crucifixion, once translated into German, made people talk and write about it.

3   The English Translation (1814)

In 1814, an English translation of Ruggieri's case history appeared on the British book market. It was published anonymously under the title *Narrative of the Crucifixion of Matthew Lovat Executed by His Own Hands at Venice, In the Month of July, 1805* in a periodical entitled *Pamphleteer.*⁵⁰ Unlike Schlegel, who had

---

47   Voigt, *Neuer Nekrolog der Deutschen*, 21: 'In dem für den Buchhandel so sehr ungünstigen J. 1807 erschien zu Gießen u. Wetzlar die zweite vermehrte Auflage der "Reise" [Reise durch einige Theile von Deutschland, M.B.] und zu Rudolstadt eine kleine Broschüre: "Geschichte der durch Mathieu Lovat zu Venedig im J. 1805 an sich selbst vollzogenen Kreuzigung, bekannt gemacht von Dr. Cesar Ruggieri, Prof. Aus dem Französischen übersetzt und mit Anmerkungen versehen". Dieses kleine Schriftchen, dessen Inhalt zwar von höchstem psychologischem Interesse, aber an sich doch eine Ephemere war, schien S. auf eigne Kosten edirt zu haben, und da es sich nicht absetzte, machte er in spätern Jahren sich und Freunden damit viel unnöthige Mühe, gab es da und dort in Kommission und erzielte doch den gehofften Absatz nicht, so daß es noch zu manchem guten Scherze Veranlassung gab'. The *Nekrolog* published biographical accounts of deceased Germans with the explicit purpose to enhance the 'national feeling' (*Nationalgefühl*) of the Germans, see the editor's preface ('Vorrede'): ibid., VIIff.

48   Ruggieri, *Mathieu Lovat's Selbstkreuzigung zu Venedig.*

49   Anonymous, 'Die Leipziger Büchermesse', *Morgenblatt für gebildete Stände*, 16 June 1821, 189–192, 190: 'Lovat's "Selbstkreuzigung" scheint nicht viel Liebhaber gefunden zu haben und wird, als wenn die Zeit ihr günstiger geworden wäre, jetzt wieder aufgeboten'.

50   C. Ruggieri, 'Narrative of the Crucifixion of Matthew Lovat Executed by His Own Hands at Venice, in the Month of July, 1805. Originally Communicated to the Public by Cesare Ruggieri, M.D. Professor of Clynical Surgery at Venice, in a Letter to a Medical Friend.

added many comments to his German translation, the English translator did not adjoin any notes. The source for the English translation was, like in the German case, Ruggieri's French edition, the *Histoire du crucifiement*. The first page of the particular issue of the *Pamphleteer* displayed a copy of the illustration showing Lovat on the cross. The subscription to the illustration claimed that the narrative was 'now first translated into English' (see illustration 7):

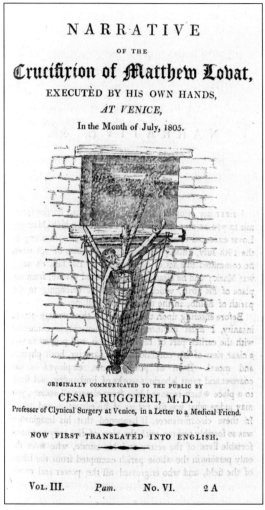

ILLUSTRATION 7   Anonymous, 'Narrative of the Crucifix-
ion of Matthew Lovat Executed by His
Own Hands at Venice, in the Month of
July, 1805' *The Pamphleteer*, 1814.

Now First Translated into English', *The Pamphleteer. Respectfully Dedicated to Both Houses of Parliament*, vol. 3, no. 6, 361–375.

The *Pamphleteer* was a London quarterly that had been launched in 1813. The declared aim of the editors was to find a remedy against the fugaciousness of the daily news delivered by the general press. In the preface to the first issue, they lament '[...] how great a proportion of that mass of information which is constantly issuing from the press, upon every topic of discussion, is consigned to undeserved oblivion by the mere vicissitude of daily occurrences'. Important arguments would get lost in this process, because '[...] like meteors rather than stars, they cease to exist the moment they cease to shine'.[51] To address this problem, the *Pamphleteer*'s aim was to keep certain news from fading away by conserving and collecting it,[52] and '[...] to present all the most accredited and best written pamphlets, but without compression or mutilation; and it will also open its repository to original compositions [...]'.[53] Accordingly, the name of the journal – *Pamphleteer* – is explained as deriving from *Pamphlets*, which '[...] burst forth upon the public, on every new object of inquiry, as stars; which, for the purpose of concentrating their rays into a more durable, as well as convenient, focus for observation, we propose to collect and combine together into distinct volumes [...]'.[54] Interestingly, the editors of the *Pamphleteer* justify their endeavour by pointing out the disadvantage of broadsheets compared to hardback books: while single pamphlets are only useful in a specific moment to a specific person and inevitably get lost afterwards, a book gains value as it '[...] occupies a place upon the shelf, and its real use is discovered perhaps many years after even the quantum of its first cost is totally out of recollection'.[55]

This statement indicates not only that the editors were very conscious about the differences in the potential of publication formats, and about the fact that the status of the book inevitably changed with the growing market of smaller publication formats. Also, their description and use of the term 'pamphlets' is telling: it brings to mind the very origins of the printing

---

51   Anonymous, 'Preface', *The Pamphleteer. Respectfully Dedicated to Both Houses of Parliament. To be Continued Occasionally, at an Average of Four or Five Numbers Annually*, vol. 1, no. 1, 1813, IIIf.

52   Ibid., V: '[...] and we claim to ourselves the merit of originality in the production of a system calculated to exalt the erratic luminaries of the day into the consequence of *fixed* stars; and, without any changes of their relative magnitudes, to give them the advantage of *permanence*'.

53   Ibid., VIf.

54   Ibid., IV.

55   Ibid., IXf.

press, and the important role of broadsheets – alternatively called pamphlets – in early modern European culture.[56] In particular in the realm of natural history, news about wondrous phenomena such as monstrous births were spread in this format,[57] medical and anatomical case histories circulated as fugitive sheets,[58] and sensationalist criminal reports were likewise disseminated in the form of broadsheets.[59] Although the *Pamphleteer*'s purpose to collect single pamphlets is thus reminiscent of the early modern endeavour of communicating extraordinary cases, its format differed significantly from early modern case collections: open to 'any great political, or moral, or scientific question' in no matter format it was published, it contributed to current public debates and addressed a broader readership rather than serving only the professional interests of a scientific elite.[60] The editors' emphasis on the original nature of their contributions as pamphlets further suggest how they had possibly made acquaintance with Lovat's case: most likely, someone had passed on to them a copy of Ruggieri's French booklet, and they considered it a 'pamphlet' worth perpetuating. As the editors had foreseen, with their publication of the English translation in the *Pamphleteer*, they allowed for an enduring distribution of the *Narrative of the Crucifixion of Matthew Lovat* in the British book trade: for many decades, British authors would cite or copy the translation of the *Pamphleteer* when discussing Lovat's case in their works.[61]

The *Pamphleteer* was also trendsetting with regard to the practice of copying the original engraving showing Lovat on the cross – the second plate showing the instruments of martyrdom had not been generally reproduced

---

56 See the classic study by Eisenstein, *The Printing Press as an Agent of Change*.

57 On the study of monsters see E. Holländer, *Wunder, Wundergeburt und Wundergestalt in Einblattdrucken des 15.–18. Jahrhunderts*, Stuttgart, Enke, 1922 and L. Daston and K. Park, 'Unnatural Conceptions: The Study of Monsters in Sixteenth- and Seventeenth-Century France and England', *Past & Present*, no. 92, 1981, 20–54.

58 See A. Carlino, *Paper Bodies: A Catalogue of Anatomical Fugitive Sheets 1538–1687*, London, Wellcome Institute for the History of Medicine, 1999. Carlino uses 'fugitive sheets' as umbrella term with reference to the German term 'fliegende Blätter' in order to denominate broadsheets and broadsides, see ibid., 1.

59 See J. Wiltenburg, 'True Crime: The Origins of Modern Sensationalism', *American Historical Review*, vol. 109, 2004, 1377–1404.

60 Anonymous, *Preface*, III.

61 From the beginning, the circulation went beyond London; for instance, the narrative also reached Scottish editors. See for instance a Scottish periodical called *The Scots Magazine and Edinburgh Literary Miscellany being a General Repertory of Literature, History, and Politics*, vol. 76, 1814, 602–606.

in foreign publications. As it was technically not possible to reproduce the original illustration without the original copper plate, the editors of the *Pamphleteer* had to make a new sketch, and, in a second step, produce a new copperplate engraving. This is why the illustration in the *Pamphleteer* varies significantly from the original illustration published in Ruggieri's editions. Two genre-related aspects help to explain why the editors considered it important to copy the picture at all: by tradition, broadsheets usually included visual representations to show quite plainly the details of the reported events, and thereby to appeal to the emotions of their readers. We thus see the kinship of the nineteenth-century popular press with the early modern sensational crime reports, as emphasised by Wiltenburg.[62] Secondly, the editors could also draw on the portrait engraving tradition in Britain that was already flourishing in the eighteenth century.[63] The rising genre of biographical narratives usually featured engraved portraits, as can be seen, for instance, in James Granger's *Biographical History of England*, first published in 1769 with many engravings and republished in countless re-editions far into the nineteenth century.[64] As we will see in the last chapter on the popular readings of Lovat's case, many other British editors would follow the example of the *Pamphleteer* in the decades to come: together with new arrangements of the narrative, they produced copies of Ruggieri's original engraving showing Lovat on the cross. Consequently, all these 'new' illustrations of Lovat's case in British publications vary slightly from the original. But it would be misleading to interpret these differences as intentional changes undertaken by the editors, as most of them are probably due to the techniques of reproduction. Despite their differences in detail, the numerous reproductions of the original illustration as well as their prominent position in British publications reveal a particular tradition of visualizing biographical accounts, which is an exclusive feature of the British representations of Lovat's case.

Viewed together, the French, German and English translation of Ruggieri's case history bespeak a broader tendency in early nineteenth-century European- print culture: the increasing production of vernacular translations

---

62   Wiltenburg, *True Crime*, 1390.

63   See the classic study by M. Pointon, *Hanging the Head: Portraiture and Social Formation in Eighteenth-Century England*, New Haven, Yale University Press, 1993.

64   J. Granger, *A Biographical History of England, from Egbert the Great to the Revolution: Consisting of Characters Disposed in Different Classes, and Adapted to a Methodical Catalogue of Engraved British Heads. Intended as an Essay Towards Reducing our Biography to System, and a Help to the Knowledge of Portraits. Interspersed with a Variety of Anecdotes, and Memoirs of a Great Number of Persons*, London, T. Davies, 1769.

which fostered the transnational exchange, both literary and scientific. In the first decades of the nineteenth century, the market for translations expanded to such an extent that some contemporaries even criticised the loss of quality due to the ubiquitous 'machineries of translations'.[65] As the different translations of Ruggieri's case history show, in many cases these '[...] translations reveal not so much the transformations of the scientists' work, as the transformations of its cultural context'.[66]

4   Journals and Reviews as Vehicles of Lovat's Case

In Britain as well as in France, Lovat's case became known to a broader readership well before the respective translations were available on the national book markets. This happened via journals and reviews, which, by the nineteenth century, had become an important part of intellectual life. Since the emergence of the first periodicals in the seventeenth century, a great diversity of periodicals had been launched, appealing to a variety of audiences.[67] Editors would include medical topics, and in particular medical case histories, in general scientific journals, but also in journals of general interest that addressed an educated readership.[68] This explains why the early circulation of Lovat's case was triggered by journals, and not primarily medical journals but journals that addressed a broader literate audience. Often, the declared purpose of these journals was to collect, reproduce or review publications that had appeared elsewhere before, or to translate contributions that had been published in foreign journals. Combining the purposes of education and entertainment, editors often mixed scientific and literary contributions and topics.

A good example of the intricate exchange of contents between publications from different countries is the *L'esprit des journaux français et étrangers par une*

---

65   See (with view to Germany) N. Bachleitner, "'Übersetzungsfabriken'. Das deutsche Übersetzungswesen in der ersten Hälfte des 19. Jahrhunderts', *Internationales Archiv für Sozialgeschichte der deutschen Literatur* (*IASL*), vol. 14, no. 1, 1989, 1–49. On the role of translation in the realm of science see also Pantin, *The Role of Translations*.

66   Ibid., 163.

67   See for instance the chapter on 'The Periodical Press' in J. Feather, *A History of British Publishing*, London and New York, Routledge, 2006, 56–61.

68   Bynum, Lock, and Porter, *Medical Journals and Medical Knowledge*, 7.

société de gens de lettres,[69] a French journal in which Lovat's case appeared in 1809. The editors present Lovat's case in their review of a German publication from the same year in which Lovat's case had been described. This German book on the 'history of the errors of the human mind'[70] contained many narratives about insane behaviour, but the French reviewers picked two of them in order to illustrate the 'strange impressions the human mind is susceptible'.[71] One is, in fact, the narrative of Lovat's self-crucifixion. The editors write that they had already read about this 'anecdote' in another French journal, and that 'the details which were published since then are almost so incomprehensible that the readers would probably take it for a fairy tale, if it had not been witnessed by respectable authorities'.[72] Over four pages, the editors give quite a detailed summary of Lovat's case, and conclude by assuring their readers that all facts were delivered by Ruggieri himself, who had taken them directly 'from the mouth of Lovat'.[73] Next to Lovat's case, they cite a comparable case of self-harm, the story of a soldier who begged his comrade to cut his body into pieces while still alive.[74] In this version, Lovat's case appeared at the same time in other French periodicals, such as the *Mercure de France*.[75] In contrast to the *L'esprit des journeaux*, this was a journal dating back to the *ancien regime,* with a long tradition of reporting news about fashion, royal life, intellectual and artistic debates as well as all sorts of anecdotes.

On the one hand, these examples highlight that soon after Ruggieri's publications, Lovat's case was transmitted across Europe as an anecdote in journals that addressed a broader public. This popularisation set in very early, at the same time as the start of the circulation of Lovat's case in medical circles, as we will see in greater detail in the following chapters. On the other hand, it highlights the important role that reviews played in the transnational dissemination

---

69   Anonymous (ed.), *L'esprit des journaux français et étrangers, par une société de gens de lettres*, Brussels, De Weissenbruch, 1809, 242–244.

70   Anonymous (ed.), *Beyträge zur Geschichte der Verirrungen des menschlichen Geistes und der Thorheiten gelehrter Männer*, Leipzig, Bruder&Hoffmann, 1809.

71   Anonymous, *L'esprit des journaux français et étrangers*, 244.

72   Ibid., 242: 'Parmi les traits plus ou moins extraordinaires, contenus dans ce recueil, nous avons retrouvé une anecdote dont un de nos journeaux avait fait quelque mention à l'époque où l'événement eut lieu. Les détails presqu'incompréhensibles qui ont été publiés depuis ce temps, auraient déterminé, sans doute, bien des lecteurs à ranger ce fait au nombre des fables, s'il n'était attesté par les autorités les moins récusables'.

73   Ibid., 243: 'Le docteur César Ruggieri, professeur de chirurgie à Venise, a écrit lui-même la relation des faits qu'il tenait de la bouche même de Lovat [...]'.

74   Ibid., 246.

75   Anonymous (ed.), *Mercure de france. Journal littéraire et politique*, vol. 38, Paris, Arthus-Bertrand, 1809, 41–43.

of Lovat's case: by providing reviews of foreign publications, journal editors reproduced parts of their content, and favourably cited remarkable cases such as Lovat's. As Hubert Steinke has shown for the medical context, reviews played an important role for both the specialisation and the widening of scientific debates, because they allowed for transnational communication. Since the middle of the eighteenth century '[t]he review journals, as a whole, fostered the establishment of neither overtly international nor explicitly national or regional realms of science and discourse'.[76]

Similar to the French case, British readers could encounter the narrative of Lovat's self-crucifixion well before the English translation was published in 1814, by reading various periodical journals, often entitled *magazines*. In 1811, several British periodicals published an identical abridged version of Lovat's case. The thematic variety of these magazines mirrors the broad spectrum of content they embraced at the beginning of the nineteenth century: they stretched from politics, social reform and economics to arts and literature.[77] For instance, Lovat's case was published in *The European Magazine and London Review*,[78] edited by the Philological Society of London since 1782. The general aim of the editors was '[...] to present to the world Biographical Anecdotes of such illustrious characters as are engaged in the great scene of political action [...] We have had it in our view to give accounts of various places and objects of public pursuit, and to describe whatever is great, new, useful, or curious, within the limits of our information'.[79] Consequently, the contributions published in the *European Magazine* ranged from amusing anecdotes, academic papers and political news to reviews of recent European publications. While Lovat's case seems to fit well in the scope of this particular magazine, it is more surprising for modern readers to see that the identical narrative was likewise published

---

76   H. Steinke, *Irritating Experiments. Haller's Concept and the European Controversy on Irritability and Sensibility, 1750–90*, Amsterdam and New York, Rodopi, 2005, 265.

77   See *The Tradesman; or, Commercial Magazine: Including Subjects Relating to Commerce, Foreign and Domestic, Together with Suggestions for New Commercial Connexions; Expositions of History and Processes of Manufactories...*vol. 8, 1811, 500; *Jackson's Oxford Journal*, vol. 16, 1811; *The Leeds Mercury*, vol. 16, 1811; *The European Magazine and London Review, Containing Traits, Views, Biography, Anecdotes, Literature, History, Politics, Arts, Manners, and Amusements of the Age*, vol. 60, 1811, 387. A similar version of the narrative was published by a journal about 30 years later: *The London Dispatch and People's Political and Social Reformer*, vol. 17, 1839.

78   *The European Magazine and London Review*, 387.

79   See the introduction to one of the early issues: Anonymous, 'Introduction', in *The European Magazine and London Review: Containing the Literature, History, Politics, Arts, Manners & Amusements of the Age*, vol. 2, 1782.

in a commercial magazine called *The Tradesman*.[80] Here, Lovat's case is again referred to as taken from 'a foreign newspaper' and appears among news concerning commercial affairs. Following a note on a 'Scotch Petition on the high Price of Grain', the narrative is introduced with the subject heading 'Extraordinary fanaticism', and is – like in *The European Magazine* – presented as a singular and deplorable case of 'religious melancholy'.[81]

The described circulation of Lovat's case in British and French periodicals highlights the 'hybrid, and overtly pluralist, intertextual format' of the publications in which Lovat's case appeared in the early nineteenth century.[82] In particular British periodicals had become more specialised and focused in their content, and editors were eager to identify and reach specific audiences, such as scientific or lay, female or juvenile readers.[83] Notwithstanding this clear trend toward specialisation, periodicals still generally sought to remain intelligible to all readers and therefore kept close to common language.[84]

Apart from mirroring the heterogeneity of the periodical press, the fact that Lovat's case appeared in several journals in the identical abridged version points to another important feature of nineteenth-century print media that we need to keep in mind when examining the European dissemination of Lovat's case: a general openness to plagiarism as well as toward contributions and contributors. As MacDonald and Murphy have remarked with view to the eighteenth century,

> [t]he press was a remarkably open medium. There were no professional reporters, and editors relied on friendly officials, self-appointed correspondents, plagiarism, and (notoriously) their own imagination for the news that they printed. Newspapers reflected the views of their editors, who wrote or rewrote the stories in them and decided what to print. Nevertheless, almost anyone might contribute articles and comments to

---

80   *The Tradesman; or, Commercial Magazine*, 500.

81   In the introduction, it says: 'Matthew Lovat, a shoemaker at Venice, presents an example of religious melancholy, equally extraordinary as deplorable [...]'.

82   L. Henson et al., 'Introduction', in L. Henson et al. (eds.), *Culture and Science in the Nineteenth-Century Media*, Aldershot, Ashgate, 2005, XVII–XXV, XVIII. See also J. Hinks, C. Armstrong, and M. Day (eds.), *Periodicals and Publishers. The Newspaper and Journal Trade 1740–1914*, London, British Library, 2009.

83   Henson et al., *Introduction*, XIX.

84   Ibid.

them, and the papers and magazines acted as a public forum for exchanging information and for debate.[85]

To some extent, this was still true at the beginning of the nineteenth century. Ruggieri's case history was hardly ever cited in one of its original editions, that is neither in his French edition of 1806 nor in his two Italian editions of 1806 and 1814. As we will see, there were few constraints regarding plagiarism: authors and editors copied existing versions of the narrative and included them in their texts, sometimes citing their sources, sometimes not.[86] For this reason, it is hardly ever possible to identify the specific editors or authors who were responsible for the reproduction of Ruggieri's case history in a certain periodical. In any case, as an effect of the transnational circulation of Lovat's case in various journals and periodicals in Germany, France and Britain, the potential readership of the narrative of Lovat's self-crucifixion was multiplied considerably.

5   The 'Interpretive Communities' of Lovat's Case: Reading and Rewriting

In the process of the European circulation of Lovat's case, an effect akin to Chinese whispers set in. Like in the children's game, where a sentence is passed on from one person to the other and is thereby transformed, the narrative of Lovat's self-crucifixion underwent minor and major changes in both its form and meaning while travelling between different kinds of publications.[87] The various ways in which editors presented, commented or only cited Lovat's case indicate how they read it: how they understood and interpreted it with an eye to a broader readership. The readers my book deals with were themselves authors, editors or writers who reproduced Lovat's case in their own works by re-writing it, and by publishing it in their books, collections or periodicals. If it is impossible to know what thousands of 'silent' readers thought about Lovat's case when reading it without reproducing it somewhere afterwards, the

---

85   M. MacDonald and T.R. Murphy, *Sleepless Souls: Suicide in Early Modern England*, Oxford and New York, Clarendon, 1990, 302.

86   On plagiarism see R. Macfarlane, *Original Copy. Plagiarism and Originality in Nineteenth-Century Literature*, Oxford, Oxford University Press, 2007.

87   In his brilliant study on a German criminal case that circulated in early twentieth-century media, Michael Hagner states that the 'circulation and transformation, the condensation and transmission of knowledge have the nature of Chinese Whispers', see Hagner, *Der Hauslehrer*, 234.

various re-writings of Lovat's case that we find in nineteenth-century publications reveal at least how numerous actors involved in publishing looked at
the case, and what they believed to be interesting for a specific or a broader
readership of their time. Therefore, the underlying assumption of the following chapters is that a medical case is neither only the product of administrative
procedures nor exclusively the product of its first author – although both play
an important role, as we have seen in the previous chapters. Rather, because it
is a narrative and therefore a readable text, it is the readers who, in the act of
interpretation, ultimately give meaning to the case and make it travel.

   With this basic assumption, I follow the insights offered by certain historians concerned with the history of publishing and reading, in particular Roger
Chartier.[88] In several works, Chartier has put forward two main arguments that
are important for my understanding of the *Storia della crocifissione* as a case
that travels between different readers. Firstly, Chartier believes that the physical form of a text governs how it is read: 'Readers, in fact, never confront abstract, idealised texts detached from any materiality'.[89] Any interpretation of a
text depends on the way in which it is presented: 'forms produce meaning, and
[...] even a fixed text is invested with new meaning and being (statut) when
the physical form through which it is presented for interpretation changes'.[90]
Chartier therefore sees the task of the historian as to '[...] reconstruct the variations that differentiate the "readable space" (the texts in their material and
discursive forms) and those which govern the circumstances of their "actu-
alisation" (the readings as concrete practices and interpretive procedures)'.[91]
The different translations examined in this chapter illustrate how, soon after
the publication of Ruggieri's original editions, Lovat's case was transmitted
in different media and presented in various new forms. In many cases, these
transformations had to do not only with the professional background of the
individual authors and editors who appropriated Lovat's case, but also with the
programme and the envisaged readership of the particular medium in which

---

88   Chartier, *Texts, Printings, Readings*; see also R. Chartier, *Forms and Meanings. Texts, Per-
      formances, and Audiences from Codex to Computer*, Philadelphia, University of Pennsyl-
      vania Press, 1995; G. Cavallo and R. Chartier (eds.), *Histoire de la lecture dans le monde
      occidental*, Paris, Seuil, 1997. Chartier's ideas have inspired many other authors working
      on a cultural history of reading practices, see for a focus on the nineteenth century for in-
      stance M. Lyons, *Le triomphe du livre. Une histoire sociologique de la lecture dans la France
      du XIXe siècle*, Paris, Promodis, 1987 and Lyons, *Reading Culture and Writing Practices in
      Nineteenth-Century France*.
89   R. Chartier, 'Laborers and Voyagers: From the Text to the Reader', *diacritics*, vol. 22, no. 2,
      1992, 49–61, 50.
90   Ibid., 50f.
91   Ibid., 50.

the narrative was reproduced. These new forms and framings produced new meanings and new publics for the case.

The second argument Chartier makes is that 'a text does not exist except for a reader who gives it signification'.[92] He therefore understands the reader's 're- ception' as an inventive process and reading as a 'creative practice': the readings and understandings of a particular text and the meanings attributed to it always depend on the readers' diverse 'appropriations' of it.[93] These appropriations in turn are shaped by the readers' cultural and social contexts. I use this notion of 'appropriation' when examining various ways in which Lovat's case was read.

Chartier further suggests distinguishing between different communities of readers who build 'interpretive communities' around certain texts. Here, Chartier borrows an expression proposed earlier by the literary scholar Stanley Fish.[94] Fish's 'interpretive communities' refer to readers who build a commu- nity because they recognise certain common interpretative principles when reading a text. In Fish's words, they follow established but always changing 'canons of acceptability', and therefore are able to produce a 'limited plural- ity' of readings.[95] The membership of such communities is continually chang- ing, and groups of readers can build 'subcommunities of communities'.[96] Borrowing Fish's term, Chartier therefore suggests that readers in 'interpretive communities' share specific modes of reading, strategies of interpretation and expectations with which they approach a text.[97] In the following chapters, I make use of this idea of interpretive communities to describe how several communities of readers shared different understandings of Lovat's case. The readers of Lovat's case, that is the various editors and authors who commented and re-wrote the narrative, can be distinguished by different interests they had in the case and by different purposes they pursued with its publication. These interests and purposes derived from their professional backgrounds, but also from considerations concerning matters of publishing or from considerations concerning the expected readership. In many cases, several of these factors played a role and overlapped, but still, one was always uppermost. The inter- pretive communities concerned with Lovat's case produced different kinds of readings, which I distinguish as 'professional readings' and 'popular readings'. By professional readings I mean those publications that are authored or ed- ited by representatives of a certain discipline or science, and that address a

---

92   Ibid.
93   Chartier, *Texts, Printings, Readings*, 156f.
94   S. Fish, *Is There a Text in This Class?*, 338–355.
95   Ibid., 249 and 342.
96   Ibid., 343.
97   Chartier, *Texts, Printings, Readings*, 158.

specialist readership and not the general reading public. These publications are epistemic genres in the sense that they are related to cognitive goals. By transmitting Lovat's case in such publications, editors used the narrative to contribute to a certain body of scientific knowledge. As far as popular readings are concerned, I examine publications that addressed a broader readership and that pursued primarily literary aims. Rather than contributing to the production of scientific knowledge, such publications aimed to morally educate and entertain the nineteenth-century reading public. In this context, editors frequently presented Lovat's case as a sensational literary narrative. Of course, the distinction between scientific and popular readings is a heuristic tool rather than a contemporary category. In the nineteenth century, many scientific publications tried to reach a broader readership, and many popular publications communicated scientific contents to a lay readership. As many studies have shown, science was not disseminated top down into popular culture; rather, it was a reciprocal exchange between both spheres. Both scientific and popular knowledge were produced in a communicative process.[98] Focusing on how Lovat's case was read by different readerships shows exactly that the boundaries between scientific and popular cultures and between epistemic and literary genres were fluid but were also becoming harder at just this time.

   Three major topics run through the various readings of Lovat's case: Religion, madness and suicide. The interest in these topics incited editors to rewrite and publish Lovat's case, and to thereby contribute to their respective interpretive community. Depending on their disciplinary background as well as on the form of the respective publications, authors and editors put different weight on these three topics, usually concentrating on one of them more than on the others. A theological perspective on Lovat's case would primarily ask for the religious motivations behind his self-crucifixion, and would inquire into his religious behaviour as described by Ruggieri. Such authors were eager to stress that Lovat's way of practising his belief was wrong and undermined

---

98   On the popularisation of science in the nineteenth century see A. Schwarz, 'Bilden, Überzeugen, Unterhalten: Wissenschaftspopularisierung und Wissenskultur im 19. Jahrhundert', in C. Kretschmann (ed.), *Wissenspopularisierung. Konzepte der Wissensverbreitung im Wandel*, Berlin, Akademie Verlag, 2003, 221–234; A. Daum, *Wissenschaftspopularisierung im 19. Jahrhundert. Bürgerliche Kultur, naturwissenschaftliche Bildung und die deutsche Öffentlichkeit, 1848–1914*, Munich, R. Oldenbourg, 1998, 221–234; P. Boden and D. Müller (eds.), *Populäres Wissen im medialen Wandel seit 1850*, Berlin, Kadmos Kulturverlag, 2009. For a broader conceptual focus see T. Shinn and R. Whitley (eds.), *Expository Science: Forms and Functions of Popularisation*, Dordrecht, Boston, and Lancaster, D. Reidel, 1985; Von Greyerz, Flubacher, and Senn, *Wissenschaftsgeschichte und Geschichte des Wissens im Dialog*.

enlightened rational religion. Other authors, by contrast, would regard Lovat's self-crucifixion primarily as a suicidal act: they would highlight the causes of this act as being either a false understanding of religion, or a mental disturbance. Authors from several professional fields shared this interest in Lovat's case as a suicide case. A third perspective on Lovat's case would regard it primarily as a case of madness: these authors were interested in finding out about the specific mental disturbance that would explain Lovat's actions according to contemporary medical and psychiatric terminology. In many cases, these three perspectives on Lovat's case – religion, madness and suicide – overlapped in the arguments put forward by the editors, the reason for this being the increasing medicalisation of both the discourse on suicide and religion in the course of the nineteenth century. Nevertheless, the disciplinary background of editors and specific national and media contexts shaped distinct ways in which the three topics were interrelated and discussed in the various rewritings of Lovat's case.

CHAPTER 4

Professional Readings: Religion

1   Saint Matthew and Origen

Because of the centrality of the self-crucifixion in Lovat's case, the narrative was often read and interpreted from a theological perspective and associated with Biblical narratives. As described in the first chapter, Ruggieri's case history was already characterised by a religious subtext that runs through the whole narrative. In the *Storia della crocifissione*, there are three main themes with religious connotations, or that Ruggieri rhetorically charged with further religious meaning: first, Lovat's self-castration; second, his attempt at self-crucifixion; and third, his religious behaviour in general. The original text of the *Storia della crocifissione* connects Lovat's actions closely with the Gospel of Matthew. His account suggests that both Lovat's self-castration and his crucifixion attempt were inspired by the Evangelist Matthew, and that Lovat was generally driven by the idea of imitating the deeds of his namesake Saint. For instance, Ruggieri reports that when Lovat tried to crucify himself for the first time and was asked for his reasons, he had told his brother that it was the festival of Saint Matthew, his namesake.[1] Ruggieri used this idea as an interpretative clue for his case history. In the second Italian edition from 1814, Ruggieri included a verse from the Latin version of the Gospel of Matthew on an extra page at the start of the publication – *A fructibus eorum agnoscetis eos.*[2] The passage refers to the warning against false prophets who were predicted to appear in sheep's clothing but turn out to be furious wolves, as reported in the respective Gospel:

> Watch out for false prophets. They come to you in sheep's clothing, but inwardly they are ferocious wolves. By their fruit you will recognise them. Do people pick grapes from thornbushes, or figs from thistles? Likewise, every good tree bears good fruit, but a bad tree bears bad fruit. A good tree cannot bear bad fruit, and a bad tree cannot bear good fruit. Every

---

1 Ruggieri, *Storia della crocifissione*, 7: 'Interrogato in varie maniere sul perchè abbia voluto crocifiggersi, non diede mai risposta ad alcuno, solo disse al indicato suo fratello, che in quel giorno correva la festa del suo Santo di nome, cioè di S. Mattio, e che non poteva ne doveva dir altro'.
2 Ibid., 2.

tree that does not bear good fruit is cut down and thrown into the fire. Thus, by their fruit you will recognise them.[3]

By citing this verse from Matthew, Ruggieri not only rhetorically plays with the strong affinity of Mattio Lovat to the Evangelist Matthew as implied in Lovat's first name, he also implicitly asks if Lovat was a false prophet.

In his 1814 Italian edition, Ruggieri includes another reference to the Evangelist Matthew. Trying to explain Lovat's amputation of his own genitals, Ruggieri hypothesises that he was afraid of carnal temptation and therefore wished to unburden himself forever of an 'enemy'. Here, Ruggieri draws a brief comparison to the Christian author Origen (185–254), stating that Origen did the same because he misunderstood the words of Matthew in his Gospel.[4] According to a complex theological tradition, Origen had in fact allegedly castrated himself in order to reach the Kingdom of Heaven.[5] The Church Father Eusebius, a devotee of Origen's ideas, was the first to spread the notion that Origen had castrated himself because he had misinterpreted a verse from Matthew.[6] The verse in question is Matthew 19:12 where Jesus says to his disciples: '[…] there are eunuchs who were born that way, and there are eunuchs who have been made eunuchs by others – and there are those who choose to live like eunuchs for the sake of the kingdom of heaven'.[7] Contemporarily as well as in the aftermath, Origen's numerous works on the exegesis of Scripture and on dogma were controversial, and his work was partly suspected of heresy. During the eighteenth century, however, Origen came to be a favourite author of many of those who were criticised as enthusiasts (*Schwärmer*), especially in Germany.[8] As an effect, the notion of self-castration as a means of salvation became known with a broader public and the association of self-castration

---

3   The Bible, Matt. 7:15–20. The citation follows *The New International Version of the Bible*, available online: http://www.biblegateway.com/passage/?search=Matthew%207&version=NIV, (accessed 17 July 2017).

4   Ruggieri, *Storia della crocifissione*, 5. The italics indicate the adjuncts in the second edition. '[…] ma non sarebbe egli più ragionevole di credere, dietro il conosciuto carattere di quest'uomo, che la di lui timida coscienza spaventata dalle tentazione delle carne, l'avesse deciso a disfarsi tutto ad un tratto e per sempre d'un formidabilissimo nemico *come ha fatto Origene per non aver bene interpretato le parole di S. Matteo?'*.

5   On Origen see C. Markschies, *Origenes und sein Erbe. Gesammelte Studien*, Berlin, Walter de Gruyter, 2007, in particular the chapter entitled 'Kastration und Magenprobleme? Einige neue Blicke auf das asketische Leben des Origenes', 15–34.

6   Ibid., 30ff.

7   The Bible, Matt 19:12.

8   See D. Breuer, 'Origenes im 18. Jahrhundert in Deutschland', *Seminar. A Journal of Germanic Studies*, vol. 21, 1985, 1–30.

with Origen became a commonplace in eighteenth-century German literature. For instance, in the 1774 German comedy by Jakob Michael Reinhold Lenz, the private teacher Läuffer castrates himself and is called 'a second Origen' by the school teacher.[9] As we shall see in the next chapters, several authors passed on the comparison of Lovat with Origen when commenting on Lovat's case.

Even more than the self-castration, Lovat's self-crucifixion had obvious Biblical associations. It could clearly be understood as an imitation of Jesus' crucifixion, an *imitatio Christi*. By reporting in great detail on the instruments that Lovat used for the self-crucifixion and the injuries he inflicted upon himself, Ruggieri conveys to the reader that Lovat's self-crucifixion was actually meant as a faithful imitation of the Biblical account of Christ's passion, even though he made clear that as a physician, he considered it to be an act of insanity.[10] For those readers interested in the religious meaning of Lovat's case, Ruggieri's text therefore inevitably raised the question of whether self-crucifixion could be taken seriously as a Christian practice. But even those readers of Lovat's case who did believe that Lovat's self-crucifixion was a religious act rather than one of insanity, had to deny it its legitimacy. Despite the prominent role of the passion of Christ in Christian theology and various accepted practices of *imitatio Christi*, self-crucifixion had never been an accepted religious practice but tended to be regarded as heretical, as explained in the first chapter.[11]

From the perspective of Christian religion, Ruggieri's case history thus raised several provocative themes that posed the question of what were considered right and accepted religious practices in post-Enlightenment Europe. Apart from the self-crucifixion and self-castration, Ruggieri's *Storia della crocifissione* described other behaviour of Lovat that readers could (and would) interpret either as individual religious practices of a very pious man, or as pathological symptoms of a disordered mind: his melancholic introspection, his voluntary fasting, and his intense reading of the Bible.[12] This religious subtext of the *Storia della crocifissione* determined the ways in which professional and

---

9   J.M.R. Lenz, *Der Hofmeister oder Vortheile der Privaterziehung. Eine Komödie*, Leipzig, Weygandsche Buchhandlung, 1774, 5.3. In the eighteenth-century German encyclopaedia by Johann Heinrich Zedler, we find an entry entitled 'eunuchs for heaven's sake'. They are described as those who, following the Gospel of Matthew 19:12, refuse to marry or, if married, behave as if they were not married, 'for the sake of the kingdom of heaven'. Anonymous, 'Verschnittener um des Himmelreichs willen', in J.H. Zedler (ed.), *Grosses vollständiges Universallexikon aller Wissenschaften und Künste*, vol. 47, Leipzig and Halle, Johann Heinrich Zedler, 1746, 1722.

10   Ruggieri, *Storia della crocifissione*, 7.

11   Bräunlein, *Passion/Pasyon*, 155.

12   Ruggieri, *Storia della crocifissione*, 16.

lay commentators would read Lovat's case. They picked up Ruggieri's theological references to the Evangelist Matthew and Origen and reflected on Lovat's religious behaviour. What made Ruggieri's case history interesting for readers concerned with theological questions, was, therefore, not only the compelling incident of Lovat's self-crucifixion, but also Ruggieri's overall description of Lovat's individual devout character. Most readers considered this individual piety as clearly exaggerated, extreme and contrary to enlightened understanding of Christian belief, which was promoted at the time. Lovat's case therefore raised the question of how to evaluate it with a view to contemporary discussions of religion, and in particular about the enthusiasts, a notion that had distinct meanings in the different national contexts.

2   A False Prophet? Lovat's Case in the Religious Critique of
       Schwärmerei

In several German publications from the first half of the nineteenth century, Lovat's case was, in various ways, framed and presented as a typical case of *Schwärmerei*, the German expression for religious enthusiasm. In particular, several German theologians dealt with the case from that perspective. Let us consider briefly two examples. In 1835, the Enlightened Catholic theologian Ignaz Heinrich Wessenberg (1774–186)[13] published a historical-philosophical study of contemporary *Schwärmerei* in which he included Lovat's case.[14] He defined the aim of his work as to,

> [...] prove as definitively and clearly as possible the boundaries between the genuine religious and patriotic sense and religious and political fanaticism; between the noble passion (*Begeisterung*) for the beautiful, right, true, good, divine and the blinded enthusiasm (*Schwärmerei*) that obscures everything; between true Christian belief that elevates the mind (*Gemüth*) and makes it strong for the holy life, and pietism and mysticism that makes it weak and intoxicates with illusions (*Einbildungen*).[15]

---

13   On Wessenberg see K. Wesseling, 'WESSENBERG[-Ampringen], Ignaz Heinrich Karl
      Joseph Thaddäus Fidel Dismas Freiherr von, katholischer Aufklärungstheologe und
      Konstanzer Generalvikar', in Traugott Bautz (ed.), *Biographisch-Bibliographisches Kirch-
      enlexikon*, vol. 13, Herzberg, Traugott Bautz, 1998, 976–988.
14   Wessenberg, *Ueber Schwärmerei.*
15   See Wessenberg's 'Kurzes Vorwort', ibid., 111f.: '[...] die Grenzlinien zwischen dem ächtre-
      ligiösen und ächtpatriotischen Sinn und dem religiösen und politischen Fanatismus,
      zwischen edler Begeisterung für das Schöne, Rechte, Wahre, Gute, Heilige und der

In his book, Wessenberg presents various cases relating to false religious ideas that he calls 'superstition' (*Aberglaube*) or 'mystic enthusiasm'. With these narratives, he clearly aims at warning his readers against a false belief. Along with the narrative of Lovat's self-crucifixion, Wessenberg gives another case of crucifixion mentioned briefly in the first chapter, namely that of Margarethe Peter, a woman from a village close to Zurich in Switzerland who believed herself to be chosen. Initially, the woman displayed extreme religious zeal and was soon regarded by some adherents as holy; later, she believed that she was receiving divine orders, and forced her family and her followers to join a cruel orgy of reciprocal torture and homicide. This collective martyrdom took place at her home and culminated in the woman being crucified by her followers, and in their arrest by the local authorities.[16] Wessenberg and several other theologians concerned with promoting a 'rational reading of the Bible' cited her case like Lovat's as daunting examples of what could happen with a misguided interpretation of Scripture.[17]

Another telling example of the employment of Lovat's case in the theological critique of enthusiasm is a German Catholic *Exempelbuch* published in 1845 by Ferdinand Ignaz Herbst, a Catholic convert who served as a priest in Bavaria. In his book, Herbst aimed to explain the doctrines of the Catholic church by means of 'remarkable examples of religious enthusiasm' (*Schwärmerei*), and Lovat's case, entitled *Matheo von Casale*, served as one of these examples.[18] Herbst was convinced that working with examples was particularly important when it came to religious enthusiasm:

> [...] religious enthusiasm, which is in relative opposition to the true religious worship, deserves to be confirmed by means of examples because of its potential to seduce unenlightened minds, and because it is

verblendenden, Alles in Dunkelheit hüllenden Schwärmerei, zwischen ächt christlichem Glauben, der das Gemüth erhebt und zum heiligen Leben kräftigt, und dem schwächenden und mit Einbildungen berauschenden Pietismus und Mystizismus mit möglichster Bestimmtheit und Klarheit nachzuweisen [...]'.

16   Ibid., 548–554: 'ɪv. Geschichte der schwärmerischen Greuelscenen zu Wildenspuch im Kanton Zürich im Jahr 1823'.

17   See for instance E. Haurenski, *Der Teufel ein Bibelerklärer? Oder Beitrag zur Entscheidung über das Zwingende einer vernunftgemässen Christenthums-und Bibelansicht sowie das Staats-und sittengefährliche des Gegenteils*, Altenburg, Johann Karl Gottfried Wagner, 1834, 179.

18   F.I. Herbst (ed.), *Merkwürdige Beispiele religiöser Schwärmerei. Gesammelt und als Supplement des kathol. Exempelbuches*, vol. 3, Regensburg, Georg Joseph Manz, 1845, 231–240: 'Fünfte Abtheilung. Vermischte Beispiele religiöser Schwärmerei. 1. Matheo von Casale'.

confirmed that the exaggeration of religious consciousness easily destroys mankind.[19]

The author considers the church the only guarantee of true religious worship, and claims that those that disobey its doctrines become enthusiasts.[20] With his book full of frightening narratives about enthusiasts, Herbst intended to show quite plainly and polemically 'the fruits of enthusiasm', and 'how rotten and full of wormholes these fruits are in their pits, no matter how beautiful they might appear from the outside'.[21]

As these two examples illustrate, the two Catholic authors labelled Lovat as a *Schwärmer* because they considered him to be a superstitious, dissident misbeliever whose behaviour was contrary to an enlightened understanding of religion and not in line with Catholic doctrine. Hence, their concern was not an inter-, but an inner-confessional demarcation: Lovat's case served them to demarcate right Catholic belief from false belief, not as a means to decry a particular Protestant attitude, as one might suspect at first sight when reading Wessenberg's allusions to pietism and mysticism. This is remarkable because, as Michael Heyd explains, in the seventeenth and eighteenth centuries, enthusiasm became increasingly subjected to criticism with different confessional implications:

> The term itself became a standard label by which to designate individuals or groups who allegedly claimed to have direct divine inspiration, whether millenarians, radical sectarians or various prophesiers, as well as alchemists, 'empirics' and some contemplative philosophers. In the Catholic camp, the confrontation with enthusiasm was less prevalent [...] since mystical experience, miracles, and spiritualist tendencies were more easily incorporated within mainstream orthodoxy. In the Protestant camp, in contrast, such claims presented a real challenge to the religious order, based as it had been since the Reformation primarily on Scripture.[22]

---

19   Ibid.: '[...] die religiöse Schwärmerei, die als relativer Gegensatz der wahren Gottesverehrung um so mehr mit Beispielen belegt zu werden verdient, je näher hier einem unerleuchteten Sinne die Verführung liegt, und je gewisser es ist, daß nicht leicht etwas der Menschheit so tiefe Wunden schlägt, als die Ausartung des religiösen Bewußtseyns'.

20   Ibid.

21   Ibid.: '[...] eine Beispielsammlung, welche zur Absicht hat, zu zeigen, wir faul und wurmstichig diese Früchte im Kerne sind, so schön sie bisweilen von außen erscheinen mögen [...]'.

22   M. Heyd, '*Be Sober and Reasonable*': *The Critique of Enthusiasm in the Seventeenth and Early Eighteenth Centuries*, Leiden, Brill, 1995, 2. On the medical critique of Enthusiasm

Considering this confessional difference, it is interesting to note that, as far as I can see, no single Protestant author used Lovat's case explicitly as a pejorative example of Catholic enthusiasm – apparently, Lovat's self-crucifixion was too extreme and too clearly beyond any Christian doctrine to serve Protestant denunciations of specific Catholic attitudes.

To fully understand some further appropriations of Lovat's case in this debate, it is helpful to briefly clarify the contemporary connotations of the term *Schwärmerei*, as well as of two other German terms that were often used alternatively, namely *Enthusiasterey*, and *fanatici*. In the important eighteenth-century German encyclopaedia, Johann Heinrich Zedler's *Grosses vollständiges Universallexikon aller Wissenschaften und Künste*, *Schwärmer* are described as 'those *fanatici* [Italian in the original, M.B.] which, because they lack the faculty of judgement, have all kinds of opinions that contradict with Christian religion and sometimes with reason itself, and thereby cause public disturbances'.[23] As to the origins of the term, the anonymous author of the entry refers to the beginnings of the Protestant Reformation: the term *Schwärmer* was firstly used for the adherents of the theologian Thomas Mün(t)zer (1488/89–1525), the leader of the Peasants' Revolt in 1525.[24] Consequently, *Schwärmer* came to describe 'types of sectarians and heretics of many kinds'.[25] What distinguishes the *Schwärmer* from other misbelievers such as the *fanatici* is, according to the author, that the *Schwärmer* tend to disturb public order, 'either out of the vitiation of their will (*Verderbnis des Willens*), in particular out of pride (*Stolz*) and pertinacity (*Hartnäckigkeit*), or else out of alleged duty (*vermeyntr Pflicht*)'.[26]

---

see in particular the Chapters 2, 3 and 7. On the critique of melancholy in the German Enlightenment period see also H.J. Schings, *Melancholie und Aufklärung. Melancholiker und ihre Kritik in Erfahrungsseelenkunde und Literatur des 18. Jahrhunderts*, Stuttgart, Metzler, 1977, 185ff. and D. Feldmann, *Die 'religiöse Melancholie' in der deutschsprachigen medizin-theologischen Literatur des ausgehenden 18. und frühen 19. Jahrhunderts*, Kiel, Diss. med., 1973.

23　Anonymous, 'Schwärmer, diejenigen Fanatici genennt', in J.H. Zedler (ed.), *Grosses vollständiges Universallexikon aller Wissenschaften und Künste*, vol. 35, Leipzig and Halle, Johann Heinrich Zedler, 1743, 1795: 'Schwärmer, werden diejenigen Fanatici genennt, welche aus Mangel der Beurtheilungskraft allerley der Christlichen Religion und bisweilen der Vernunft selbst, widersprechende Meinungen hegen, und dadurch öffentliche Unruhen anrichten'.

24　On Thomas Mün(t)zer see D. Heinz, 'MÜNTZER (Münzer)', in Traugott Bautz (ed.), *Biographisch-Bibliographisches Kirchenlexikon*, vol. 6, Herzberg, Traugott Bautz, 1993, 329–345.

25　Anonymous, *Schwärmer, diejenigen Fanatici genennt*, 1795: 'Weil der Nahme eines Schwärmers vielerley Gattungen von Sectirern und Ketzern zukommt, so kann der Ursprung derselben nicht genau bestimmt werden'.

26　Ibid.: 'Es erhellet hieraus der Unterscheid zwischen ihnen und den Fanaticis, von welchen im IX Bande, S. 212 gesagt worden; da nehmlich die letzteren bey ihren ungereimten

In such cases, it would be legitimate for state authorities to intervene.[27] The main characteristic of a *Schwärmer* is, however, that his ideas do not follow any recognisable logic: 'one cannot depict a system of the teachings of these people, because it would be against the nature of the *Schwärmerey* to establish any coherence between their absurd doctrines'.[28] *Fanatici* are defined as misbelievers as well; however, they are different from the *Schwärmer* in that they are concerned with 'incoherent imaginations of various kinds', while the *Schwärmer* are concerned exclusively with divine inspiration (*göttlichen Eingebungen*).[29]

According to the *Zedler*, *Enthusiastery* is also characterised by divine inspiration.[30] The author of the article highlights that in origin, '*Enthusiastery* has a positive meaning, and denotes a divine impact and impulse in the human mind'.[31] However, the term came to be understood in a negative sense, and was associated with insane fury (*Raserey*) and devil's work.[32] *Enthusiasterey* is presented as a particularly complex problem, because its identification requires a clear distinction between imagination on the one hand, and natural effects on the other hand: *Enthusiasterey* is defined as 'a weakness of the mind, if someone has a too vivid imagination combined with a weak faculty of judgement, so that his imagination makes him believe to feel divine forces in his soul, yet they are but natural forces'.[33] Moreover, a 'melancholic temper' enhances

---

Einbildungen stehenbleiben, die Schwärmer hingegen noch weiter gehen, und entweder aus Verderbnis des Willens, besonders durch Stolz und Hartnäckigkeit, oder auch aus vermeynter Pflicht, ihre Irrthümer zu Stöhrung der Ruhe und zu allerley Verwirrungen anwenden'.

27   Ibid.
28   Ibid., 1796: '[...] daß man kein Systema von den Lehren dieser Leute geben könne, massen es wider die Natur der Schwärmerey seyn würde, einen Zusammenhang ihrer widersinnigen Lehren zu bestimmen'.
29   Anonymous, 'Fanatici', in J.H. Zedler (ed.), *Grosses vollständiges Universallexikon aller Wissenschaften und Künste*, vol. 9, Leipzig and Halle, Johann Heinrich Zedler, 1734, 212: 'Der Fanaticismus und die Enthusiasterey, so nahe sie einander kommen, sind doch darinnen von einander unterschieden, daß letzterer nur mit göttlichen Eingebungen zu hun hat, jener aber in allerhand nicht zusammenhängenden Einbildungen bestehet [...]'.
30   Anonymous, 'Enthusiasterey', in J.H. Zedler (ed.), *Grosses vollständiges Universallexikon aller Wissenschaften und Künste*, vol. 8, Leipzig and Halle, Johann Heinrich Zedler, 1734, 1285–1290.
31   Ibid., 1285: 'Die Bedeutung ist also seinem Ursprunge nach gut, und zeigt eine göttliche Wirkung und Regung in dem menschlichen Gemüthe an'.
32   Ibid., 1286.
33   Ibid.: '[...] ist die Enthusiasterey eine Schwachheit des Verstandes, wenn ein Mensch eine allzulebhafte Imagination und dabey ein schwaches Judicium hat, so daß er sich durch seine Einbildungskraft allerhand göttliche Würckungen in seiner Seelen vorstellet, welche doch nur natürliche Würckungen sind'.

Enthusiasterey.[34] Finally, readers are advised against two common responses to *Enthusiasterey*: the first is to deny the existence of divine forces in honest believers altogether and to dismiss their claims as 'enthusiastic dreams' – something that only 'atheists, naturalists and their adherents' would do. The other warning is that one should not lapse into 'a rough or subtle *Enthusiasterey*, out of naivety related to simple-mindedness towards God'.[35] Finally, *Enthusiastery* is summarised as something 'that sometimes really exists, but that sometimes is only feigned'.[36]

Considering the fact that the English term 'enthusiasm' does not carry the plural meanings inherent in the German terms, it is important to be aware of these subtle differences when examining the German appropriations of Lovat's case. Most German authors referred to Lovat as a *Schwärmer*, the term that combined divine inspiration and religious zeal with public disturbance. This explains Wessenberg's above cited reference to patriotic sense and political fanaticism. In the pre-revolutionary German states, clergymen frequently considered religious enthusiasts on the same level as the new threat from political fanatics. Those considered as *Schwärmer* not only threatened an Enlightened understanding of religion, they also represented a danger for the political, social and moral order. Hence, although Lovat's self-crucifixion implied violence only against himself, the act itself was considered a disturbance of public and religious order. Notwithstanding its Italian origin, this public aspect in Lovat's case made it a useful case for those authors in the German states whose concern was to promote a rational religion that would sustain political and public order as well as political cohesion.

Educationists also presented Lovat's case as a deterrent example of aberrant religious education, for instance, an extensive discussion of Lovat's case that was published in 1831 in *Der Correspondent für Volksschullehrer. Eine pädagogische Zeitschrift*.[37] The aim of this pedagogical journal was to advise parents and school teachers in educational matters, and to thereby promote national

---

34   Anonymous, *Enthusiasterey*, 1288.

35   Ibid., 1289: 'Man hat bey dieser Sache zwey Abwege zu vermeiden; den einen gehen die Atheisten, Naturalisten und ihr Anhang, diese leugnen alle göttliche Würckungen in denen Seelen derer Gläubigen, u. halten dasjenige, was christliche Lehre von denen Gnadenwürckungen Gottes in denen Sellen derer Gläubigen lehren, rechtschaffene Gläubige auch von ihrer eigenen Empfindung vorgeben, vor enthusiastische Träume. Der andere Abweg ist, daß man nicht selbst in eine grobe oder subtile Enthusiasterey aus einer mit Einfalt verknüpfter Treuherzigkeit gegen Gott verfalle'.

36   Ibid., 1286: 'Man hat diesen Unterschied von der Enthusiasterey zu mercken, daß sie manchmal etwas würckliches ist, manchmal aber nur auf ein verstelltes Wesen hinausläuft'.

37   *Der Correspondent der Volksschullehrer. Eine pädagogische Zeitschrift*, vol. 1, 1831. The journal had only been just launched to appear in 25 issues.

education (*Volksbildung*). Serialised in three issues during January 1831, the anonymous author presents Lovat's case under a heading 'about the consequences of a false religious education. An instructive narrative for parents and educators'.[38] In accordance with the notions of eighteenth- and nineteenth-century pedagogy, the central argument of the narrative is the importance of education for the sane development of individuals. To this end, the author transforms Lovat's case into a pedagogical story (*belehrende Erzählung*). The subject of his text is not an insane patient, but an originally innocent child. Gradually, the reader learns how this innocent child – Lovat – went astray, due to the negative influence of his parents, religious educators, masters and his social environment.

Convinced that 'it is parents and educators who, in the earliest youth, lay the foundations for men's vices and virtues, fortune and misfortune',[39] the author considers religious education as the most important part of child education, and believes that everything depends on how and when religious doctrines are taught.[40] The reader is warned about a false religious education that produces 'hypocrites or even dangerous enthusiasts (*Schwärmer*)',[41] and Lovat is introduced as a 'remarkable example of how disadvantageous sensations that have been excited in young days can become'.[42] Therefore, the story puts great emphasis on Lovat's youth and place of birth. Inventing details that are not contained in Ruggieri's original case history, the author describes how Lovat's parents struggled to feed their children although they worked hard as farmers;[43] and how Lovat, characterised by his friendly manner, his gentle heart and vivid mind in contrast to his brothers and sisters, was his mother's favourite.[44] Lovat's father, by contrast, disliked him because of his weak body, which made him useless for any kind of work except for tending sheep. According to the author, Lovat was permanently under threat of corporal punishment and was told that

---

38   Anonymous, 'Von den Folgen eines unrichtig geleiteten Religions-Unterrichtes. Eine belehrende Erzählung für Aeltern und Erzieher', *Der Correspondent der Volksschullehrer. Eine pädagogische Zeitschrift*, vol. 1, 1831, 3–21.

39   Ibid., 3: 'Zu des Menschen Tugenden und Laster, Glück und Mißgeschick wird von den Aeltern und Erziehern oft schon in der frühesten Jugend der Grund gelegt. [...]'.

40   Ibid., 4.

41   Ibid., 4: 'Gewöhnlich wird bey einem unrichtig geleiteten Religions-Unterrichte ein versteckter Heuchler, wohl gar gefährlicher Schwärmer erzogen'.

42   Ibid.: 'Der Schuhmacher Mathäus Lovat ist ein auffallendes Beispiel, wie nachtheilig in der Jugend stark erregte Gefühle für den Menschen werden können'.

43   Ibid., 5.

44   Ibid.

he was useless, which made him feel discontent with his situation, averse to other people and disposed to loneliness.[45]

According to the author's narrative, the religious education that Lovat received from his parents was likewise disadvantageous for Lovat's development. The parents were very pious people, regularly attended services and used to fast for many days, partly because of poverty and partly out of duty. Accordingly, they taught their children a very physical way of practising belief, telling them 'about the gentle consolations of religion, and about the duties that we have by divine doctrine towards God, towards our self and our fellow man'.[46] When Lovat was subjected to violence by his master, his parents reminded him that earthly pain was nothing and that he would receive all the more recompense in heaven the more he suffered during his lifetime.[47] As a result, Lovat prayed excessively, chastened himself, went to church and meditated on the saints. The author concludes that 'Lovat withdrew from society and spent his youth mostly dreaming and lost in introspective thoughts. He lacked the inner power to fling off restraints and to overcome his fate with courage'.[48]

This pedagogical narrative also relates Lovat's individual religious education to the general religious atmosphere in the North Italian village of Casale where he spent his childhood. A meagre and isolated place in a romantic position in the mountains, the village is described as a place of poor education where superstition had reigned for centuries. Hindered by the Venetian government, 'no ray of enlightenment could enter the lonely village'.[49] People were not familiar with 'holy and divine prayers', as these had been replaced by 'empty formulas and practices of repentance'. The author concludes that '[t]his false direction of religious sense that every innocent man has, should later become the cause of Lovat's great mental confusion'.[50] Besides the parents, the author blames Lovat's religious educators for Lovat's fate. His personal confessor added insult to injury. He neither consoled Lovat nor did he

45   Ibid.
46   Ibid., 6: 'Aber tiefes Stillschweigen herrschte dagegen über die gottähnlichen Gesinnungen und Empfindungen, über die sanften Tröstungen der Religion und über die Pflichten, welche uns die göttliche Lehre gegen Gott, gegen uns selbst und gegen unsere Mitmenschen auflegt'.
47   Ibid., 8.
48   Ibid.: 'Lovat zog sich aber ganz in sich selbst zurück, und verlebte seine Jünglingsjahre meistens träumend und in Selbstbetrachtungen verloren. Ihm mangelte die innere Kraft, seine Fesseln zu zersprengen und sich kühn über sein Schicksal zu erheben'.
49   Ibid., 5: 'In das einsame Dörfchen konnte kein Strahl von Aufklärung dringen; weil sie die venetianische Regierung mehr zu unterdrücken als zu befördern besorgt war'.
50   Ibid., 6: 'Diese falsche Richtung des, in jedem unverdorbenen Menschen befindlichen religiösen Sinnes, wurde später die Ursache zur großen Geistesverirrung des Lovat'.

tell him that his self-destructive ideas were wrong. Instead, he declared that Lovat's thoughts were influenced by the devil and told him to pray, fast and chasten himself.[51] Consequently, Lovat meditated intensively on the life stories of martyrs and longed to become a saint himself.[52] Then he fell ill and his enthusiasm (*Schwärmerey*) increased. He chastened himself for all his physical desires and struggled with sinful dreams.[53] According to the author, it was the example of Origen, which Lovat came to know 'by chance' when he was 44 years old that encouraged him to mutilate himself in order to 'forever destroy the source of all sinful thoughts'.[54] Similarly, the author considers Lovat's two attempts at public self-crucifixion as motivated by some false interpretations of verses from the Bible.[55] The author concludes that because Lovat was not made familiar with the one, superior Christian religion, he necessarily became a dreamer and an enthusiast.[56] Therefore, he hopes that,

> His [Lovat's, M.B.] great aberrations may serve parents and educators as an exemplary warning; that they should not declare godliness and religious feelings to be only a matter of emotions, but that they also seek to act upon the reason and the hearts of children, in order to bring up rational, useful citizens, and not crippled enthusiasts or useless dreamers.[57]

This and the examples cited above show that the reason why Lovat's case provoked German theologians and educationists to comment and rewrite it in their works was the contemporary call for an enlightened and rational religion, opposed to individual mystical and superstitious beliefs that were attributed to the so-called enthusiasts.[58] In consequence of the German Enlightenment, a

---

51 Ibid., 8.
52 Ibid., 9f.
53 Ibid., 10.
54 Ibid.: 'Dieses Beyspiel begeisterte den vier und vierzigjährigen Lovat so, daß er sich fest vornahm, eine gleiche Verstümmelung an seinem Körper vorzunehmen, und so die Urquelle aller unreinen Gedanken auf immer zu vernichten'.
55 Ibid., 11.
56 Ibid., 21.
57 Ibid.: 'Mögen seine großen Verirrungen Aeltern und Erziehern zum warnenden Beispiele dienen, daß sie nicht Gottesfurcht und religiösen Sinn zur alleinigen Sache des Gefühls machen; sondern, daß sie auch suchen, auf den Verstand, und das Herz der Kinder einzuwirken, um vernünftige, nützliche Bürger des Staates, und keine verkrüppelten Schwärmer oder unnütze Träumer zu erziehen'.
58 J.G.A. Pocock, 'Enthusiasm. The Antiself of Enlightenment', in L.E. Klein and A.J. La Vopa (eds.), *Enthusiasm and Enlightenment in Europe, 1650–1850*, San Marino, CA, Huntington Library, 1998, 7–28.

rational reading of the Bible, meaning a historical-critical understanding of its texts and their genesis, was propagated.[59] In this context, the notion that Lovat had literally interpreted the Gospel of Matthew as a call for self-castration and self-crucifixion was therefore a provocation. Authors referred to Lovat's self-crucifixion and self-castration as deterrent examples that illustrated to what self-destructive deeds a wrong interpretation of the Bible could lead.

While the German readings of Lovat's case from the first half of the nineteenth century are thus characterised by their framing of Lovat's case as a case of enthusiasm, this notion is strikingly absent from the contemporary British and French religious readings of the case. The reason for this is not that enthusiasm was not an issue in the other countries, but that the terms to designate it varied. Jan Goldstein has compared the English and French lexical status of the two terms 'enthusiasm' and 'imagination'.[60] She finds that while in eighteenth-century Germany and Britain '"enthusiasm" functioned as a powerful term of opprobrium which conjured up everything antithetical to, and rejected by, enlightened rationality',[61] French authors preferred the term 'imagination' over 'enthusiasm' to discredit unenlightened and irrational behaviour of believers:

> As inhabitants of a country that had for the most part repelled the Protestant Reformation, the French had never had their word *enthousiasme* so thoroughly saturated with the particular set of pejorative connotations that derived from hostility to the religious claims of Protestant sectaries. As a result, the French generally used the term "imagination" and its cognates to do the work – or the dirty work – that "enthusiasm" performed for their British and German contemporaries.[62]

The suggested distinction between the terms 'enthusiasm' and 'imagination' should not, however, be rigidly drawn: as we have seen before, a German encyclopaedia considered 'a too vivid imagination' the cause of enthusiasm. But insane imagination in fact served French authors as a medical explanation for Lovat's mental disorder, while in British readings of Lovat's case the notion of the religious 'eccentric' prevailed.[63]

---

59   On reading the Bible in this period see A. Polaschegg and S. Martus (eds.), *Das Buch der Bücher – gelesen. Lesarten der Bibel in den Wissenschaften und Künsten*, Bern, Lang, 2006; A. Polaschegg and D. Weidner (eds.), *Das Buch in den Büchern. Wechselwirkungen von Bibel und Literatur*, Munich, Wilhelm Fink, 2012.

60   Goldstein, *Enthusiasm or Imagination*.

61   Ibid., 29.

62   Ibid., 32.

63   On medical concepts of imagination see E. Fischer-Homberger, 'On the Medical History of the Doctrine of Imagination', *Psychological Medicine*, vol. 9, 1979, 619–628 and

3   A Pious Madman? Lovat's Case in the Medical Critique of
       Schwärmerei

Enthusiasm was not only a controversial issue for theologians and educationists, physicians were likewise concerned with it.[64] The medical critique of enthusiasm had its roots in ancient medicine, which had linked enthusiasm to
melancholy or madness.[65] In the seventeenth century, the medicalisation of
the critique of enthusiasm was even employed in the theological discourse.
As Heyd argues, '(i)n designating religious eccentrics and non-conformists as
"mentally sick", the critics of enthusiasm imperceptibly redefined religious
orthodoxy in medical terms of health and mental balance, rather than, or at
least, side by side with, theological terms of correct faith'.[66]

   This is exactly what we find in several of the German appropriations of Lovat's case: parallel theological and medical arguments, and in particular an
equation of the notion of *Schwärmerei* and a diagnosis of insanity. An interesting example of how the notion of *Schwärmerei* was applied to Lovat's case
from early on and how it was linked to the emerging idea of a mental medicine
('psychische Medizin') in Germany, is a long philosophical essay on 'The power
of enthusiasm' (*Die Gewalt der Schwärmerey*) in Lovat's self-crucifixion that
was published in 1812 in a journal entitled *Beyträge zur Beförderung einer
Kurmethode auf psychischem Wege* ('Contributions to the Promotion of Psychological Treatment').[67] The editor of the journal was the German physician
Johann Christian Reil (1759–1813),[68] who, because of his various publications
on mental therapies, is generally considered one of the leading figures of
early psychiatry in Germany.[69] Within the German historiography of psychia-

---

        G.S. Rousseau, 'Science and the Discovery of the Imagination in Enlightened England',
        Eighteenth Century Studies, vol. 3, no. 1, 1969, 108–135.

64   Heyd, *The Critique of Enthusiasm*, Chapters 2, 3 and 7.

65   Ibid., 44ff.

66   Ibid., 10. See Chapter 7: 'The new medical discourse and the theological critique of enthu-
        siasm', 191ff.

67   J.C. Reil and J.C. Hoffbauer, *Beyträge zur Beförderung einer Kurmethode auf psychischem
        Wege*, vol. 2, Halle, In der Curt'schen Buchhandlung, 1812, 157–185.

68   On Reil see R. Mocek, *Johann Christian Reil (1759–1813). Das Problem des Übergangs von
        der Spätaufklärung zur Romantik in Biologie und Medizin in Deutschland*, Frankfurt, Pe-
        ter Lang, 1995; M.J. Bandorf, 'Reil, Johann Christian', in Historische Kommission bei der
        Bayerischen Akademie der Wissenschaften (ed.), *Allgemeine Deutsche Biographie*, vol. 27,
        Munich, Duncker & Humblot, 1888, 700–701.

69   H. Schott and R. Tölle, *Geschichte der Psychiatrie. Krankheitslehren, Irrwege, Behandlungs-
        formen*, Munich, C.H. Beck, 2006, 55ff. Reil is associated with the so-called 'Romantische
        Medizin', a group of German physicians and philosophers who were influenced by the
        natural philosophy of Joseph von Schelling, see R. Wöbkemeyer, *Erzählte Krankheit. Medi-
        zinische und literarische Phantasien um 1800*, Stuttgart, Metzler, 1990, 90–131.

try, Reil has even been labelled the 'German Pinel', i.e. the founding father of German psychiatry, and is said to have invented the German term 'Psychiatrie' in 1808.[70] The author of the essay on Lovat's case was, however, not Reil himself but his co-editor Johann Christoph Hoffbauer (1766–1827).[71] As a Kantian philosopher, Hoffbauer had published extensively on logic, moral philosophy as well as on legal and medical aspects of what he called 'diseases of the soul', or 'psychology'.[72] Important German psychiatrists of the late nineteenth century (Richard Krafft-Ebing, for example) retrospectively considered Hoffbauer and Reil, among others, as representatives of the 'philosophical-psychological direction' in early German psychiatry which, in their view, had hindered the development of psychiatry into a genuine 'natural science' (*Naturwissenschaft*).[73] Hoffbauer had a special interest in religious *Schwärmerey*, as can be seen from a 'psychological study of madness' that he published in 1807, which explains his particular interest in Lovat's case.[74]

With their journal, Hoffbauer and Reil explicitly sought to follow the model of the *Magazin für Erfahrungsseelenkunde*. This was a late eighteenth-century journal edited by the German writer Karl Philipp Moritz with the purpose of establishing an 'empirical psychology' through the collection of authentic case reports.[75] Like that project, Reil and Hoffbauer's aim was to collect case

---

70   A. Marneros and F. Pillmann (eds.), *Das Wort Psychiatrie ... wurde in Halle geboren: von den Anfängen der deutschen Psychiatrie*, Stuttgart, Schattauer, 2005. For the first time, Reil used the term 'Psychiaterie' in J.C. Reil and J.C. Hoffbauer, *Beyträge zur Beförderung einer Kurmethode auf psychischem Wege*, vol. 1, Halle, In der Curt'schen Buchhandlung, 1808, 161.

71   On Hoffbauer see C. von Prantl, 'Hoffbauer, Johann Christoph', Historische Kommission bei der Bayerischen Akademie der Wissenschaften (ed.), *Allgemeine Deutsche Biographie*, vol. 12, Munich, Duncker & Humblot, 1880, 567–568.

72   See for instance J.C. Hoffbauer, *Untersuchungen über die Krankheiten der Seele und die verwandten Zustände*, Halle, Bey Joh. Gottfr. Trampens Erben, 1802–1807; J.C. Hoffbauer, *Die Psychologie in ihren Hauptanwendungen auf die Rechtspflege nach den allgemeinen Gesichtspunkten der Gesetzgebung; oder, Die sogenannte gerichtliche Arzneywissenschaft nach ihrem psychologischen Theile*, Halle, Schimmelpfennig, 1808.

73   R. von Krafft-Ebing, *Lehrbuch der Psychiatrie: auf klinischer Grundlage für praktische Ärzte und Studierende*, Saarbrücken, Verlag Dr. Müller, 2007, 40. See the chapter 'Geschichte der Psychiatrie vom Ende des 18. Jahrhunderts ab', 38ff.

74   J.C. Hoffbauer, *Psychologische Untersuchungen über den Wahnsinn und die übrigen Arten der Verzückung und die Behandlung derselben*, Halle, Bey Hemmerde und Schwetschke, 1807. See the Chapters XXXVI–XXXIX, 373ff., concerning the effects of *Schwärmerei*, its relation to insanity and its supposed incurability.

75   On this project see for instance A. Gailus, 'A Case of Individuality. Karl Philipp Moritz and the Magazine for Empirical Psycchology', *New German Critique*, no. 79, 2000, 67–105, and Y. Wübben, 'Writing Cases and Casuistic Reasoning in Karl Philipp Moritz' Journal

narratives that dealt with melancholy or madness and explored the human soul.[76] The *Beyträge zur Beförderung einer Kurmethode auf psychischem Wege* had five principal aims: first, to provide examples of psychological healings; second, to present experiments in psychology; third, to make observations about the psychological effects of external causes on the body; and fourth, to communicate attempts to establish a mental therapy. Lovat's case is included in the fifth section in which the editors write about new international medical writings and incidents relevant to their concept of a *Psychische Medizin*.[77]

In his appropriation of Lovat's case, Hoffbauer proposes a specific tool of analysis, as suggested by the title: the power of enthusiasm (*Die Gewalt der Schwärmerey*).[78] His text represents a philosophical-medical critique of enthusiasm viewed through the lens of Lovat's case. Hoffbauer considers Lovat's case a perfect example of his general observation that in many cases, enthusiasm not only 'repressed reason' but in which 'reason even served enthusiasm'.[79] This idea consequently dominates Hoffbauer's interpretation of Lovat's case. He repeatedly insists on the fact that Lovat, in spite of his obvious insane actions, proceeded with a striking acuteness of mind during both his self-mutilation and his self-crucifixion. For instance, as regards Lovat's amputation of his genitals, he argues that this act cannot be regarded as an 'excess of an irrational passion' because Lovat had prepared the remedies for his wounds with

---

of Empirical Psychology', in *Early Science and Medicine*, vol. 18, 2013, 471–486. See also Chapter 7.

76   The kinship between the two journals is emphasised by S. Dickson, 'Die internationale Rezeption der Fallgeschichten im Magazin zur Erfahrungsseelenkunde', in S. Dickson, S. Goldman and C. Wingertszahn (eds.), *'Fakta, und kein moralisches Geschwätz'. Zu den Fallgeschichten im 'Magazin für die Erfahrungsseelenkunde' (1783–1793)*, Göttingen, Wallstein, 2011, 256–276, 259 and 267.

77   Reil and Hoffbauer, *Beyträge zur Beförderung einer Kurmethode auf psychischem Wege*, vol. 1, 2: 'Die Zeitschrift soll I. Beyspiele von psychischen, wenn auch nicht Curen, doch Heilungen mit Versuchen, diese zu analysieren, enthalten; II. Versuche in den zum Behufe der psychischen Medicin noch mehr zu bearbeitenden Fächern der Psychologie liefern; III. Beobachtungen über die Einwirkung äusserer Ursachen auf den Körper, in so fern sie psychisch sind; und IV. Versuche einer psychischen Therapeutik mittheilen, und außerdem V. von den neuern psychologischen und medicinischen Schriften, in so fern sie für die psychische Medicin wichtig sind, Nachricht geben, und auf das Wichtige in ihnen aufmerksam machen, auch von allen Ereignissen, die für die psychische Medicin wichtig sind, Bericht erstatten'.

78   Ibid., 157–185.

79   Hoffbauer, *Die Gewalt der Schwärmerey*, 157: 'Das [sic!] die Schwärmerey die Vernunft unterdrückt, heisst zu wenig sagen. In vielen Fällen wenigstens muss die Vernunft der Schwärmerey selbst dienen, und ihr mit Anstrengungen dienen, die ihr sonst fremd wären, oder deren sie sonst nicht gewachsen seyn würde'.

the highest care – in Hoffbauer's words, Lovat acted as his own physician.[80] The reason for Lovat's self-mutilation was, in the author's view, not his wish to deaden carnal desire, but his longing for sanctity, as this would be probable '(f) or an enthusiast who has the head full of saints [...]'.[81]

In contrast to Ruggieri's account that Lovat felt offended by people's mockery and withdrew from social life, Hoffbauer presumes that Lovat, like a typical enthusiast, craved recognition and was therefore rather pleased to be persecuted.[82] In his eyes, Lovat's main aim was to cause a public stir. Therefore, by crucifying himself, he created a spectacle for the people in order to make himself immortal through this singular death.[83] Amour-propre (*Eitelkeit*) and ambition (*Ehrsucht*) incited Lovat's craziness. Pointing to the public dimension of both the self-mutilation and the attempted self-crucifixion, Hoffbauer claims that it would be the aim of all enthusiasts to make their intentions public.[84] This emphasis on publicity is in line with the classic definition of the term *Schwärmer* in Zedler's dictionary, which combined divine inspiration and religious zeal with public disturbance, as we have seen before. Hence, Hoffbauer's reading of Lovat's case follows a specific 'logic of the enthusiast'[85] that he identifies at work in Lovat. He finds that his case resembles those of other enthusiasts but is singular at the same time. It is typical in that it shows the enthusiasts' frequent 'insistence on their senseless intentions, their ruinous ambition and so forth'; and it is singular because it reveals a unique interplay of insanity and reason: 'how the most absurd madness can go along with sober-mindedness and an inventive spirit [...] this case shows probably in a unique way'.[86]

---

80   Ibid., 165: 'Man kann diese That nicht als den plötzlichen Ausbruch einer ohne Ueberlegung handelnden Leidenschaft, die den Menschen wie einen Windstoß hinreisst, betrachten. Denn so wie Lovat jene Operation selbst vorgenommen hatte, war er sein eigener Arzt [...]'.

81   Ibid., 166.

82   Ibid.

83   Ibid., 174f.: 'So sauer liess Lovat es sich werden, dem Volke ein Schauspiel zu geben, dass er keinen anderen Zweck haben konnte, als sein Andenken durch den Tod zu verewigen, den vor ihm sich kein Anderer gegeben hatte'.

84   Ibid., 177f.: 'Diese Eitelkeit oder Ehrsucht habe ich Lovat's Tollheit, ohne mich auf einen Beweis derselben einzulassen, zum Grunde gelegt. Denn von dem Augenblicke an, wo er vor unsern Augen handelt, war alles darauf berechnet, nicht allein, was er sich vorgenommen anzuführen, sondern es auch zur Kunde der Welt – denn das war ihm, und ist jedem Schwärmer, dieser Art, das grössere oder kleinere Publikum, in dem er lebt – zu bringen'.

85   Ibid., 168: 'nach der Logik des Schwärmers [...]'.

86   Ibid., 176: 'Ich übergehe mehrere Bemerkungen, weil die Geschichte des Schwärmers nur zu oft auf sie führt, wie über die Beharrlichkeit in ihren sinnlosen Vorsätzen, ihrer wahnwitzigen Ehrsucht u. d. gl.; nur wie die sinnloseste Tollheit mit der ruhig-sinnendsten Erfindsamkeit gepaart seyn kann [...] zeigt diese Geschichte, wie vielleicht keine andere'.

A second idea that Hoffbauer sees exemplified in Lovat's case is therefore that men can demonstrate the highest degree of prudence (*Besonnenheit*) in their action without being self-conscious (*seiner selbst mächtig*).[87] This, Hoffbauer says, is a crucial issue for contemporary law (*Rechtspflege*), since 'so far, one was used to deduce from the thoughtfulness of an action the proof that it was done by free will (*Freyheit*)'.[88] Hoffbauer then discusses at great length the role of the free will in human action more generally, the nature of 'heroic passions' in suicides and crimes, and the effects of penalties imposed by the state.[89] Turning back to Lovat's case only after several pages, Hoffbauer recommends that everybody should read Schlegel's annotated translation because of its great psychological interest.[90] In line with this interest, Hoffbauer criticises Ruggieri for not having included Lovat's personal letter in his original text, presuming that 'perhaps, there is a lot to be revealed by it'.[91] Hoffbauer was thus not interested in Lovat's letter as a proof of authenticity for the facts told by Ruggieri, but he was interested to read Lovat's own words and writing.[92] This statement suggests that Hoffbauer was the very author Ruggieri referred to in his second Italian edition of 1814, when he decided to include a full copy of Lovat's letter at the request of a 'foreign author'.[93]

Although Hoffbauer based his essay on Schlegel's German translation, his narrative does not follow the original structure of Ruggieri's case history.

---

87   Ibid., 178f.: 'Dass nähmlich der Mensch die grösste Besonnenheit, die sinnendste und ruhigste Überlegung, bey der Vollführung einer That beweisen kann, ohne dass man berechtigt ware, ihn seiner selbst mächtig zu betrachten, oder ihm diese Handlung zu rechnen wollte, würde ihn an Unsinn übertreffen'.

88   Ibid., 179: 'Denn es ist bekannt, dass man bisher gewohnt gewesen, in der Bedachtsamkeit und Ueberlegung, welche jemand bei der Verübung einer Handlung gezeigt, einen Beweis zu finden, dass der Beschluss zu derselben mit Freyheit gefasst, oder wo dies auch nicht sein sollte, mit Freyheit unterhalten sey?'

89   Ibid., 179–184.

90   Ibid., 185.

91   Ibid., 162: 'Vielleicht hätte man vieles, wenn auch nicht in ihm, doch aus ihm lesen können, was uns Hr. R...Geschichtserzählung nicht sagt'.

92   Guthmüller suggests that in France, this reading of the patient's language as symptoms of mental disorder increases only by the middle of the nineteenth century, see M. Guthmüller, 'Der Traum im psychopathologischen Fallbericht des 19. Jahrhunderts: Maurice Macario, Alfred Maury, Sante de Sanctis', in R. Behrens, N. Bischoff, and C. Zelle (eds.), *Der ärztliche Fallbericht. Epistemische Grundlagen und textuelle Strukturen dargestellter Beobachtung*, Wiesbaden, Harrassowitz, 2012, 171–200, 173.

93   Ruggieri, *Storia della crocifissione*, 13: 'Ho creduto bene di qui unire copia della carta sudetta tal quale fu estesa da Mattio colla stessa sintassi ed ortografia perchè non pochi m'hanno tacciato d'inesatezza per non averlo che ricordato quando pubblicai la prima volta questo singolarissimo caso di pazzia'.

Explicitly, Hoffbauer decided to present the plot (*Geschichtserzählung*) in a different form.[94] His narrative starts with the day of Lovat's self-crucifixion, and not with Lovat's biographical background. Unlike the *Storia della crocifissione* and other typical medical case histories, the death does not mark the end. Instead, Hoffbauer turns back to a reconstruction of Lovat's past and adds several passages in which he discusses in depth the psychological significance of Lovat's self-crucifixion. He then develops his ideas about more general legal-philosophical problems, in particular on the question of how to integrate a philosophical and psychological dimension in contemporary criminal law.[95] Hoffbauer thus transforms the narrative structure in a way that best served him to discuss his own professional interests.

On the whole, Hoffbauer's reading of Lovat's case presents him as a typical enthusiast, in the specific 'German' sense of *Schwärmerey*, and in a medicalised understanding of it. Tellingly, as a philosopher, Hoffbauer does not feel qualified to comment on the specifically medical aspects of Lovat's case.[96] But his 'logic of the enthusiast' is based not on a religious critique, such as the later theological critique proposed by Herbst and Wessenberg that we have examined before, but on the opposition of reason and unreason in the framework of German *psychische Medizin*. Hoffbauer's appropriation of Lovat's case is, therefore, exemplary for how the medical and the theological critique of enthusiasm overlapped in the discussions of cases such as Lovat's. It illustrates what Lawrence Klein and Anthony La Vopa have described as the 'the obvious shift in the discourse of anti-enthusiasm from theological polemic to new languages of science and medicine'.[97]

Hoffbauer's philosophical essay is also illustrative for how in the debates on a *Psychische Medizin* in early nineteenth-century Germany, the disciplinary fields of religion, medicine, psychology, philosophy and law were deeply intertwined. Because they required a combination of knowledge from different fields, authors employed cases like Lovat's to underline the need and sense of a *psychische Medizin* as opposed to medical approaches that focused primarily

---

94   Hoffbauer, *Die Gewalt der Schwärmerey*, 158: 'Allein, auch wenn ich, was ich wünschte, diese Schrift als meinen Lesern bekannt, voraussetzen dürfte, so hätte ich mich doch der Mühe nicht überheben dürfen, der darin enthaltenen Geschichtserzählung eine andere Form zu geben'.

95   Ibid., 175–185.

96   See ibid., 185. Hoffbauer says here that he leaves it up to the physician to comment on the rapid healing of Lovat's wounds in relation to his state of mind. At present, he says, 'this is an issue of only little clearness in psychology and physiology'.

97   L.E. Klein and A.J. La Vopa, 'Introduction', in L.E. Klein and A.J. La Vopa (eds.), *Enthusiasm and Enlightenment in Europe, 1650–1850*, San Marino, CA, Huntington Library, 1998, 1–6, 4.

on somatic aspects, and to establish a canon of knowledge for it. Several related questions arose in the debates of such cases: How should one define the relation of body and soul? How should one consider the role of the free will in insane actions? What are the inner motivations, that is to say the moral causes, for insane or criminal actions? A journal such as the *Beyträge zur Beförderung einer Kurmethode auf psychischem Wege*, shaped by the specific interests of its editors, namely a physician and a philosopher, achieved to integrate these different fields of knowledge to a large extent. The way in which Hoffbauer employed Lovat's case in his and Reil's journal therefore confirms a specific function many case narratives fulfilled in this period: to serve as instruments of scientific innovation and to prepare new and interdisciplinary fields of knowledge.[98]

In the course of time, the medical critique of enthusiasm separated itself more clearly from the theological critique to become more and more autonomous. Increasingly, physicians used the adjectives 'religious' or 'pious' in a newly developed psychiatric terminology to describe a specific condition of insanity, a self-contained diagnosis, namely 'religious madness', in German called *religiöser Wahnsinn* or *Religionswahnsinn*. In German psychiatry, the making of this disease category by physicians was, at least initially, strongly influenced by the described religious and medical critique of enthusiasm. The example of Karl Wilhelm Ideler's allusions to Lovat's case helps to explain the continuing influence of the notion of enthusiasm in the psychiatric discussions of Lovat's case, which are the subject of the next chapter. Ideler (1795–1860), the son of a Protestant priest and a physician by profession, was appointed the director of the psychiatric division of the Berlin Charité hospital in 1828. From 1840 onwards, he was professor and director of the new psychiatric clinic.[99] Similar to Reil and Hoffbauer, Ideler stood in for an interdisciplinary concept of the 'science of the soul' (*Seelenlehre*) on the basis of philosophy and anthropology. His main idea was that psychiatric research should primarily focus on individual biographies and the psychological 'development' (*Entwickelung*) of patients.[100] Later psychiatrists therefore labelled him, together with Reil and Hoffbauer, a *Psychiker,* in a pejorative way.[101] Like most future German psychiatrists, Ideler

---

98   Pethes, *Vom Einzelfall zur Menschheit*, 76.

99   On Ideler see H. Schipperges, 'Ideler, Karl Wilhelm', in Historische Kommission bei der Bayerischen Akademie der Wissenschaften (ed.), *Neue Deutsche Biographie*, vol. 10, Berlin, Duncker & Humblot, 1974, 116–118.

100   Ideler published a book on the biographies of mentally disordered patients, see K.W. Ideler, *Biographien Geisteskranker in ihrer psychologischen Entwickelung dargestellt*, Berlin, Schroeder, 1841.

101   Krafft-Ebing, *Lehrbuch der Psychiatrie*, 40.

was strongly influenced by the earlier works of the French alienists. Tellingly, he came to know Lovat's case when he translated a book into German which, as we will see, played an important role for the circulation of Lovat's case in France: Charles Marc's 1840 study *De la folie considérée dans ses rapports avec les questions medico-judiciaires*.[102]

Ideler was so fascinated by Lovat's case that he included it in his own influential study *Versuch einer Theorie des religiösen Wahnsinns* ('Essay on Theory of Religious Madness') published in 1848.[103] In this study, Ideler develops a systematic approach for the classification of 'religious madness' (*religiöser Wahnsinn*). He introduces Lovat's case in the section entitled 'religious madness in its individual forms', in a subchapter about 'actions contrary to reason as a consequence of religious madness'.[104] Such actions (*vernunftwidrige Handlungen*), Ideler argues, require a separate discussion since they are different from other kinds of madness. In the case of the 'pious madmen' (*fromme Geisteskranke*), their mind and behaviour are opposed to the laws of nature even more than in other cases of madness because they long for the supernatural. Their 'ludicrous actions' (*aberwitzige Handlungen*) are directly linked to their general beliefs, and have therefore to be understood in relation to them.[105] Consequently, Ideler distinguishes different types of such ludicrous actions: self-mutilation, self-crucifixion, homicide and malicious arson, and presents several exemplary cases to illustrate each of them. These narratives are taken from various

---

102   C.C.H. Marc, *De la folie considérée dans ses rapports avec les questions medico-judiciaires*, vol. 1 Paris, J.-B. Baillière, 1840; K.W. Ideler, *Die Geisteskrankheiten in Beziehung zur Rechtspflege von C.C. Marc, Leibarzte des Königs der Franzosen etc.etc. Deutsch bearbeitet und mit Anmerkungen begleitet. Ein Handbuch für Gerichts-Aerzte und Juristen*, Berlin, Voss'sche Buchhandlung, 1843–1844. Marc's narrative is on 251–258.

103   K.W. Ideler, *Versuch einer Theorie des religiösen Wahnsinns. Ein Beitrag zur Kritik der religiösen Wirren der Gegenwart. Erster Theil: Die Erscheinungen des religiösen Wahnsinns*, Halle, Schwetschke und Sohn, 1848 and K.W. Ideler, *Versuch einer Theorie des religiösen Wahnsinns. Ein Beitrag zur Kritik der religiösen Wirren der Gegenwart. 2. Theil: Die Entwickelung des religiösen Wahnsinns*, Halle, Schwetschke und Sohn, 1850.

104   Ideler, *Die Erscheinungen des religiösen Wahnsinns*, 186–205.

105   Ibid., 186: 'Daher ist das Leben der Wahnsinnigen eine Kette von verderblichen Handlungen, und im vorzüglichen Sinne gilt dies von den frommen Geisteskranken, weil ihre Verstandesbethörung in eine übersinnliche Welt hinüberschweifend, sich mehr, als bei jeder anderen Seelenstörung in den schneidensten Widerspruch mit den Naturgesetzen stellt, und in der Voraussetzung von Wundern schwärmend, durch sie unmittelbar wirken zu können wähnt. Hierbei muss besonders in Erwägung gezogen werden, daß die aberwitzigen Handlungen der Geisteskranken jedesmal im innigen psychologischen Zusammenhange mit ihrer gesamten Denkweise und Gesinnung stehen, und daher als nothwendige und praktische Konsequenzen anzusehen sind, daher sie auch nur in Verbindung mit jener gedacht richtig verstanden werden können'.

journals and they all relate to people who hurt themselves or others because of their desire to imitate the Passion of Christ. As to castration, Ideler calls this a frequent form of self-mutilation of enthusiasts,[106] and he mentions Origen and his devotees as much-cited models of such martyrs.[107] As to self-crucifixion, Ideler distinguishes between less and more serious forms of the imitation of Christ, and presents Lovat as a very serious case. He too compares Lovat's self-crucifixion with that of Margarethe Peter in Switzerland,[108] and briefly cites further cases of homicide motivated by religious zeal, as well as arson provoked by divine inspiration.[109] For Ideler, self-crucifixion represents a typical action of enthusiasts among others, which he considered as possible manifestations of religious madness. That Ideler was inspired by the theological debate on enthusiasm is not only revealed by several direct references, but also by the frontispiece of his book. Here, we find the same Biblical verse referring to Matthew 7:16, which Ruggieri had used for the frontispiece of his second Italian edition of the *Storia della crocifissione* in 1814: 'By their fruit you will recognise them [the prophets]'.[110] Apparently, the picture of the false prophets fitted perfectly the idea of the enthusiast who disguises himself as a very pious man but is denounced by others as an insane misbeliever. Because later German psychiatrists frequently engaged with Ideler's *Versuch einer Theorie des religiösen Wahnsinns* when trying to classify different forms of religious madness, Ideler's contribution triggered further readings of Lovat's case in German psychiatric publications in the second half of the nineteenth century.

---

106   Ibid., 192.
107   Ibid., 193.
108   Ibid.
109   Ibid., 200.
110   On Ideler's frontispiece, it says: 'An seinen Früchten sollt ihr den Baum erkennen'.

CHAPTER 5

Professional Readings: Madness

Focusing on how European psychiatrists appropriated Lovat's case in their publications, this chapter is concerned with the construction of the disease category of 'religious madness' through case narratives such as Lovat's. The relationship between madness, understood as a category of human experience, and religion, broadly conceived as a way to understand the world, changed significantly between the seventeenth and the nineteenth centuries in European societies. The traditional religious view of madness, which considered it either as a demonic or divine sign, was gradually replaced by a medical view of madness, which considered it as an illness. While for centuries religion had the 'status as the major element of the conceptual framework of madness', the rise of the psychiatric science made religious mania 'the occasion for an extremely severe form of psychopathology', as a recent contribution to the history of psychiatry puts it.[1]

Several historians of psychiatric science and culture have emphasised the important and ambivalent role of religion in the making of 'modern madness' in nineteenth-century Europe.[2] On the one hand, they have shown how Christian ideas and practices have, at various levels, shaped the formation of the psychiatric profession. Not only was the management of mental asylums in the nineteenth century often shared between physicians and religious nursing orders, a situation which produced rivalries and struggles of competence – as we have seen in the first chapter, the Venetian asylum San Servolo, where Lovat died, was also directed by an Italian Catholic nursing order called

---

1   P. Huneman, 'From a Religious View of Madness to Religious Mania: the Encyclopédie, Pinel, Esquirol', *History of Psychiatry*, vol. 28, no. 2, 2017, 147–165, 148.
2   A. Goldberg, *Sex, Religion and The Making of Modern Madness. The Eberbach Asylum and German Society 1815–1849*, Oxford, Oxford University Press, 1999 and H. Guillemain, *Diriger les consciences, guérir les âmes. Une histoire comparée des pratiques thérapeutiques et religieuses, 1830–1939*, Paris, La Découverte, 2006. On the 'invention' of psychiatry in Germany more in general see D. Kaufmann, *Aufklärung, bürgerliche Selbsterfahrung und die 'Erfindung' der Psychiatrie in Deutschland, 1770–1850*, Göttingen, Vandenhoeck & Ruprecht, 1995 and D. Kaufmann, 'Wahnsinn und Geschlecht. Eine erfahrungsseelenkundliche Fallgeschichte aus der Entstehungszeit der bürgerlichen Gesellschaft in Deutschland', in C. Eifert et al. (eds.), *Was sind Frauen? Was sind Männer? Geschlechterkonstruktionen im historischen Wandel*, Frankfurt, Suhrkamp, 1996, 176–195. On French psychiatry see J. Goldstein, *Console and Classify. The French Psychiatric Profession in the Nineteenth Century*, Chicago, University of Chicago Press, 2001.

fatebenefratelli.[3] Christian ideas and certain religious practices of consolation also served as a model for the development of the so-called *traitement morale*. This was an early psychological treatment of mental diseases propagated by several European asylum reformers in the early nineteenth century, such as the French physician Philippe Pinel, the Italian Vicenzo Chiarugi, and the Quaker tukes in York. In Goldstein's words, '[...] the moral treatment meant the use for the cure of insanity of methods that operated upon the intellect and emotions, as opposed to the traditional methods of bleedings and purging applied directly to the lunatic's body. While it did not entail a total abandonment of the old repertory of physical remedies, it did entail an acknowledgement of their grave insufficiency'.[4] In the framework of the moral treatment, a right exposure to religious belief and practices was considered a therapy against mental disturbances.[5]

But the early specialists of mental diseases did not regard religion only as therapeutic and helpful. In particular in France, the first physicians who specialised in the treatment and classification of mental diseases, the so-called alienists (*aliénistes*), held differing opinions about the impact of religious belief on mental diseases. According to Goldstein, a cautious attitude generally prevailed, and the advocates of a strong position of the clergy in mental asylums and of religion as a therapeutic means were in the minority.[6] The alienists increasingly criticised certain religious habits from a medical perspective as having negative effects on the health condition of people.[7] There was hardly any publication in which they did not discuss the problem of religion as a cause or at least an expression of mental disorder. In order to provide evidence for the strong influence of religion in certain mental disorders, the alienists frequently referred to case narratives when they reported on extreme religious behaviours in their publications.

These case narratives derived either from the alienists' own psychiatric practice, or from the experience of other physicians who had published the cases

---

3   See for this aspect Guillemain, *Médecine et religion au XIXe siècle* and L. Soeur, 'La place de la religion catholique dans les asiles d'aliénés au XIXe siècle', *Revue Historique*, vol. 289, no. 1, 1993, 141–148.

4   Goldstein, *Console and Classify*, 65.

5   Soeur, *La place de la religion catholique*, 144. On the role of religion in the medical discourse concerning melancholy and enthusiasm see J. Andrews, 'Cause or Symptom? Contentions Surrounding Religious Melancholy and Mental Medicine in Late-Georgian Britain', *Studies in the Literary Imagination*, vol. 44, no. 2, 2011, 63–91.

6   See Goldstein, *Console and Classify*, 226.

7   See C. Crignon-De Oliveira, 'La mélancolie entre médecine et religion: d'une pathologie des comportements religieux à une pratique pathologique de la religion', *Gesnerus*, vol. 63, 2006, 46–60.

they had observed, as in Lovat's case. The construction of 'religious madness' as a disease category was, in fact, not only the result of a theoretical discussion, but was closely related to the emerging psychiatric practice. In German mental asylums, for instance, physicians worked with this diagnosis from the early nineteenth century onwards, as historian Karoline Grossenbach has shown. She examines files of patients from a German asylum who were labelled by their physicians as suffering from religious madness (*Religionswahnsinn*).[8] The physicians identified and described various individual religious practices as symptoms of this disease, such as an excessive reading of the Bible and devotional texts, loud preaching in the streets, or reflecting upon religious issues in an introspective manner.[9] Grossenbach claims that if the historian takes into account the perspective of individual patients, such behaviour appears not necessarily as an illness, but rather as an expression of individual religious experiences, religious crises, or subjective ways to understand the world, in her case in rural areas in pre-revolutionary Germany. By diagnosing religious madness, physicians in mental asylums thus tended to pathologise those individual expressions of belief that differed from accepted social norms and values. According to Grossenbach, her findings suggest an advancement of secularisation in terms of a repression of individual religious worldviews.

This chapter does not examine patient files that derive from psychiatric practice but various publications in which nineteenth-century psychiatrists, in particular in France and Germany, classified mental diseases. Although they reproduce numerous case histories reporting about deviant religious behaviour, among them Lovat's, the psychiatrists' focus is not on the individual cases per se but on the broader disease category they are trying to define. So the purpose of this chapter is not to discuss whether the religious behaviours described by psychiatrists were individual expressions of belief or pathological symptoms. Rather, I seek to show how religious madness became a specific mental disease only through the narrative description of and reference to various cases that illustrated and confirmed its specific characteristics. For various reasons, the psychiatrists found Lovat's case especially helpful for this purpose.

---

8 See K. Grossenbach, 'Fromme Quergänger in der Psychiatrie des Vormärz: Religionswahnsinn bei Patienten des großherzoglich-hessischen Hospitals Hofheim', *WerkstattGeschichte*, vol. 33, 2002, 5–21.

9 Ibid., 15. See also E. Saurer, 'Religiöse Praxis und Sinnesverwirrung. Kommentare zur religiösen Melancholiediskussion', in R. van Dülmen (ed.), *Dynamik der Tradition. Studien zur historischen Kulturforschung IV*, Frankfurt, Fischer, 1992, 213–239.

1   Lovat's Case in the Organisation of Proto-Psychiatry in Paris

In July 1811, Cesare Ruggieri personally brought his French edition, the *Histoire du crucifiement*, to Paris. He handed it over to the physician Charles Chrétien Henry Marc, who disseminated it in the *Société médicale d'Émulation*.[10] The context of this Parisian medical society is important because it ensured that the French alienists would intensively debate Lovat's case in their works throughout the nineteenth century. The *Société Médicale d'Émulation* contributed to what Goldstein calls the 'proto-organisation of psychiatry', that is the informal endeavour of a group of Parisian physicians during the first half of the nineteenth century to establish a new medical speciality which focused exclusively on the study of mental diseases.[11] The society was initiated in 1796 by a group of physicians under the guidance of the influential physician Jean-Nicolas Corvisart (1755–1821), and embraced physicians and surgeons from different medical institutions in Paris. In line with the general trend toward specialisation in medicine at the time, many of them were about to specialise in particular fields of medical science.[12] The society's programme as set out in its two journals was to embrace all 'human sciences' (*sciences humaines*), and to cultivate an understanding of the medical sciences in the plural.[13] Accordingly, members were expected to be interested in the 'entirety of human knowledge' (*connoissances humaines*).[14] In 1798, the society included about 60 resident members, among others the physicians Philippe Pinel, Xavier Bichat, Jean-Louis Alibert, Pierre Gean Georges Cabanis and Charles Marc. Among the many correspondent members, there were notable German and Italian

---

10   The following biographic details on Chales Marc are taken from A. Jubinal, *Notice biographique sur le Docteur Charles-Chrétien-Henri Marc,* Paris, Laurent Thoinon et Cie, 1865. For further details see the biographic dossier of the *Bibliothèque de l'académie nationale de médecine*, MS 552, 1424, as well as F. Fouzia, *Charles-Chrétien Henri Marc 1771–1840. Un pionnier de la psychiatrie médico-légale en France*, Université de Caen, 1993, Bibliothèque de l'académie nationale de médecine, MS 76237.

11   Goldstein, *Console and Classify*, 121: 'By the proto-organisation of psychiatry, I mean that purely informal and officially unrecognised organisation that began to take shape in the opening decade of the nineteenth century and sufficed until the founding of the first formal organisation of French psychiatrists, the Société médico-psychologique, in 1852'.

12   On the emergence of medical specialties at the beginning of the nineteenth century in Paris see Ackerknecht, *Medicine at the Paris Hospital*, 163–180.

13   La Société medicale d'Émulation (ed.), *Mémoires de la société medicale d'émulation, séante à l'école de médecine de Paris. Pour l'an Ve de la république*, Paris, Chez Maradan, 1798, 1xf.

14   J.-B.-É. Graperon (ed.), *Bulletin des sciences médicales. Publié au nom de la société médicale d'émulation de Paris,* vol. 1, Paris, Chez Crochard, 1807, 1x.

physicians, such as Georg Friedrich Hildebrandt and Christoph Hufeland, and the Italian physicians Valeriano-Luigi Brera, Vincenzo Malacarne and Antonio Scarpa.[15] Tellingly, the Italian physicians had all been, at various times, teachers or colleagues of Cesare Ruggieri, which suggests that the international medical networks were tight, especially between Paris and Padua.

Like other scientific societies founded in the years after the French Revolution,[16] the *Société médicale d'Émulation* was inspired by the idea that medical science should be revived after it had been 'buried' by the Revolution. In the first issue of the society's first journal, the *Mémoires de la société medicale d'émulation*, Xavier Bichat said that the society's intention was 'to proceed unvariedly on the guideline of experience and observation. Hippocrates is still our eternal model, like he was for our erudite masters'.[17] The objectives of the *Société medicale d'Émulation* also related to the project of unifying surgery and medicine, as was the case in the Venetian society described in the second chapter.[18] As Toby Gelfand has shown, the medical elite in Paris had been concerned with this project since the second half of the eighteenth century. Institutionally, the union of surgery and medicine in medical education was achieved by the foundation of the *École de Santé de Paris* in 1794.[19] According to Gelfand, the 'assimilation of the surgical elite as a medical specialty' played a major part in turning Paris medicine into a modern professional corpus.[20]

Ruggieri was interested in joining this particular circle by presenting a piece of work. Tellingly, he did not only present the *Histoire du crucifiement* to the Society, but also another case history of his, the *Storia di una blennorea* (1809).[21]

---

15   See the two lists of members included in La Société medicale d'Émulation, *Mémoires de la société medicale d'émulation, séante à l'école de médecine de Paris. Pour l'an Ve de la république*, XIII–XX, and La Société medicale d'Émulation (ed.), *Mémoires de la société médicale d'émulation, séante à l'école de médecine de Paris. Pour l'année 1816*, Paris, Chez Crochard, Gabon, 1817, V–XXIII.

16   For a summary of the main changes and the term 'Paris School' see D.B. Weiner and M.J. Sauter, 'The City of Paris and the Rise of Clinical Medicine', *Osiris, 2nd Series*, vol. 18, 2003, 23–42.

17   La Société medicale d'Émulation, *Mémoires de la société medicale d'émulation, séante à l'école de médecine de Paris. Pour l'an Ve de la république*, II and X.

18   Ibid., 1.

19   From 1800 onwards called *Société de l'École de Médecine*, up to 1821.

20   Gelfand, *Professionalizing Modern Medicine*, 191.

21   Ruggieri, *Storia di una blennorrea*. A short summary of this case appeared in the September issue of the *Bulletin* in 1811: Anonymous, 'Histoire d'une blennorrhée accompagnée d'ulcères, produite par le LÉCHEMENT d'un chien (traduit de l'italien)', in M. Alard and C.C.H. Marc (eds.), *Bulletin des sciences médicales. Publié au nom de la société médicale d'émulation de Paris, séant à l'école de médecine, et rédigé par M. Alard, secrétaire général, et par M. Marc, adjoint à la rédaction*, vol. 8, Paris, Chez Crochard, 1811, 174–179.

Very likely, Ruggieri's submission of these two case histories essentially constituted his application for membership.[22] By 1814 he had definitely become a corresponding member, as was announced in the title of the second Italian edition dating from that year.[23] Applicants for external membership were expected to regularly correspond with the society and to deliver work in the form of *observations* or *mémoires*.[24] Like the works of the resident members, these contributions were discussed in the Society's meetings which took place twice a month.[25] The contributions arrived via correspondence either in the form of manuscripts or prints; they were carefully registered and conserved by the Society's archivist, and eventually prepared for publication in the Society's journal, the *Mémoires de la société medicale d'émulation*.[26] However, members repeatedly complained that, once discussed during the meetings of the Society, many texts disappeared into the archive without being published – a concern that Ruggieri also had with respect to the Venetian society. This is why in 1807, the Society launched a second journal that was to appear twice a year, entitled *Bulletin des sciences médicales*.[27] It published the contributions of corresponding members (*Les mémoires, les notices, les observations*) either complete or in part. Because of the importance that the editors attributed to them, they were commented and furnished with 'analogical cases' (*faits*) in order to provide new insights or 'more certain methods'.[28]

It is in this *Bulletin des sciences médicales* that Lovat's case appeared, soon after Charles Marc had presented Ruggieri's *Histoire du crucifiement* in July 1811 to the Society.[29] The minutes of this particular session are not preserved,[30] but

---

22   The archive conserves a register in which the members had to sign each session they attended. It does not seem that guests had to sign, there is therefore no evidence of Ruggieri's participation in one of the sessions of July 1811, see BIU, Registres diverses provenant de la société médicale d'émulation. Registre de présence aux séances (1797–1868), MS 2193.

23   Ruggieri, *Storia della crocifissione*.

24   La Société Médicale d'Émulation, 'Règlement de la société médicale d'émulation de Paris', in J.-B.-É. Graperon (ed.), *Bulletin des sciences médicales. Publié au nom de la société médicale d'émulation de Paris, séant à l'école de médecine*, vol. 1, Paris, Chez Crochard, 1807, 8f.

25   See ibid., 14f.

26   See ibid., 12f.

27   Graperon, *Bulletin des sciences médicales*.

28   See ibid., VIII.

29   Alard and Marc, *Bulletin des sciences médicales*. The contribution is on 5–17 and belongs to the section entitled No. XLVI, Juillet 1811.

30   Société Médicale d'Émulation, Registres divers provenant de la société médicale d'émulation. Tome Ier. Procès-verbaux du 7 février 1810 au 19 octobre 1831, MS 2191. This register includes only a few minutes regarding the year 1810, and then proceeds with september 1811. The collection of the correspondance discussed during the sessions starts

the printed version of Marc's oral contribution indicates how the Society discussed Lovat's case. In the *Bulletin*, the narrative is presented under the category of 'medicine'[31] and is entitled 'Religious melancholy. Report made for the Société médicale d'émulation, by the doctor Mr. Marc, in a booklet which is entitled: HISTOIRE DU CRUCIFIEMENT...'.[32]

Marc first addresses his colleagues and explains the circumstances of how he came to know Lovat's case:

> about two years ago, I told you that a Venetian had crucified himself in a mood of melancholy. I had found this fact mentioned in a German medical journal, and I regretted that I was not able to give you further details. The doctor Mr. Ruggieri, who is in Paris at the moment, has handed on to you a copy of this very rare text, in which he exposes the circumstances of this incident, and I hurry to give you an account.[33]

In what follows, Marc's report is a precise summary of Ruggieri's *Histoire du crucifiement*. He remains true to its original structure and details, but replaces the first-person narrator with the third person, such as 'Mr. Ruggieri presumes that...', 'Mr. Ruggieri has continuously observed that...', or 'this is at least what Ruggieri presumes...'.[34] In contrast to many of the later appropriations of

---

in 1811, but does not contain any file regarding Ruggieri's case history, see BIU, Société médicale d'Émulation, Procès-verbeaux des séances de la société, Carton 1: 1811–1831 and 1837, MS 2194.

31   The different categories of the *Bulletin* are: Anatomy and physiology; medicine and surgery; pharmacy, physics, chemistry and natural history; legal medicine and varieties.

32   C.C.H. Marc, 'Mélancolie religieuse. Rapport fait à la société médicale d'émulation, par M. le docteur MARC, sur une brochure ayant pour titre: Histoire du crucifiement exécuté par sa propre personne, par Mathieu Lovat; communiquée au public, dans une lettre de César RUGGIERI, docteur en médecine et professur de clinique chirurgicale à Venise, écrite à un médecin de ses amis', in M. Alard and C.C.H. Marc (eds.), *Bulletin des sciences médicales publié au nom de la société médicale d'émulation de Paris, séant à l'école de médecine, et rédigé par M. Alard, secrétaire général, et par M. Marc, adjoint à la rédaction*, vol. 8, Paris, Chez Crochard, 1811, 5–17. The contribution belongs to the section entitled No. XLVI, Juillet 1811.

33   Ibid., 5f.: 'Messieurs, Je vous fis part, il y a environ deux ans, qu'un Vénitien s'était crucifié dans un acccès de mélancolie. J'avais trouvé ce fait simplement mentionné dans un journal de médecine allemand, et je regrettai de ne pouvoir vous en donner les détails. M. le docteur Ruggieri, présentement à Paris, vous ayant remis un exemplaire de l'écrit extremêment rare, dans lequel il expose les circonstances de cet événement, je m'empresse de vous en rendre compte'.

34   Ibid., 6, 14, and 17.

Lovat's case, Ruggieri's authority as an author thus remains present through-out Marc's account. Because Marc also repeats the direct citation of Lovat's own words, Lovat's voice is also conveyed.[35] Remarkably, Marc calls Lovat a 'modern Origen', so we can presume that it was his report that incited Ruggieri to include this notion when he added a reference to Origen in his 1814 Italian edition.[36] The illustrations were mentioned but not reprinted in the *Bulletin*, which explains why they never reappeared in French publications.[37]

In the final part of his account, Marc critically reviews Ruggieri's medical explanations. He repeats Ruggieri's diagnosis that Lovat suffered from pellagra without any further comment, which suggests that this diagnosis did not mean anything to him, or that he even sought to de-contextualise the narrative from its original Italian context to make it more adaptable to the contemporary debates of the French alienists. As to Ruggieri's hypothesis that the insensibil-ity of insane persons can be explained by the lack of neural fluid, he calls this 'too hypothetical to be commented on'. But he agrees with Ruggieri on the point, made by the physiologist Erasmus Darwin, that martyrs of all religions experience tortures with inexplicable pertinacity because 'their sensitive fac-ulty is absorbed by the contemplation of heavenly goods'.[38] He therefore com-pares Lovat's self-crucifixion with other practices of self-harm motivated by religion:

> it is enough to take a look at the immense history of errors of the human
> mind. There, you will see Indians, pushed by religious delirium, who hang
> themselves on hooks that go through their chairs; the Mussulmen who
> slit themselves with stabs of a knife; you will see the captive Iroquois, ab-
> sorbed by the idea of glory, supporting harms that are a thousand times
> stronger than the ones of crucifixion, with an insensitivity which cannot
> be entirely pretended. I thought I had to adjunct these little reflections to

---

35   See ibid., 12.
36   Ibid., 7: 'Mathieu Lovat ne tarda pas d'acquérir une sorte de célébrité dans son village;
      mais elle eut des suites funestes: les plaisanteries amères dont tout le monde accabloit
      l'Origène moderne lui devinrent insupportables [...]'.
37   Ibid., 16.
38   Ibid.: 'Cette dernière opinion, quoiqu'adoptée par un grand nombre de physiologistes,
      me semble trop hypothétique pour qu'on doive s'y arreter; il n'en est pas de même par la
      première, qui est aussi, comme l'observe M. Ruggieri, celle de Darwin. Cet illustre physi-
      ologiste en dérive la fermeté inexplicable avec laquelle ce grand nombre de martyrs de
      toutes les religions, et dont la faculté sensitive s'absorboit dans la contemplation des
      biens célestes, a pu vaincre les tortures et les supplices'.

Mr. Ruggieri's contribution, a piece of work that everybody will read with the greatest interest.[39]

Referring in this way to the broader history of religious fanaticism, Marc concludes that Lovat's behaviour is 'indeed unique in its details, but definitely not as far as its genre is concerned'.[40] For Marc, Lovat's individual case represents the broader category of 'religious melancholy' in connection with a 'religious delirium': he subsumes Ruggieri's original diagnostic suggestions (*pellagra, delirium melancholicum* and *mania cum studio*) under the terms *mélancolie religieuse* and *délire religieux*, thereby highlighting the pathological character of excessive religion.

The new form in which the narrative appeared denied the case its uniqueness in several ways. Firstly, in the framework of the *Bulletin,* Ruggieri's booklet was turned from a monograph into a journal article, the form it had when it was first published in Amoretti's miscellanea. This meant that the case appeared among many other *observations, mémoires* and pieces of work delivered regularly by the members of the society. As such, the narrative no longer stood by itself but represented a broader disease category. Secondly, as the *Bulletin* propagated the collective work of a medical society rather than promoting the scientific reputation of individual physicians, Ruggieri's authority as the author was clearly reduced. Instead, another physician used Lovat's case to display his scientific skills. By reporting on Lovat's case, Charles Marc advertised himself as someone eager to gather and to communicate noteworthy cases to the *Société Médicale d'Émulation* as well as to the broader medical community.[41]

Marc was interested in Lovat's case first and foremost because of his specialisation in legal medicine and psychiatry. He had studied medicine and law

39   Ibid., 17: 'Pour s'en convaincre, il suffit de jeter un léger coup-d'oeil sur l'histoire immense des travers de l'esprit humain, [sic!] On y verra les Indiens, poussés par un délire religieux, se suspendre à des crocs qui pénètrent dans leurs chairs; des Musulmans se déchirer eux-mêmes à coups de couteau; on y verra l'Iroquois captif, absorbé par la seule idée de la gloire, endurer avec une insensibilité qui ne peut être entièrement feinte, des douleurs mille fois plus atroces que celles du crucifiement. J'ai cru devoir ajouter ce peu de réflexion au travail de M. Ruggieri, que personne ne lira sans le plus grand intérêt'.

40   Ibid.: 'Ces divers considérations diminueront sans doute, chez le médecin, l'étonnement qu'inspire, au premier abord, l'action de Matthieu Lovat; mais si elle est unique par ses détails, elle ne l'est certainement pas par son genre'.

41   His colleagues occasionally complemented Marc on his translations and publications that he arranged for the society, see J.-B.-É. Graperon (ed.), *Bulletin des sciences médicales. Publié au nom de la société médicale d'émulation de Paris, séant à l'école de médecine,* vol. 2, Paris, Chez Crochard, 1808, 367f.

in Erlangen, Germany, and became an active participant in the medical reform discussions taking place in Paris in the years after the French Revolution.[42] He assumed several important posts as a physician in Paris,[43] and over time, established close contacts with the circle of the Parisian *aliénistes*. Marc's publications mirror how his professional interests gradually moved from physical towards mental diseases and their juridical consequences (*médecine légale*).[44] Consequently, he became involved in several important criminal cases. In 1835, for instance, Marc was a medical consultant in the case of Paul Rivière, the famous family murderer whose case Michel Foucault was to edit in 1973.[45] Marc's last book, entitled *De la folie considérée dans ses rapports avec les questions medico-judiciaires* and published shortly before his death in 1840, demonstrates his specialisation in legal medicine and mental diseases.[46]

Another reason why Marc presented Lovat's case to the Parisian society is that he spoke up for the exchange of knowledge between savants of all countries.[47] The fact that he was familiar with two scientific cultures, the German and the French, turned him into a scientific mediator in the circle of the *Société médicale d'Émulation*. As the minutes of the Society's meetings suggest,

---

42   See Jubinal, *Notice biographique sur le Docteur Charles-Chrétien-Henri Marc*. For further details see the biographic dossier of the *Bibliothèque de l'académie nationale de médecine*, MS 552 (1424) as well as Fouzia, *Charles-Chrétien Henri Marc 1771–1840*.

43   In 1816, Marc became a member of the sanitary council (*conseil supérieur de santé* and *conseil de salubrité*), and in 1821, a member of the *Académie de médecine*. Private physician of the Orléans family since 1815, Marc was appointed personal physician (*premier médecin*) of king Louis Philippe (1830–1848) when he ascended the throne after the July Revolution in 1830, see Fouzia, *Charles-Chrétien Henri Marc*.

44   For a detailed bibliography see Jubinal, *Notice biographique sur le Docteur Charles-Chrétien-Henri Marc*, 20–22. From 1812 onwards, Marc formed part of the editorial staff of the newly founded *Dictionnaire des sciences médicales. Par une société de médecins et de chirurgiens*, working in particular for the sections on public sanitary and legal medicine (*Hygiène publique* and *médecine légale*). Together with Étienne Esquirol, he later initiated the first journal of juridical medicine, called *Annales d'hygiène publique et de médecine légale*, see Goldstein, *Console and Classify*, 175.

45   Foucault, *Moi, Pierre Rivière*. Together with other famous forensic doctors, Marc had published a medical certificate on Rivière's mental condition in the *Annales d'hygiène publique et de médecine légale* in 1836, see C.C.H. Marc, 'Consultation délibérée à Paris sur l'état mentale du Pièrre Rivière', *Annales d'hygiène publique et de médecine légale*, vol. 15, no. 1, 1836, 202–205: The text dates from the 25. December 1835 and is signed by Esquirol, Marc, Orfila, Pariest, Rostan, Mitivié and Leuret.

46   Marc, *De la folie considérée dans ses rapports avec les questions medico-judiciaires*, vol. 1, 347–361.

47   He expressed this idea explicitly much later in his introduction to the journal, C.C.H. Marc, 'Introduction', *Annales d'hygiène publique et de médecine légale*, vol. 1, no. 1, 1829, XXXVIII–XXXIX.

Marc was not only a very active participant of the discussions.[48] Because he was also able to read several languages, he reported regularly about foreign medical publications, and translated them or had them translated.[49] This agency of Marc as a mediator of scientific cultures explains his promotion of Lovat's case, which was decisive for its further circulation among the French psychiatrists.

More generally, the fact that the distribution of Lovat's case in France happened via a medical society points to the importance of case histories within scientific societies in Europe at the time. As Philip Rieder has argued, many of them promoted a 'practical medicine' based on empirical cases.[50] However, the example of the *Société médicale d'Émulation* also shows that different views on the status and the use of case histories in medicine co-existed. On the one hand, there were physicians who were primarily interested in the classification and description of disease entities and therefore questioned the use of single case histories. Philippe Pinel, for instance, was concerned with introducing reliable methods into medical science. He searched for a 'true descriptive method', which would allow him to generalise findings and to overcome the limitations of individual cases (*les histoires particulières qu'on trouve dans les recueils d'observations*), as they would only deliver 'isolated facts'.[51] Pinel called on 'French medicine' to advance towards clinical observation in hospitals, and towards the identification of species instead of the pure collection of particular facts, to 'finally proceed on the same level with all the other parts of natural history'.[52] Although Pinel intensively referred to case histories

---

48   The archive is conserved in the *Bibliothèque interuniversitaire de Santé* in Paris: BIU, So-
      ciété médicale d'Émulation, Procès-verbaux des séances de la société, Carton 1: 1811–1831
      et 1837, MS 2194. See for instance BIU, Société médicale d'Émulation, Registres divers
      provenant de la société médicale d'émulation. Tome Ier. Procès verbaux du 7 février 1810
      au 19 octobre 1831, MS 2191, 24.

49   Marc's language skills embraced Latin, French, German and Dutch, see Fouzia, *Charles-
      Chrétien Henri Marc*, 7.

50   Rieder, *La médecine pratique*.

51   P. Pinel, 'Mémoire sur la manie périodique ou intermittente par Ph. Pinel, professeur à
      l'école de médecin de Paris', in La Société medicale d'Émulation (ed.), *Mémoires de la
      société médicale d'émulation, séante à l'école de médecine de Paris. Pour l'an Ve de la ré-
      publique*, Paris, Chez Maradan, 1798, 95: 'Les histoires particulières qu'on trouve dans les
      recueils d'observations, ne sont que des faits isolés, où la vraie méthode descriptive est
      également négligée, et les auteurs n'ont eu guère d'autre but que de faire valoir certains
      remèdes, comme si le traitement de toute maladie, sans la connoissance exacte de ses
      symptomes et de sa marche, n'étoit pas aussi dangereux qu'illusoire'.

52   Ibid., 118: 'Le moment peut-être est venue où la médecine française, dégagée des entraves
      que lui donnoient l'esprit de routine, l'ambition de parvenir son association avec des in-
      stitutions religieuses, et sa défaveur dans l'opinion publique, peut désormais affirmer sa

in his principal work *Traité medico-philosophique sur l'aliénation*, he was not interested in individual cases per se, but used them as examples to illustrate broader categories.[53] His main concern was to turn the art of medical observation into a proper system, a task that concerned many other contemporary French physicians.[54]

On the other hand, other members of the *Société médicale d'Émulation* defended the traditional value of collecting and sharing individual and rare cases. The two journals contain numerous individual case histories reporting extraordinary surgical operations, tumours, cancer or venereal diseases. We also find several cases describing hermaphrodites[55] and other 'monstrosities', that is deformed foetuses or deformed living bodies, such as children with two heads.[56] In this regard, the *Société médicale d'Émulation* was in line with earlier scientific societies such as the Royal Society of London.[57] However, while the collection of rare cases had absorbed naturalists and physicians throughout the early modern period, a new relation developed between scientific curiosity

marche, porter une sévérité rigoureuse dans l'observations des faits, les généraliser, et marcher ainsi de front avec toutes les autres parties de l'histoire naturelle'.

53   On Pinel's use of case histories see C. Frey, 'Am Beispiel der Fallgeschichte. Zu Pinels "Traité medico-philosophique sur l'aliénation"', in J. Ruchatz, S. Willer and N. Pethes (eds.), *Das Beispiel. Epistemologie des Exemplarischen*, Berlin, Kadmos Kulturverlag, 2007, 263–278.

54   See for instance A. Courbon-Pérusel, *Essai sur la manière d'observer les maladies. Dissertation présentée et soutenue à l'école de médecine de Paris*, Paris, Migneret, 1803. Much later, in 1819, Pinel co-published the article on 'Observation (histoire des maladies)', in A.J.L. Jourdan et al. (eds.), *Dictionnaire des sciences médicales. Par une société de médecins et de chirurgiens*, vol. 37, Paris, Panckoucke, 1819, 29–35.

55   See for instance La Société medicale d'émulation, *Mémoires de la société medicale d'émulation, séante à l'école de médecine de Paris. Pour l'an Ve de la république*, 243–247: 'Quelques considérations sur l'hermaphrodisme, suivies de l'extrait d'une observation du cit. GIRAUD, sur une conformations des parties sexuelles; par L.M. Moreau'; *Bulletin des sciences médicale*, vol. 8, 49–56: 'RÉFLEXION sur les prétendus hermaphrodites, par M. le docteur LARMET, membre de la société médicale; suivies de l'examen anatomique de la conformation d'une femme qui sembloit tenir aux deux sexes, par M. CYVOC, médecin à Belley'.

56   See for instance Alard and Marc, *Bulletin des sciences médicales*, vol. 8, 249–251: 'DESCRIPTION d'un foetus difforme, communiquée au docteur MUGGETTI, directeur du cabinet pathologique de Bologne, etc., par M. MORESCHINI. EXTRAIT'; A.-E. Tartra (ed.), *Bulletin des sciences médicales. Publié au nom de la société médicale d'émulation de Paris, séant à l'école de médecine, et rédigé par M. Alard, secrétaire général, et par M. Marc, adjoint à la rédaction*, vol. 6, Paris, Chez Crochard, 1810, 6–33: 'Mémoire sur un ENFANT BICEPHALE, dont le squelette, les viscères et les vaisseaux sanguins, conservés par l'injection, existent dans le cabinet anatomique du grand hopital du Saint-Esprit de Rome...'.

57   On this society see P.F. da Costa, *The Singular and the Making of Knowledge at the Royal Society of London in the Eighteenth Century*, Newcastle upon Tyne, Cambridge Scholars Publishing, 2009.

and popular voyeurism at the beginning of the nineteenth century. Particularly in Paris, physicians and their case histories played an important role in a new public enterprise of exposing otherness.[58] A famous example is the so-called *Vénus Hottentotte*, a South African women called Saartjie Baartman who was brought to Paris via London in 1815. Due to her appearance, she was displayed in public gardens to physicians as well as to the public. After her death, her body was dissected, parts of it were conserved and a copy was displayed in the *Musée de l'homme* until 1974. Similarly, the authors of several case histories in the *Bulletin* referred to the current exhibitions of the 'monsters' they described in public places in Paris.[59]

In contrast to the Venetian society and its model the *Société Royale de Paris*, the *Société médicale d'Émulation* did not pursue the collective enterprise of making general observations of environmental factors in relation to disease.[60] Rather than focusing on epidemic diseases, it put weight on the collection of single cases, which reported on medical problems of individual patients. This explains why Ruggieri believed it particularly promising to present his two case histories to this society. His *Histoire du crucifiement*, but equally his *Storia di una blennorea* touched medical problems (mental diseases and venereal diseases respectively) that members frequently discussed at the Society's meetings in that period. Moreover, both cases corresponded to the Society's interest in the reciprocity of the physical and the moral in pathology. Goldstein in fact argues that the *Société Médicale d'Émulation* promoted a new conception of medicine, which consisted in the interplay between the physical and the moral part of men: the society understood medicine as 'anthropology', and '[o]ne result of the new conception of medicine was to make central to the medical enterprise the investigation of what would later be called "psychiatric" subjects [...]'.[61]

Other medical journals also played an important role for the early transmission of Lovat's case in France. After its publication in the *Bulletin*, Marc's report was immediately reproduced in a periodical called *Bibliothèque médicale*, 'a

---

58   See for this and other expositions of humans the catalogue by P. Blanchard et al. (eds.), *Exhibitions: L'invention du sauvage*, Paris, Actes Sud, 2011.

59   See for instance the reference to the exhibition of a 'monstrous child' in the Marais quarter in Paris in 1811, Alard and Marc, *Bulletin des sciences médicales*, vol. 8, 289: 'On montre en ce moment au public, sur le boulevard du Temple, un enfant monstreux, agé d'un an, qui est né à Chevreuse, près Versailles'.

60   On this medical society see Gillispie, *Science and Polity in France*, 194–203. On the making of general observations see Mendelsohn, *The World on a Page*.

61   Goldstein, *Console and Classify*, 49f.

periodical collection of extracts of the best works of medicine and surgery'.[62]
The editors regarded their journal as a 'public deposit' (*dépôt public*) of current
medical knowledge that made it possible to follow the progress of its auxil-
iary sciences, at a time when medical science extended in all its specialisa-
tions.[63] Their aim was to provide extracts of the most valuable and the most
recent works in order to 'stimulate the curiosity of the reader rather than sat-
isfying it'.[64] In addition, the reader finds work by ancient authors because, as
the editors claim, 'science enlightens itself always by means of comparison'.[65]
The editors explicitly address a foreign readership, which would find in the
periodical 'a truthful picture of the current state of French medicine'.[66]

For the editors of the *Bibliothèque médicale*, the *Société médicale d'Émulation*
was the most important medical society of the period. Tellingly, they considered its members the first propagators and the principal supporters of the
'medicine of observation' (*la médecine d'observation*).[67] Reporting regularly on
the Society's journals, they also included a three-page extract of Marc's report
in a volume published in 1811.[68] In it the editors deliberately transgressed a specific rule of the *Bibliothèque médicale* only to give accounts of printed works on
the basis of originals, never on the basis of reports published by other journals.
However, 'the horrible singularity of the case in question as well as the rarity of
the brochure which contains its details, determines us to make an exception'.[69]
By introducing Lovat as 'an extraordinary as well as deplorable example of religious melancholy brought to its highest degree', the editors passed on Marc's

---

62   Société de Médecins (ed.), *Bibliothèque médicale ou recueil périodique d'extraits des meil-
      leurs ouvrages de médecine et de chirurgie. Par une société de médecins*, vol. 1, 1803.

63   Ibid., 3f.

64   Ibid., 4: '[...] c'est exiter la curiosité du lecteur et non la satisfaire'.

65   Ibid., 5: 'La science s'éclaire toujours par des rapprochements; et l'on peut même dire,
      dans ce sens, qu'elle s'enrichit des erreurs comme des vérités'.

66   Ibid.: 'Enfin l'étranger, souvent injuste dépréciateur de ce qu'il ne connoit pas, pourra voir,
      dans un tableau fidèle, l'état de la médecine française, et apprendre à l'estimer à sa juste
      valeur'.

67   Société de Médecins (ed.), *Bibliothèque médicale ou recueil périodique d'extraits des meil-
      leurs ouvrages de médecine et de chirurgie. Par une société de médecins*, vol. 33, 1811, 282.

68   Ibid., 378ff.: 'Bulletin des sciences médicales, par la société médicale d'émulation de Paris
      – Cahier de juillet 1811, I. Rapport fait à la société médicale d'émulation; par M. Marc,
      D.M., sur une brochure ayant pour titre: Histoire du crucifiement executé sur sa propre
      personne, par Mathieu Lovat, communiquée au public dans une lettre de César Ruggieri,
      D.M., professeur de clinique chirurgicale à Venise'.

69   Ibid., 378: 'L'horrible singularité du fait dont il s'agit ici, et la rareté de la brochure qui en
      contient les détails, nous déterminent à faire une exception à la règle que nous nous som-
      mes prescrite, de ne jamais rendre compte des ouvrages imprimés, d'après les rapports
      qui en auroient été publiés dans d'autres journaux'.

classification, but they no longer conveyed the diagnosis of pellagra.[70] In the following decades, the *Bibliothèque médicale* became the most important source for French authors referring to Lovat's case. For this reason, they all missed this important original diagnosis.

By including Ruggieri's case histories in their 'public deposit' of current medical knowledge, the editors of the *Bibliothèque médicale* introduced it into the broader contemporary debate on the utility of individual cases – alternatively called in French *observations particulières*, *histoires particuliers* or most often *faits* – for the advancement of the medical sciences. Like the journals of the *Société médicale d'Émulation,* the *Bibliothèque médicale* emphasised empiricism and direct observation: the only doctrine they would adhere to, declare the editors, is 'the severe doctrine of observation'.[71] However, they also problematise the relation between the observation of single cases and the necessity to generalise findings. They are concerned that 'maybe our century focuses too much on the exclusive study on individual cases (*faits*); maybe we have neglected the search for general truths which must be their consequences'. Against the general aversion against systems (*la méthode systématique*), they insist that 'one should not deny the most beautiful prerogative of the thinking being, this is the faculty of generalising facts and ideas'.[72]

In these first appropriations of Lovat's case in the Parisian medical context, the narrative to a great extent maintained its original form. In both, the *Bulletin des sciences médicales* and the *Bibliothèque médicale*, it was still recognisable as the medical case history that had originally been communicated in the form of the *observatio* by a Venetian surgeon. The two periodicals ensured, however, that the transmission of Lovat's case no longer depended on the private distribution of a rare pamphlet: now, it was easily accessible to the whole

---

70   Ibid.: '*Mathieu Lovat*, cordonnier à Venise, offre un exemple aussi extraordinaire que déplorable de mélancolie religieuse portée en plus haut degré', and 380: 'Pendant le traitement, ont eut lieu de faire une observation assez remarquable, c'est que pendant les intervalles lucides que lui laissoit son délire mélancolique, il souffroit cruellement de ses plaies, tandis que, dans les autres moments, il ne paroissoit éprouver aucune douleur'.

71   Ibid., 6: 'Fidèles à la plus rigoureuse impartialité, les rédacteurs déclarent qu'ils sont étrangers à toute espèce d'école et de secte médicales; la sévère doctrine de l'observation est la seule dont ils fassent profession'.

72   Ibid., 46: 'Peut-être que le siècle où nous vivons est trop porté à l'étude exclusive des faits, et peut-être négligeons-nous trop la recherche des vérités générales qui en doivent être les conséquences. [...] Peu s'en faut aujourd'hui que la médecine, réduite à la seule inspection des phénomènes, au seul instinct des observations, ne rejette comme suspecte toute vérité générale; peu s'en faut que pour être mis en rang des grand médecins, la première condition ne soit de renoncer à la plus belle prérogative de l'être pensant, à la faculté de généraliser les faits et les idées'.

French-speaking medical community. If Ruggieri had deliberately chosen the *Société médicale d'Émulation* as the most suitable vehicle for his case history in France, in the following decades, Lovat's case was to become more and more detached from its original context, circulating independently from its origin in a variety of French psychiatric publications.

2   Lovat's Case in the Making of Religious Madness in French Psychiatry

Marc had introduced the narrative of Lovat's self-crucifixion as a case of religious melancholy. As this was one of the most important categories that came to be revised in the creation of psychiatric knowledge,[73] Lovat's case piqued the interest of the *aliénistes*. Together, they formed an important interpretive community for Lovat's case, which was mainly restricted to Paris. However, the narrative also reached physicians based at other places in France via networks and publications. In the process of being passed on, Lovat's case underwent significant transformations as regards both its narrative form and its meanings. By integrating it into specific lines of argument and by putting Lovat's case next to other case narratives, the alienists emphasised different aspects of the narrative. While they all used Lovat's case to sustain the classification of religious madness, they stressed different elements of the case and built 'subcommunities' in their broader interpretive community.[74]

The key themes and the most important disease categories that the French alienists associated with Lovat's case were: voluntary fasting, *lypémanie* (melancholy), *monomanie* (monomania), *folie mystique* (mystical insanity) and *monomanie orgueilleuse* (haughty monomania), all of which are closely connected and sometimes mixed up. Authors gave priority to one or the other aspect and accordingly framed Lovat's case in different ways. However, one important aspect of Lovat's case got lost along the way: Ruggieri's idea that Lovat was a victim of the local disease pellagra. In the physicians' search for a broader pattern and the general knowledge to which Lovat's individual case

---

73   On the concept of melancholy between medicine and religion see Crignon-De Oliveira, *La mélancolie entre médecine et religion.*

74   The use of case histories as an example has been discussed with view to Pinel's study by Frey, *Am Beispiel der Fallgeschichte* and with view to Emil Kraepelin's textbooks by Y. Wübben, 'Ordnen und Erzählen. Emil Kraepelins Beispielgeschichten', *Zeitschrift für Germanistik*, vol. 2, 2009, 381–395.

could be connected, we clearly see the nature of the case that oscillates between the particular and the general, as described by Ankeny.[75]

3   An Example of Voluntary Fasting

One interpretive subcommunity of Lovat's case focused on his voluntary fasting as a specific symptom of mental disorder, picking up some remarks made by Ruggieri in the *Storia della crocifissione*. Here, Ruggieri suggests that Lovat's food abstinence during his stay in the Clinical School and at San Servolo was voluntary and motivated by his individual religious convictions. Firstly, Ruggieri emphasises that already in his youth, Lovat was considered 'quite a pious man, because he talked about nothing but church, sermons, saints, and fasts etc'.[76] Reporting on Lovat's stay in the Clinical School, Ruggieri then relates that Lovat wanted to leave the hospital 'because, having recovered, he said that he did not want to stay and eat his bread without doing anything; one day, he decided to stop eating'.[77] Ruggieri's emphasis on Lovat's voluntary fasting is further enhanced by the before-mentioned report of Lovat's stay in San Servolo included in Ruggieri's text.[78] These observations, written by the physician Portalupi, resemble a hagiographical account of a fasting saint. Portalupi reports that after eight days in the hospital, Lovat 'began to refuse any kind of food and drinks, and to become taciturn'. For seven days, it was impossible to make him drink 'even one swallow of water'. Encouraged by another patient, Lovat then started to eat again for about fifteen days; then he stopped, 'for a perfect food abstinence' for the next eleven days. He then repeated longer and shorter periods of fasting several times, but never for more than twelve days. During these abstinences, Lovat was force-fed with clysters; however, as the author remarks, Lovat's body 'did not appear affected, neither as regards his physical strength nor his outer appearance'.[79]

---

75   Ankeny, *Using Cases to Establish Novel Diagnoses*.

76   Ruggieri, *Storia della crocifissione*, 5: '[...] un Uomo assai pio, perchè non parlava che di Chiesa, di prediche, di Santi, e di digiuno ec'.

77   Ibid., 16: 'Quindi voleva partire assolutamente dello Spedale, che essendo guarito, diceva non voler stare collà a mangiare il pane senza far niente, anzi un giorno s'era prefisso di non voler mangiare'.

78   Ibid., 18–20.

79   Ibid., 18f.: '[...] ne' primi otto giorni mostrossi docile e tranquillo; quindi incomminciò a rifiutare qualunque sorta di cibo e di bevanda, e ad essere taciturno: ad onta di tuti li tentativi sì di persuasione che di violenza, non fu possibile fargli prendere neppure un sorso d'aqua per il corso di sette giorni; in questo intervallo s'ebbe ricorso a' clisteri nutrienti, a' quali non dimostrava avversione. In capo al settimo giorno, per l'importunità di un'

In his 1816 book *Nouvelles recherches sur les maladies de l'esprit* ('New Research on Mental Maladies'), the physician Andrey Matthey was obviously inspired by Ruggieri's remarks on Lovat's voluntary fasting.[80] He included the case in a chapter on 'the actions of the brain in the delirium in general, and in the different species of mental diseases'.[81] As to religious melancholy, Matthey explains that in this condition, the 'brain only receives the impressions produced by the brain itself; it seems that the most common sensations of the inner neural extremities as well as the exterior sensations no longer affect the melancholic'. This is why the affected 'do not feel hunger, or are able to resist to it by force of their own will'.[82] The first example Matthey gives to illustrate these general explanations is the case (*histoire de la maladie*) of a melancholic soldier who refuses to eat. This soldier reads the Bible intensively and dreams of an angel who tells him that he does not need to eat because of a special drink he receives. After the soldier has almost starved himself to death and has been unsuccessfully force-fed in a hospital, he has a vision of the devil and finally dies of starvation.[83] Matthey's second example is Lovat's case. He writes that 'the horrible case (*fait*) of which the professor Cesare Ruggieri has given us the details shows to which degree of rapid courage and insensitivity religious melancholy can lead'.[84] By means of the first example, two aspects of Lovat's case become more significant than the others: Lovat's refusal to eat

---

altro pazzo suo vicino, s'indusse a prendere qualche ristoro; in seguito al quale continuò a mangiare giornalmente per il corso di circa quindici giorni, e quindi incominciò di nuovo a rifiutare ogni cibo, persistendo per il corso di undici giorni in un perfetto digiuno; s'ebbe ricorso di nuovo a' clisteri nutrienti, dei quali non si potè far uso che una volta al giorno. Nel corsi di questi undici giorni non ebbe verun scarico alvino, ed una sol volta separò incirca due libbre di orina; in un si fatto disordine dell'animale economia non apparve alterato il suo fisico si nelle forze, che nell'esterio aspetto. Digiuni cosi severi li replicò più fiate, protratti a lungo or più ed or meno con egual successo, non però oltre li dodici giorni'.

80   A. Matthey, *Nouvelles recherches sur les maladies de l'esprit, précédées de considerations sur les difficultés de l'art de guérir*, Paris and Geneva, Paschoud, 1816.

81   Ibid., 179: 'L'ACTION DU CERVEAU DANS LE DÉLIRE EN GÉNÉRAL, ET DANS LES DIVERSES ESPÈCES D'ALIÉNATION MENTALE'.

82   Ibid., 186f.: 'Revenons au délire partiel. [...] Dans la mélancolie religieuse ou le délire mystique, au contraire, le cerveau ne perçoit plus que les impressions nées dans son sein même; les sentiments les plus habituels des extrémités nerveuses internes, et les sensations extérieures semblent ne plus frapper le mélancolique: il ne sent plus le besoin impérieux de la faim, ou du moins il acquiet le pouvoir d'y résister par la force seule de sa volonté, que l'idée dominante rend souvent invincible'.

83   Ibid., 186–195.

84   Ibid., 195: 'L'horrible fait dont le professeur César Ruggieri nous a transmis les détails, montre jusqu'à quel degré de courage féroce et d'insensibilité peut porter la mélancolie religieuse [...]'.

as well as his eagerness to read Scripture. Matthey thus uses Lovat's case to identify the denial of food consumption and an intensive reading of religious texts as typical features of religious melancholy.

Matthey was based in Geneva, but due to his Paris education, he had close contacts with the Parisian alienists and was a corresponding member of the *Société médicale*. His work was submitted in a competition on the nature of mental diseases (*aliénation mentale*) proposed by the Medical Society of Marseille in 1812.[85] His book aimed at distinguishing different species of mental diseases, revising the established classifications, basing his definitions primarily on published cases. He had found most of them in the *Annals of Insanity* published by William Perfect in 1800, in which more than one hundred 'curious and interesting cases in the different species of lunacy, melancholy, or madness' were collected.[86] While Matthey's case collection addressed a medical readership, he explicitly considered case histories (*histoires particulières*) both a means of deterrence and of moral improvement, and therefore also of use for a broader public.[87]

A similar emphasis on Lovat's voluntary fasting is presented in an 1822 book by the alienist Jean-Pierre Falret, a student of Étienne Esquirol and member of the *Société médicale d'Émulation*.[88] In *De l'hypochondrie et du suicide*, Falret deals with hypochondria and suicide from the perspective of mental diseases.[89]

---

85   Ibid., v–vi. The title of the 'concours ouvert' was: 'Sur la nature et le siège des diverses espèces d'aliénation mentale'. As a result of his contribution, Matthey was accepted as a member of this society. The first part of the publication, on 'the difficulties of the art of healing', was concerned with a different subject and written for another occasion.

86   W. Perfect, *Annals of Insanity, Comprising a Selection of Curious and Interesting Cases in the Different Species of Lunacy, Melancholy, or Madness with the Modes of Practice in the Medical and Moral Treatment, as Adopted in the Cure of Each*, London, Chalmers, 1800.

87   Matthey, *Nouvelles recherches sur les maladies de l'esprit*, IX: 'Au surplus, je pense que la lecture de ces histoires particulières peut être utile sous plus d'un rapport, et au plus grand nombre des lecteurs. On sait qu'à Lacédémone, on cherchoit à préserver les jeunes Spartiates de l'ivrognerie, en mettant sous leurs yeux le dégoutant spectacle des Ilotes abrutis par l'ivresse. C'est ainsi que la folie peut fournir d'utiles lecons de sagesse à quiconque sait rentrer en lui-même, et désire sincèrement régler son esprit et devenir meilleur'.

88   On Falret see Goldstein, *Console and Classify*, 262. Falret was an advocate of a strong influence of religious staff in mental asylums, see his text J.-P. Falret, *De l'utilité de la religion dans le traitement des maladies mentales et dans les asiles d'aliénés. Extrait des annales médico-psychologiques, article intitulé: Visite à l'établissement d'aliénés d'Illenau et conditions générales sur les asiles d'aliénés*, Paris, Bourgogne et Martinet, 1845. Goldstein even speaks of Falret's '"clericizing" of psychiatric treatment', Goldstein, *Console and Classify*, 228.

89   J.-P. Falret, *De l'hypochondrie et du suicide. Considérations sur les causes, le siège et le traitement de ces maladies, sur les moyens d'en arreter les progrès et d'en prévenir le développement*, Paris, Croullebois, 1822.

In the second part of his study, he emphasises the 'necessity of a good collection of observations on insanity' and provides eighty 'particular observations as evidence for the general ideas presented above'.[90] These observations are partly made by him and partly taken from other journals, and they all focus on 'suicidal delirium' (*délire-suicide*).[91] Falret copies the version of Lovat's case from the *Bibliothèque médicale*, but mentions both Marc's report and Ruggieri's original case history. He directs the reader's focus on Lovat's voluntary abstinence as a symptom of mental disorder by means of two narrative tricks: he introduces Lovat's case under the headline 'ascetic melancholy followed by suicide'[92] and presents another case immediately before, entitled 'Voluntary death from abstinence, described by the victim himself'.[93] This much-cited case is about a man who starved himself to death. During his fasting, the man wrote a diary on his sufferings, which was first published by the German physician Hufeland. Tellingly, Charles Marc translated and published the case narrative in the *Bibliothéque médicale* in 1820.[94]

The emphasis on voluntary fasting as articulated in Matthey's and Falret's appropriations of Lovat's case indicates an important tendency in the construction of psychiatric knowledge: an increasing medicalisation of behaviour that, from a Christian perspective, could also be considered as religious practices. Voluntary fasting had always been an important Christian practice of penitence, in particular in medieval female spirituality.[95] As Caroline Walker Bynum has shown, thanks to the 'notion of imitatio Christi as fusion with the suffering physicality of Christ'[96] as well as due to a distinct eucharistic piety, food had a religious significance for believers.[97] As food was predominantly a female concern, in particular women practiced food-abstinence as a means to 'cultivate closeness to God'.[98] Cases of male saints who practiced fasts and ecstatic eucharistic devotion were less common.[99]

---

90   Ibid., 288ff: 'Observations particulières a l'appui des idées générales précédemment exposées [...]'. The 'Essai sur le suicide' begins on 1.
91   Ibid., 289.
92   Ibid., 330–333: 'Observation quatorzième. Mélancolie ascétique suivie de suicide'.
93   Ibid., 316–325.: 'Observations douzième. Mort volontaire par abstinence, décrite par la personne même qui en a été la victime'.
94   Ibid., 316f.
95   C.W. Bynum, *Holy Feast and Holy Fast. The Religious Significance of Food to Medieval Women*, Berkeley, University of California Press, 1987; C.W. Bynum, 'Fast, Feast, and Flesh: The Religious Significance of Food to Medieval Women', *Representations*, vol. 11, 1985, 1–25.
96   Ibid., 207.
97   Bynum, *Holy Feast and Holy Fast*, 73f.
98   Ibid., 298. See the chapter entitled: 'Food as a female concern', 73ff.
99   See the chapter 'Men's Lives and Writings: A Comparison', ibid., 94ff.

In contrast to this religious view, physicians regarded voluntary fasting as a medical problem because it threatened the health of patients. Early modern physicians had traditionally associated voluntary fasting with the humoral concept of melancholy. In the eighteenth century, an increasing interest in the psychological effects of eating and digestion set in, as well as in therapies that focused on diets.[100] As Elizabeth Williams has shown, starting from Philippe Pinel, nineteenth-century alienists elaborated this medical view on voluntary fasting and paid great attention to eating behaviour in their observations of patients suffering from mental disorders. For this reason, they described and collected cases of voluntary fasting.[101] To what extent the alienists were concerned with eating habits depended on whether they believed the origin of mental disorders to be the brain or the stomach, thus it depended on where they positioned themselves in the debate between so-called cerebralists and so-called visceralists.[102] Although Pinel emphasised the moral causes of mental diseases, he fundamentally remained true to the ancient medical view that saw the origin of mental diseases in the 'epigastric region'.[103] Thus, he identified 'neuroses seated in the lower regions of the body',[104] and related distinct eating behaviour to different mental conditions, for instance he saw the resistance to food as a frequent behaviour of melancholics.[105] Pinel's student Esquirol followed this path, emphasising moral rather than physiological causes of mental diseases; nevertheless he associated refusal of food with melancholy and regarded it as especially dangerous. He proposed force-feeding as an inevitable and effective means in such cases.[106] In the long run, focusing increasingly on the brain, the alienists came to consider eating disorders as an effect and not as a cause of mental illnesses.[107] With the rise

---

100   E.A. Williams, 'Neuroses of the Stomach: Eating, Gender, and Psychopathology in French Medicine 1800–1870', *Isis*, vol. 98, no. 1, 2007, 54–79, 54.

101   See for instance Pinel's case history on a fasting Catholic, P. Pinel, *L'aliénation mentale ou la manie. Traité médico-philosophique*, Paris, Chez Richard, Caille et Ravier, 1800, 59–61. For a later approach see E. Desportes, *Du refus de manger chez les aliénés*, Thesis, Faculté de Médecine de Paris, 1864.

102   Until the middle of the nineteenth century, this dichotomic view was supported by Xavier Bichat's 'two lives doctrine', which implied the independence of these two regions, see Williams, *Neuroses of the Stomach*, 56.

103   Ibid., 58f.

104   Ibid., 55.

105   Ibid., 59.

106   Ibid., 62f.

107   On the relation between the stomach and the mind see J. Kennaway and J. Andrews, '"The Grand Organ of Sympathy": "Fashionable" Stomach Complaints and the Mind in Britain, 1700–1850', *Social History of Medicine*, https://academic.oup.com/shm/article-abstract/doi/10.1093/shm/hkx055/4080244/The-Grand-Organ-of-Sympathy-Fashionable-Stomach?redirectedFrom=fulltext, (accessed 6 October 2017).

of neurology in the second half of the nineteenth century, eating disorders were primarily located in the nervous system and considered 'diseases of the will'.[108] So, whereas in earlier centuries voluntary fasting could be considered a religious practice or even an expression of holiness, it became a psychiatric theme in the course of the nineteenth century. This is why for Falret and Matthey, it made sense to present Lovat's case primarily as one of voluntary fasting: as a symptom of mental disorder, Lovat's voluntary fasting confirmed the pathological character of excessive religion.

4   From *lypémanie* to *monomanie*

Another interpretive community discussed Lovat's case as one of *monomanie* (monomania), a new classification of a specific mental disorder proposed by Jean-Étienne Esquirol, the famous student of Pinel. As Goldstein argued, Esquirol played a major role in the education of the second generation of French *aliénistes* in Paris by establishing a circle of disciples.[109] Before becoming employed in 1812 as an ordinary physician at the Salpêtrière hospital for female patients, he had run a private institution (*maison de santé*) for patients suffering from mental diseases. From 1825 up to his death in 1840, Esquirol served as chief physician at the Charenton hospital. While at an institutional level, Esquirol's main aim was to create a therapeutic community of patients and physicians in a family atmosphere, he also revised and elaborated the classificatory system previously established by Pinel, proposing various new disease categories, among them that of *monomanie*.[110]

To introduce his main new classifications of mental diseases, Esquirol published several articles in the influential *Dictionnaire des sciences médicales*:[111]

---

108   Williams, *Neuroses of the Stomach*, 56.
109   On the following see the chapter 'The Politics of Patronage' in Goldstein, *Console and Classify*, 120–151.
110   P. Pinel, *Traité medico-philosophique sur l'aliénation mentale*, Paris, Brosson, 1809.
111   This dictionary, promoted in the subtitle as a project for a 'society of physicians and surgeons', was published by Panckoucke from 1812 onwards. The editors were a group of physicians that have already been introduced as core members of the *Société médicale d'Émulation*: among them Philippe Pinel, Jean-Louis Alibert, and Charles Marc. Their aim was to display the current state of French medicine by assigning well-known physicians and surgeons who had rendered outstanding scientific contributions to medical science, see a review of the project: Anonymous, 'Variétés médicales, dictionnaire des sciences médicales par une société de médecins et de chirurgiens, avis des editeurs', *Bibliothèque médicale ou recueil périodique d'extraits des meilleurs ouvrages de médecine et de chirurgie. Par une société de médecins*, vol. 35, 1812, 129–131. On the publisher Panckoucke see

an 1814 article on *démonomanie*[112] as a variety of religious melancholy, in 1819 one on monomania[113] and another on melancholy.[114] Departing from Pinel's idea of a *manie sans délire*, Esquirol used *monomanie* to refer to all kinds of so-called 'partial deliria'. Such disorders were generally recognisable in terms of an *idée fixe*, 'a single pathological preoccupation in an otherwise sound mind'.[115] Moreover, he replaced the traditional term melancholy with *lypémanie*, thereby detaching it from its traditional connection with humoral theory and from its complex cultural connotations.[116]

Esquirol first examined Lovat's case in an article on suicide in the 1821 *Dictionnaire des sciences médicales*.[117] He presented the case in the version of the *Bibliothéque médicale* as a telling example of suicide caused by *lypémanie*, commenting that 'Marc has introduced us to the following observation, published by the doctor Ruggieri, pharmacist [sic!] in Venice. The observation demonstrates the whole influence of *lypémanie* on the determination to commit suicide'.[118] Esquirol compared Lovat's case with two other cases of suicide induced by partial deliria, in order to sustain his *monomania* concept.

In 1838, Esquirol republished this article on suicide unchanged in his influential book *Des maladies mentales*.[119] In this way, Lovat's case was included in one of the most cited studies in the history of French psychiatry and

---

R. Darnton, *The Business of Enlightenment. A Publishing History of the Encyclopédie, 1775–1800*, Cambridge, MA, Harvard University Press, 1979, 72–80.

112   J.-E. Esquirol, 'Démonomanie', in A.J.L. Jourdan et al. (eds.), *Dictionnaire des sciences médicales. Par une société de médecins et de chirurgiens*, vol. 8, Paris, Panckoucke, 1814, 294–316.

113   J.-E. Esquirol, 'Monomanie', in A.J.L. Jourdan et al. (eds.), *Dictionnaire des sciences médicales. Par une société de médecins et de chirurgiens,* vol. 34, Paris, Panckoucke, 1819, 34–115.

114   J.-E. Esquirol, 'Mélancolie', in A.J.L. Jourdan et al. (eds.), *Dictionnaire des sciences médicales. Par une société de médecins et de chirurgie*ns, vol. 32, Paris, Panckoucke, 1819, 147–183.

115   See Goldstein, *Console and Classify*, 155f.

116   Ibid., 156.

117   J.-E. Esquirol, 'Suicide', in A.J.L. Jourdan et al. (eds.), *Dictionnaire des sciences médicales. Par une société de médecins et de chirurgiens*, vol. 13, Paris, Panckoucke, 1821, 213–283.

118   Ibid., 223f.: 'M. le docteur Marc a fait connaître l'observation suivante, publiée par le docteur Ruggièri [sic!], pharmacien à Venise. Elle prouve toute l'influence de la lypémanie sur la détermination au meurtre de soi-même'.

119   J.-E. Esquirol, *Des maladies mentales considérées sous les rapports médical, hygienique et médico-légal* [...] *Accompagnées de 27 planches gravées*, Paris, Chez J.-B. Baillère, 1838, 268f. For a recent edition see J.-E. Esquirol, *Des maladies mentales (1838)*, vol. 1, ed. Thérèse Lempérière, Toulouse, Privat, 1998. With this book, Esquirol intended to consolidate his lifelong studies in the field of mental diseases without however aiming at all-embracing explanations or systems, see ibid., v.

determined the ways in which future authors framed it. For instance, Charles Marc, who had presented the *Histoire du crucifiement* in the *Bulletin des sciences médicales* in 1811, later applied Esquirol's term *monomanie* to Lovat's case when he reproduced his own first report about it in his last book *De la folie* in 1840.[120] While he kept his original title *mélancolie religieuse*, Marc now introduced Lovat's case as an example of *monomanie religieuse*. Consistent with the emphasis he had put on Lovat's lack of sensitivity to pain in his first report, he included the case in a discussion about the role of sensitivity in mental diseases (*sensibilité percevante*), and used it to illustrate the 'loss of the perceptive sensitivity' in a condition of insanity:

> The concentration of perceiving sensitivity from the exterior to the interior is much more evident with insane people who are exposed to impressions which take intense possession of their imagination. These impressions absorb their imagination – so to speak – in a similar manner as in religious monomania. Matthieu Lovat was affected by this condition, on which I was instructed to make a report to the *Société médicale d'émulation* of Paris. The case on which this report is based, is so extraordinary in its details, and so conclusive in favour of what has just been said, that I think I ought to present it here with the same terms that I have used to make it known.[121]

Marc's second and revised appropriation of Lovat's case demonstrates the great success of Esquirol's monomania concept. In the meantime, the label had been imposed upon all kinds of cases that roughly fitted in the clinical picture of a partial deliria he established. And it likewise reflects the changing contexts for Lovat's case by the 1840s: from a rare medical booklet, it had become a much-cited 'psychiatric' case that functioned as a touchstone in the heated French controversy about *monomanie*.

---

120   Marc, *De la folie considérée dans ses rapports avec les questions medico-judiciaires*, 347–361.
121   Ibid., 347f.: 'La concentration de la sensibilité percevante de l'extérieur vers l'intérieur, est beaucoup plus évidente encore chez les fous en butte à des conceptions qui s'emparent vivement de leur imagination, qui l'absorbent, pour ainsi dire, ainsi que cela se voit surtout dans la monomanie religieuse. Telle était celle dont Matthieu Lovat fut atteint, et sur laquelle je fus chargé de faire un rapport à la Société médicale d'émulation de Paris. Le fait qui a donné lieu à ce rapport, est si extraordinaire par ses détails, et si concluant en faveur de ce qui vient d'être dit, que je crois devoir l'exposer ici avec les mêmes termes, qui m'ont servi à le faire connaître'.

5   An Example of *monomanie*: Partial or Full Insanity?

Monomania was one of the key terms that served the French alienists to sustain a position as a new medical speciality. In particular, it played an important role in their attempt to strengthen their position as a profession in relation to the law.[122] In this 'boundary dispute', jurists as well as physicians criticised the concept of monomania.[123] Critics argued that there was no such thing as 'partial' delirium; instead, they considered the fixation on one single object the result of a general disorder of the intellectual faculties. Both defenders and detractors of *monomanie* used case histories as a means to support their arguments, and Lovat's case became one of the most cited in the debate.

At stake was the question of the relationship between mental diseases and criminal responsibility.[124] The core problem that physicians, jurists and philosophers discussed was: Is someone, who is able to show signs of reason in a condition of insanity, certifiably sane and thus responsible for his actions, or is he *non compos mentis* and thus not accountable in law?[125] To be sure, the juridical concept of mental incapacity was not a novelty to the nineteenth century. Insanity had served as an excuse for murder already in the early modern period.[126] At that time, however, insanity was a legal and a community judgement, and 'medical knowledge was not required to identify the insane'.[127] The development of criminal psychology in the eighteenth and nineteenth centuries, shaped in particular in Germany (*Kriminalpsychologie*), led to a change and brought about a new perspective on the delinquent, focusing on the psychological motives of an individual rather than only on criminal actions.[128] As the new experts of mental diseases, physicians increasingly provided medical views on criminal cases, and thereby gained influence in the courtroom. Consequently, cases of certifiable insanity increased, and the juridical term

---

122   See for this topic Goldstein's chapter on 'Monomania' in *Console and Classify*, 152–196.

123   Ibid., 166.

124   See for instance Martschukat, *Von Seelenkrankheiten und Gewaltverbrechen im frühen 19. Jahrhundert*, 223–247.

125   Ibid., 228, my translation: 'War ein Mensch, der angeblich sogar in der aktiven Phase der Krankheit Zeichen von Verstandesbeherrschung offenbarte, zurechnungsfähig und somit seiner Taten schuldig, oder war er unzurechnungsfähig und stand außerhalb des Zugriffsrechts der peinlichen Gerichtsbarkeit?'

126   Ruggiero, *Excusable Murder*.

127   Ibid., 113.

128   Y. Greve, 'Die Unzurechnungsfähigkeit in der "Criminalpsychologie" des 19. Jahrhunderts', in M. Niehaus and H.W. Schmidt-Hannisa (eds.), *Unzurechnungsfähigkeiten. Diskursivierungen unfreier Bewusstseinszustände seit dem 18. Jahrhundert*, Frankfurt, Peter Lang, 1998, 107–132.

'mental incapacity' was informed by new ideas of disease.[129] Medical case histories played a key role in the debate and were an important instrument in sustaining arguments.[130]

Alongside other mental disorders, physicians considered monomania a condition of certifiable insanity and used it frequently in the insanity defence. After Esquirol had cited Lovat's case in his article on suicide in 1821, the case became established in alienists' publications as an example of religious monomania. Although Lovat's crucifixion attempt had not been a criminal action in the narrow sense, several jurists chose Lovat's case to attack the whole monomania doctrine. For instance, Elias Regnault, a young lawyer in Paris who, in a book of 1828, questioned the competence of physicians in juridical questions concerning mental diseases.[131] His book was a comprehensive critique of the medical classifications of insanity and strongly attacked the monomania concept.[132] Lovat's case served Regnault to deny the existence of partial delirium.

Regnault dedicates a whole chapter to voluntary self-mutilations as a form of partial suicide (*suicide partiel*) associated with certain mental diseases.[133] He criticises physicians for considering such acts of mutilation as proof of insanity and using them in an undifferentiated manner to create a new genre of insanity.[134] For Regnault, the physician's main fault is that they mistake the symptoms of insanity for insanity itself.[135] In this way, he says, they have turned penitents, hermits, monks and other believers into madmen by considering their self-destructive behaviour as proof of an insane mind.[136] For Regnault, there is no insanity in such behaviour because it is voluntary and motivated: 'the one who acts out of religious conviction has of course wrong ideas about what God asks from him, but he is always able to reject this way of life; he still has his free will and reason'.[137] Those who are really insane, by contrast, do not have clear motives and are pushed by a 'mechanical movement against their

---

129   Ibid., 116.
130   M. Niehaus and H.W. Schmidt-Hannisa, 'Einleitung', in M. Niehaus and H. Schmidt-Hannisa (eds.), *Unzurechnungsfähigkeiten. Diskursivierungen unfreier Bewusstseinszustände seit dem 18. Jahrhundert*, Frankfurt, Peter Lang, 1998, 7–13, 9.
131   E. Regnault, *Du degré de compétence des médecins dans les questions judiciaires relatives aux aliénations mentales*, Paris, B. Warée, 1828. Lovat's case is on 135–138.
132   Ibid., VII.
133   Ibid., 123ff.: Chaptre IV: 'De la douleur et des mutilations volontaires'.
134   Ibid., 124.
135   Ibid., 123.
136   Ibid., 124.
137   Ibid., 126: 'Quoi qu'il en soit, celui qui agit ainsi par conviction religieuse, a, sans contredit, des idées fausses sur ce que la Divinité exige de lui; mais il est toujours maître de renoncer á ce genre de vie; il conserve la liberté et la raison'.

will'.[138] Acting out of free will or out of inner necessity are, for the jurist Regnault, the parameters that distinguish sanity from insanity.[139]

To illustrate his argument, Regnault gives two examples. The first is a medical case history that had been published in the *Mémoires* of the *Académie royale de médecine* a few years earlier. A man called Trubert suffered from a hernia (i.e. a large swelling in the nether regions caused by a rupture). He turned introspective and melancholic, and developed an *idée fixe* of getting rid of this hernia with an operation. Before asking medical advice, he twice tried to operate on himself.[140] The example of Trubert serves Regnault to demonstrate how physicians have identified cases of insanity where he himself sees no insanity at all. In Regnault's view, Trubert had a rational motive, which was to be relieved of his pains. Trubert's painful attempts to operate himself were therefore due to ignorance but not due to the absence of reason.[141] Regnault's second example is Lovat's case which he had read about in Falret's book. It explicitly serves him as a comparison to show the difference between 'a real madman [Lovat, M.B.], and a man who reasons badly, that is incompletely [Trubert, M.B.]'.[142] In Regnault's opinion, Lovat's self-mutilations had 'no motive at all', or rather an 'insane motive', while Trubert's self-operations were reasonable and motivated: 'Trubert, if he had only been more educated, would have asked a surgeon to carry out the operation instead of himself; while Lovat, given his educational background, necessarily had to accomplish his horrible idea'.[143]

---

138   Ibid., 125: 'C'est un mouvement machinal qui les entraine malgré eux'.

139   Ibid., 126.

140   The narrative is on 126–134. Such an operation of the hernia was a controversial issue because it meant a (self-)castration. At the end of the eighteenth century, charlatans had been accused of carrying out such operations in series, even in cases in which it was medically not necessary. See the article C.C.H. Marc, 'Castration. Considérée sur le rapport de la médecine légale e de la hygiène publique', in A.J.L. Jourdan et al. (eds.), *Dictionnaire des sciences médicales. Par une société de médecins et de chirurgiens*, vol. 4, Paris, Panckoucke, 1812, 278.

141   Regnault, *Du degré de compétence des médecins*, 131f.: 'Je conçois que les médecins aient voulu expliquer par la manie tout acte dont ils ne pouvaient autrement rendre compte; c'était s'épargner les difficultés de l'analyse; mais dans ce fait, tout est si facile à expliquer, la conduite de Trubert peut si bien se raisonner, que je m'étonne qu'on ait voulu l'attribuer à la folie'.

142   Ibid., 133f.: 'Si l'on veut comparer cette observation avec l'observation suivante, on appréciera sans peine toute la différence qui existe entre un fou et un homme qui raisonne mal, c'est-à-dire incomplétement'.

143   Ibid., 138: 'La comparaison de ces deux faits suffit pour distinguer les actes de la folie de ceux de la raison. Dans un cas, c'est un ignorant qui se mutile, mais pour se guérir; les souffrances qu'il s'impose ont pour but de le élivrer de souffrances plus cruelles: c'est le cas de toutes les opérations chirurgicales. Dans l'autre, c'est un être privé de raison qui se

Regnault thus used Lovat's case for his purpose of deconstructing the mono-mania concept that, in his view, undermined juridical debates in the court-room. In his chapter on monomania, he pointed to the general impossibility of classifying mental diseases: '[...] the naturalists have classified the different bodies of nature. The physicians sought to classify the subtleties of madness, that is, a thing which is as little possible to be classified as the clouds'.[144] Reg-nault's attack provoked harsh protest from physicians, who in their reviews of the book, claimed that he was wrong because he had no clinical experience of mental diseases.[145] As a telling example of the problem in question, reviewers picked up on Lovat's case only. A reviewer in the *Journal universel des sciences médicales*, for instance, took up Lovat's case to affirm the possibility of reason-ing in a condition of insanity:

> in a grammatical sense, he [i.e. Matthieu Lovat, M.B.] definitely did not reason. Nevertheless, howsoever we look at the behaviour of this man, he succeeded and did not fall short of his aim. Which name can we give to this long sequence of actions deriving from the human mind? We can, I believe, call it the reasoning of a madman, or, if you want, *folie raison-nante*, even if the words seem to resist.[146]

The author finally refers to Origen's presumed self-castration in order to dem-onstrate the difficulty of judging Lovat's self-mutilation as an insane action: 'Was Origen insane? [...] We can, *à priori et à posteriori*, exclude for one of the greatest geniuses of Christianity insanity and crime'.[147]

---

coupe les parties génitales sans aucune espèce de motif, qui se met en croix par un motif délirant. Trubert, un peu plus éclairé, se serait probablement adressé à un chirurgien, au lieu de se confier à lui-même, tandis que Lovat, quelle que fut d'ailleurs son éducation antérieure, n'aurait pas pu ne pas exécuter son horrible idée'.

144   Ibid., 19f.: 'Les naturalistes ont classé les différents corps de la nature. Les médecins ont voulu classer les nuances de la folie, c'est-à-dire des choses aussi peu suceptibles d'être classées que les nuages'.

145   See the reviews cited by Goldstein, *Console and Classify*, 185ff.

146   *Journal universel des sciences médicales, quatorzième année*, vol. 63, 1829, 69: 'A coup sur, dans le sens grammatical, il ne raisonnait pas. Néansmoins, de quelque facon qu'on re-garde la conduite de cet homme, il allait à son but, et ne l'a pas manqué. Quelle dénomi-nation donner à cette longue suite d'actions de l'entendement humain? On peut, je crois, l'appeler raisonnement d'un fou, ou, si l'on veut, folie raisonnante, quoique les mots pa-raissent se repousser'.

147   Ibid., 82: 'Origène était-il fou? [...] On peut, à priori et à posteriori, redouter, pour un des plus grands génies de la chrétienté, ou la folie ou le crime'.

So the principal reason why Lovat's case challenged the monomania controversy was that it questioned the idea of a partial disorder that was implied in
the concept of monomania. It was clear to all authors that Lovat somehow had
to be considered insane. However, many hesitated to declare him fully insane
because there seemed to be too much reasoning in his actions. In the French
monomania controversy, therefore, Lovat's case served to negotiate the blurred
boundaries of partial insanity as well as of certifiable and incertifiable insanity.

6   An Example of *folie mystique*

Like the German authors in the debate of enthusiasm, the French alienists
were concerned with the question of how to distinguish between 'sane' and
'insane' religion. Their focus was, however, less on religious orthodoxy than
on the specific kind of madness related to it. Reading case histories of religious fanatics, they tried to identify specific mental disorders and labelled the
protagonists with medical diagnoses. Some authors underlined the proximity
of religious exaltation and certain conditions of insanity. For instance Félix
Voisin, another member of the Esquirol circle,[148] published in 1826 a study on
'the moral and physical causes of mental diseases', in which he dedicated a
whole chapter to the 'influence of fanaticism and superstition'.[149] Voisin's main
concern was to demonstrate the similarity between a religious man (*homme
religieux*) and a man affected by insanity (*homme frappé d'aliénation*). He argues that while religious belief can have very positive effects on human character, a man turns into an 'unhappy frenetic' (*malheureux frénétique*) as soon
as he surpasses a certain degree of religious exaltation.[150] According to Voisin,
such people suffer from 'pious manias' (*manie pieuses*).[151] He claims that they
should therefore not be punished for their actions but rather be excused and
subjected to moral treatment.[152] Voisin cites Lovat's case from the short version
of the *Bibliothèque médicale* to show that 'sometimes, these poor insane people

---

148   Goldstein, *Console and Classify*, 363f. Together with the alienist Falret, Voisin ran a private
       asylum in a Parisian suburb. Like Falret, Voisin was an adherent of Gall's phrenology; not-
       withstanding this clear commitment to physiology, he was also an advocate of the moral
       treatment in which emphasis was put on the spiritual dimension in men, see ibid., 262.

149   F. Voisin, *Des causes morales et physiques des maladies mentales: et de quelques autres af-
       fections nerveuses telles que l'hystérie, la nymphomanie et la satyriasis,* Paris, Chez J.-B-
       Baillière, 1826, 33: 'Institutions religieuses. Influence du fanatisme et de la superstition'.

150   Ibid., 40f.

151   Ibid., 36.

152   Ibid., 63.

direct the furore of their fanaticism toward themselves',[153] and to demonstrate 'the most astonishing conformity'[154] between religious exaltation and insanity. Voisin concludes that both those affected by religious exaltation and those affected by insanity '[...] live under the force of an exclusive feeling; they have an *idée fixe*, and they submit religion to the caprices of imagination and to the disorder of the passions'.[155] He finally refers to the Convulsionists, equating their behaviour with the condition of delirium and calling them *véritable monomanes*.

Voisin was not the only author to associate Lovat's case with the Parisian Convulsionists from the early eighteenth century. With their public display of the convulsions they experienced from religious exaltation, they had provoked a heated debate between political, medical and religious authorities on the supernatural or natural nature of the phenomenon.[156] The reason why the alienists were interested in the Convulsionists was the question why these individuals voluntarily inflicted pain upon their bodies, and how they could bear such great physical pain. The physicians' main concern in this debate was to find natural explanations for a phenomenon that, on the part of believers and a broader public, had been traditionally associated with miraculous healings and stigmatisation. In 1829 Francois-Emmanuel Fodéré (1764–1835), professor of legal medicine in Strasbourg,[157] published an essay on mental disorders 'which have as their main characteristic the insensibility, and which cannot be explained with the simple knowledge about the organism'.[158] Among the subjects which he calls 'truly extraordinary and worth of piety',[159] he discusses the Convulsionists and their alleged lack of sensitivity to pain. He reproduces Lovat's case from the *Bibliothéque médicale* and calls Lovat's self-crucifixion an

---

153   Ibid., 43: 'C'est quelquefois sur eux-mêmes que ces pauvres malades exercent les fureurs de leur fanatisme'.
154   Ibid., 46f. '[...] parce que j'ai cru trouver entre les aliénés qui les ont fournies et certains fanatiques la plus frappante conformité [...]'.
155   Ibid., 62f.: 'Comme les aliénés, d'abord ils vivent sous l'empire d'un sentiment exclusif; ils ont une idée fixe, et ils asservissent la religion aux caprices de l'imagination et aux dérèglements des passions'.
156   On the convulsionist see for instance Goldstein, *Enthusiasm or Imagination*; and Maire, *Les convulsionnaires de Saint-Médard*.
157   Goldstein, *Console and Classify*, 163f.
158   F.-E. Fodéré, *Essai théorique et pratique de pneumatologie humaine, ou recherches sur la nature, les causes et le traitement des flatuosités et des diverses vésanies, telles que l'extase, le somnambulisme, la magi-manie, et autres qui ont pour phénomène principal l'insensibilité, et qui ne peuvent s'expliquer par les simples connaissances de l'organisme*, Strasbourg, Février, 1829. The term vésanie was borrowed from Philippe Pinel and referred to non-organical mental disorders, see Williams, *Neuroses of the Stomach*, 59.
159   Ibid., 123f.: '[...] des sujets vraiments extraordinaires et dignes de pitié [...]'.

'act of mystical insanity (*folie mystique*)'.[160] Fodéré puts Lovat's case in historical perspective when writing:

> one must remark that the end of the eighteenth century and the begin-
> ning of the current one was the period in which there was the greatest in-
> credulity in Italy, and in which the beliefs of the people were suppressed
> (*les croyances contrariées*); this has brought them to the point of fanati-
> cism, a constant effect of contradiction and persecution.[161]

Fodéré thus suggests that religious fanaticism increased in Italy precisely because of a general decline of religious sentiment in that period. He is one of
the few authors who tried to historicise Lovat's self-crucifixion with view to the
original Italian social and religious context.

The alienists' views on the proximity of insanity and religion also influenced scholars who were concerned with the exploration of the human un-
conscious. Consider the example of Alfred Maury, known as the originator of
a science of dreams in the middle of the century, who discussed Lovat's case
in his works.[162] Maury was not a physician and had no clinical experience, but
he was an erudite autodidact interested in mental pathology and a friend of
many of the alienists in Paris.[163] In a long article on 'the ecstatic mystics and
the stigmatics' published in 1855,[164] Maury defines the mystic as someone 'who
searches for divinity by a secret communication with the invisible',[165] and he
clearly looks at mystics from the perspective of pathology.[166] For Maury, 'the
mystic in a state of ecstasy is a *halluciné*', and 'can always be put into the category of monomaniacs'.[167] He explicitly turns against 'unenlightened' people
who mistake the 'illusions of a brain in the state of delirium for serious lessons

---

160   Ibid., 131.
161   Ibid.: 'Or, il faut noter que la fin du dix-huitième siècle et le commencement de celui-ci
      avaient été l'époque où il y avait le plus d'incrédulité en Italie, et où les croyances du
      peuple avaient été le plus contrariées, ce qui les avait portés jusqu'au fanatisme, effet con-
      stant de la contradiction et des persécutions'.
162   On Maury see J. Carroy, 'Observer, raconter ou ressuciter les rêves? "Maury guilotiné"
      en question', *Communication*, vol. 84, 2009, 137–149 and J. Carroy, 'L'étude de cas psy-
      chologique et psychanalytique (xɪxe siècle-début du xxe siècle)', in J.-C. Passeron and J.
      Revel (eds.), *Penser par cas*, Paris, ЕНЕSS, 2005, 201–228.
163   Carroy, *Observer, raconter ou ressuciter les rêves*, 138.
164   A. Maury, *Les mystiques extatiques et les stigmatisés*, Paris, Martinet, 1845–1855.
165   Ibid., 1: 'Le mystique cherche la divinité par un commerce secret avec l'invisible'.
166   Ibid.
167   Ibid., 2: 'Le mystique extatique est un halluciné. [...] Non pas qu'il soit proprement aliéné,
      qu'il puisse même être toujours rangé dans la catégorie des monomanes [...]'.

of religion [...]'.[168] He argues that stigmatics represent 'the highest degree of Christian ecstasy',[169] and sees the phenomenon of receiving stigmata and crucifixion attempts in close relation, as acts of penitence.[170] Maury attributes such phenomena to Italy and Spain, where mysticism is most distinctive and gives a series of historical examples for the self-infliction of the pain of crucifixion.[171] His examples are mainly hagiographical reports about Italian nuns who, as a result of their identification with Christ, experienced Christ's passion. Voluntarily or involuntarily, some of them thereby allegedly imitated the posture of the Crucified with their bodies.[172] Maury also reproduces medical cases on similar phenomena, among them Lovat's. Altogether, he calls his examples 'cases of *catalepsie extatique* in which the sick, under the power of a religious preoccupation, display the posture of Christ on the cross'.[173] Like Fodéré, Maury puts Lovat's self-crucifixion, which he calls *un accès de frénésie religieuse*, into historical perspective when stating that 'the times had changed; the poor ecstatic was considered a madman'.[174] Implicitly, he thus suggests that some process of secularisation had taken place by Lovat's time in Italy, which made that such phenomena were coming to be considered from a medical viewpoint rather than from a religious one.

The striking parallels between legends of saints and medical case histories in Maury's article illuminate again the increasing medicalisation of religious behaviour in psychiatric discourse. If in Maury's text Lovat's case is equated with hagiographical cases, this is not because Maury considers Lovat's behaviour a mystical expression of belief. Rather, his study argues that saints and mystics themselves were insane monomaniacs.

7   An Example of *monomanie orgueilleuse*

A smaller interpretive subcommunity of Lovat's case read it as an expression of a *monomanie orgueilleuse* (haughty monomania). Behind this category stood

---

168   Ibid., 3: '[...] confondant ainsi les chiméres d'un cerveau en délire avec les graves enseignements de la religion [...]'.

169   Ibid.: 'Je m'attacherai surtout aux stigmatisés, à la stigmatisation qui est certainement le plus haut degré de l'extase chrétienne'.

170   Ibid., 18.

171   Ibid., 18f.

172   Ibid., 18–20.

173   Ibid., 20: 'Les médecins on noté plusieurs cas de catalepsie extatique dans lesquels les malades, sous l'empire d'une préoccupation religieuse, affectaient la pose du Christ en croix'.

174   Ibid., 20f.: 'Mais les temps avaient changé; le pauvre extatique fut reconnu pour un fou. On le guérit de ses blessures; toutefois il finit par mourir d'étisie'.

the idea that the religious and political Zeitgeist played a crucial role in the development of certain mental disorders, or at least the ways in which these mental disorders were expressed, a common idea among French alienists from the middle of the nineteenth century onwards.[175] In 1845, Gerard Marchant, a student of Esquirol at the Charenton and later alienist in Toulouse, published his 'research on the insane'.[176] In this collection of articles, he is concerned with promoting the study of the insane (*la science des aliénés*) as a necessary endeavour for understanding mankind.[177] Like Voisin, Marchant tries to investigate the 'fluent boundaries' between reason and insanity, and argues that one must only enhance the 'tableau of the passions' in order to see them convert into insanity.[178] In his chapter on 'hallucinations, illusions and wrong ideas (*idées fausses*)' produced by the passions, Marchant claims that 'the form of delirium borrows a lot from the dominant ideas of the age'.[179] He observes that contemporary asylums are '[...] full of kings, emperors, princes and all kinds of dignitaries [...] We do not exaggerate if we say that, from those insane that we met, the number of those who called themselves Napoleon reaches fifty'.[180] In addition, Marchant remarks, 'Gods, prophets and saints are not uncommon among the insane'.[181]

To illustrate these general observations, Marchant reports at length on a 'highly interesting lunatic' which serves as a comparison for Lovat's case. In 1841, a farmer called Paulin from the south of France came to Paris where he was admitted to a mental asylum because of his 'insane actions'. Paulin had left his family with the purpose to fight against Parisian irreligion. According to Marchant, he believed himself to be chosen for this project because of a white

---

175   On this phenomenon see L. Murat, *L'homme qui se prenait pour Napoléon: Pour une his-toire politique de la folie*, Paris, Gallimard, 2011.

176   Goldstein, *Console and Classify*, 146.

177   G. Marchant, *Recherches sur les aliénés*, Toulouse, Bonnal et Gobrac, 1845, VIIf.

178   Ibid., 69ff.: 'Analogies et différences entre la raison et la folie'; ibid., 77: 'La 1re [vérité, M.B.], c'est que les limites entre la raison et la folie sont flottants, et par conséquent d'une ap-préciation souvent difficile. [...] La seconde, c'est qu'il suffit de grossir les traits, d'aviver les couleurs et d'éxagérer les ombres du tableau des passions, pour le convertir en celui de la folie'.

179   Ibid., 47: 'Et comme la forme du délire emprunte beaucoup aux idées dominantes de l'époque [...]'.

180   Ibid.: 'Les maisons de fous sont peuplées de rois, d'empereurs, de princes et de dignitaires de tout genre. On y rencontre, à chaque pas, le superbe dédain des hommes, le ton de mépris de la suffisance et les protections hautaines de la médiocrité ignorante. [...] Nous n'exagérons pas en portant à plus de cinquante le nombre d'aliénés que nous avons con-nus se disant Napoléon'.

181   Ibid.: 'Les dieux, les prophétes, les saints ne sont pas rares parmis les fous'.

strand of hair. Like Lovat, Paulin was convinced that he had to die on the cross like Jesus. He called himself a saint and distributed his *mémoires*, in which he explained his motives and depicted himself on a cross.[182] When briefly citing Lovat's case in a later passage, Marchant remarks that 'apparently, Paulin had also made such attempts to commit suicide, in the very same way, before he was admitted to the Bicêtre [hospital]'.[183]

Marchant puts Lovat's and Paulin's case in the broader framework of cases in which individuals believed themselves to be important political or religious figures. In this way, their belief of being the redeemer is put on the same level as the conviction of being Napoleon or another famous person. In this way, the two cases illustrate just one variety of a more general model of disease, a form of a partial delirium described by Pinel and consequently by many other alienist alternately as *monomanie orgueilleuse*, *délire des grandeurs*, or, in the second half of the century, *mégalomanie*.[184] As Laure Murat has shown in her study on the reciprocity between contemporary political events and mental disorders in nineteenth-century Paris, several authors, primarily physicians but also novelists, described the *monomanie orgueilleuse* as *mal du siècle*, that is a malady produced by the age and its political and religious upheavals.[185]

8   (Not) an Example of Pellagra?

While the alienists charged Lovat's case with different meanings, Ruggieri's original diagnosis that Lovat suffered from pellagra got lost very early in their readings of the case. Already in the abridged version of the *Bibliothèque médicale*, the reference to pellagra was eliminated. This ignorance is perplexing since pellagra was not unknown to French physicians. At the beginning of the nineteenth century, pellagra was first identified as a disease specific to the

182 Ibid., 47f.

183 Ibid., 52: 'Il paraitrait que le malade dont nous avons cité l'observation, Paulin, aurait également fait des tentatives de suicide, et par le même moyen, antérieurement à son admission à Bicêtre'.

184 See the titles: A. Foville, *Note sur la mégalomanie ou lypémanie partielle, avec prédominance du délire des grandeurs*, Paris, Imprimerie de l'Étoile, 1888; É. Nicoulou, *Essai sur la mégalomanie*, Bordeaux, Mourau, 1886.

185 Murat, *L'homme qui se prenait pour Napoléon*, 172. On the tendency to 'imitate' Napoleon and how this phenomenon changes during the nineteenth century see M. Pohlig, 'Individuum und Sattelzeit oder: Napoleon und der Triumph des Willens', in C. Jaser, U. Lotz-Heumann, and M. Pohlig (eds.), *Alteuropa – Vormoderne – Neue Zeit. Epochen und Dynamiken der europäischen Geschichte (1200–1800)*, Berlin, Duncker & Humblot, 2012, 265–282, 278ff.

Italian region of Lombardy,[186] but by the middle of the century, the disease had also been observed in French regions and had become an issue for public health policies.[187] French physicians collected and published individual cases of pellagra in order to discuss its characteristic traits,[188] but like in Italy, there was great uncertainty as regards the explanations of causes and possible therapies. In a thesis from the year 1819, the author stated that 'the ideas on pellagra are not at all fixed yet, and we have invented multiple contradicting theories, this is why there is the greatest disorder in everything regarding the therapies of this disease, and the treatment is not based on solid ground'.[189]

Although some of the French alienists mentioned above participated in the French debate on pellagra, none of them associated Lovat's case with it. Esquirol, for instance, referred to the presentation of Lovat's case in the *Bibliothèque médicale*, but could not know about the pellagra hypothesis and consequently neglected it when reporting on Lovat's case.[190] However, in his book *Des maladies mentales* from 1838, Esquirol wrote that 'skin diseases (*les dartres répercutées*) require great attention in the study of madness'.[191] He tells that in the meantime, he had studied the phenomenon of pellagra in Italy, and shows himself familiar with Italian publications on the subject. Following their medical explanations, he briefly describes the different stages of the disease development. Emphasising that one third or even half of those suffering from pellagra commit suicide, he applies his category *lypémanie suicide* to

---

186   As far as I can see, the first French monograph on *pellagra* was published in 1805 by a physician from Caen who was doyen of the faculty of medicine in Paris: T. Levacher de La Feutrie, *Recherches sur la pellagre, affection cutanée endémique dans la Lombardie*, Paris, Crapart, Caille et Ravier, 1805.

187   See for instance L. Marchant, *Étude de la pellagre des landes...rapport au conseil central de salubrité du département de la Gironde*, Bordeaux, impr. de P. Faye, 1840; J.-B.V. Théophile Roussel, *De la pellagre, de son origine, de ses progrès, de son existence en France, de ses causes et de son traitement curatif et préservatif*, Paris, Bureau de l'Encyclopédie médicale, 1845; P.-P. Cazaban, *Recherches et observations sur la pellagre, dans l'arrondissement de Saint-Sever (Landes)*, Paris, Rignoux, 1848.

188   J.-B.V. Théophile Roussel, *Histoire d'un cas de pellagre observé à l'hôpital Saint-Louis, dans le service de M. Gibert*, Paris, impr. de Moquet et Hauquelin, 1842.

189   A.J.L. Jourdan, *Dissertation sur la pellagre, présentée et soutenue à la faculté de médecine de Paris, le 18 décembre 1819, pour obtenir le grade de docteur en médecine*, Paris, Didot Jeune, 1819, 16: 'Comme les idées ne sont point encore fixées sur la pellagre, et qu'on a imaginé plusieurs théories opposées les unes aux autres pour s'en rendre raison, le plus grand désordre règne dans tout ce qui concerne la thérapeutique de cette maladie, et le traitement n'est pas établi sur des bases fixes'.

190   Esquirol, *Des maladies mentales*, 268f.

191   See ibid., 181f.: 'Les affections de la peau meritent une grande attention, dans l'étude de la folie. Souvent les dartres répercutées ont causé cette maladie'.

these cases.[192] The reason why Esquirol did not apply these insights to Lovat's case is probably not only due to his specific source, but to the way in which he compiled his book. The cases he cited derived from different periods and contexts. He did not review them in the light of his novel findings but included them unchanged.[193]

Esquirol's case is typical: French alienists generally recognised that pellagra could cause mental disorders, but only few of them investigated in depth the specific relation between the diseases' physical and mental symptoms. The alienist Alexandre Brière de Boismont, a member of the Esquirol circle and the *Société médicale d'Émulation*, published the first comprehensive study dedicated to the problem of the so-called *folie pellagreuse* in 1834.[194] His study on pellagra includes numerous medical observations that he had collected in Italian hospitals.[195] Brière complains that French physicians tend to ignore foreign scientific findings and therefore have neglected the study of pellagra, a disease that nevertheless would affect thousands of people in France.[196] Generally Brière believes that the most efficient means to curb the spread of pellagra were legal prescriptions regarding sanitation.[197] Brière was an advocate of the physicians' involvement in interdiction procedures at court, and as such a supporter of the concept of monomania.[198] In his book, he therefore considers religious monomania (*monomanie religieuse*) as the most frequent mental disorder to appear with pellagra in Italy. For Brière, this 'is not at all surprising, because religion is the basis of the Italian people's education, which they suck up from their infancy, so to speak'.[199] Curiously, while other authors blamed incredulity and a decrease of piety as a source of religious fanaticism in Italy around 1800, Brière blames the strong influence of religious education. On the

---

192   This passage is in paragraph three, 'Des climats, des saisons, des ages et des sexes considérés comme causes du suicide', ibid., 283ff. The reference to *pellagra* is on 291.

193   See the editorial remarks in Esquirol, *Des maladies mentales (1838)*, III.

194   A. Brièrre de Boismont, *La pellagre et de la folie pellagreuse, observations recueillies au grand hôpital de Milan. Mémoire lu à l'académie des sciences dans sa séance du 30 novembre 1830*, Paris, Baillière, 1834.

195   Ibid., 60.

196   See ibid., V.

197   Ibid., VIII.

198   On Boismont see Goldstein's register in *Console and Classify*, 387. According to Goldstein, Boismont changed his mind in the 1850s when he came to argue in favour of more spiritualist positions and refused the idea of partial deliria, see ibid., 191 and 272.

199   Brièrre de Boismont, *La pellagre et de la folie pellagreuse*, 23f.: 'Obs. 6. Trosième degré, délire religieux. L'espèce d'aliénation mentale qu'on observe le plus fréquemment dans la pellagre, est la monomanie religieuse. Cette variété de la folie n'a rien de surprenant, la religion faisant la base de l'éducation des Italiens, quil la sucent, pour ainsi dire, avec le lait'.

basis of numerous observations entitled *délire religieux*,[200] Brière sketches a
general picture of religious delirium.[201] Among other things,

> the insane has a sombre physiognomy, is depressed, expressing fear and
> desperation; he does not want to talk to anybody, escapes from society,
> seeks for solitude, closes his hands, murmurs prayers, points his eyes
> up to heaven, stares at the ground, accuses himself of his sins, asks for
> priests, wishes to confess, believes himself to be condemned, persecuted
> by divine vengeance, implores heavenly mercy, sings Mass, preaches, or
> believes himself to be a religious man, priest, God, an apostle.[202]

Finally, the affected tend to suicidal monomania (*monomanie-suicide*).[203] Thus,
rather than speculating on the actual causes of pellagra-related mental disorders, Brière describes the religious behaviour of those affected. Many features
of this view of the disease are not only similar to what Ruggieri described for
Lovat, but his description is strikingly similar to the picture Ruggieri sketched
in his lexical article on pellagra. The fact that Brière did not refer to Lovat's
case in his important study on pellagra again confirms that the French alienists
did not associate Lovat's case with this disease, although it would have fitted
perfectly into this debate.

It seems that the only French author who related Lovat's case with pellagra did not belong to the alienists' interpretive community, but was a specialist on skin diseases – Jean-Louis Alibert, at that time chief physician at the
Saint-Louis hospital for patients suffering from skin diseases in Paris, included
Lovat's case in his important *Monographie des dermatoses ou précis théorique et
pratique des maladies de la peau* (1832).[204] Alibert's famous illustrations of skin
diseases show that dermatology was asserting its status as a proper medical

---

200   See the observations on ibid., 23–26.

201   Ibid., 44ff.: Considérations générales.

202   Ibid., 55: 'Le malade a la physionomie sombre, abbatue, exprimant l'angoisse et le dése-
      spoir; il ne veut parler à personne, fuit la société, cherche la solitude, joint les mains, mar-
      motte des prières, lève les yeux au ciel, regarde fixement la terre, s'accuse de ses péchés,
      demande des prêtres, veut se confesser, se croit damné, poursuivi par la vengeance di-
      vine, implore la miséricorde céleste, chante la messe, preche, ou bien il se croit religieux,
      prêtre, dieu, apotre. La monomanie-suicide est très-fréquente à cette époque'.

203   Ibid., 56.

204   J.-L. Alibert, *Monographie des dermatoses ou précis théorique et pratique des maladies de
      la peau*, Paris, Daynac, 1832. Alibert had published several editions of this text before in
      which he also referred briefly to Ruggieri's case history, see J.-L. Alibert, *Précis théorique et
      pratique sur les maladies de la peau*, vol. 2, Paris, Chez Caille et Ravier, 1818, 186.

specialism.[205] As a student of Pinel, Alibert was convinced that physicians, in particular those specialising in skin diseases, should apply the same method as naturalists in order to identify diseases.[206] His intention was therefore to write 'natural history with the diseases of mankind'.[207] In Alibert's classification, pellagra is one of the subspecies of eruptions of the skin (*Dermatoses Eczémateuses*).[208] Alibert describes the external symptoms of the 'pellagra of Lombardy', presuming that they were primarily caused by the effects of sunlight on malnourished bodies.[209] He emphasises that neural afflictions influence physical behaviour, either by producing 'convulsive movements' or 'constant immobility', often leading to chronic delirium, 'the most sombre melancholy' and suicide.[210] Alibert mentions in passing that 'several scientific journals have told the history of a fanatic, called Matteo Lovat... who made fatal attempts to nail one of his hands down to a cross he had constructed, and to subject himself to the martyrdom of Christ'.[211]

The disappearance of pellagra in the alienists' readings of Lovat's case shows that whether a certain diagnosis associated with a case is transmitted or not, does not only depend on whether the disease raises the interest of contemporaries in a given context. It also matters that once an interpretive community is influential enough and has established a certain reading of the case, this interpretation remains relatively stable and unquestioned. Lovat's case helped the French alienists to negotiate, differentiate and shape the boundaries of the disease category of religious madness. The narrative of Lovat's self-crucifixion accompanied their publications all the way from what Goldstein has described as the 'proto-organisation of psychiatry'[212] in the early nineteenth century up to its formal organisation as a professional group, the foundation of the *Société*

---

205   For this aspect see L.S. Jacyna, 'Pious Pathology. J.L. Alibert's Iconography of Disease', in C. Hannaway and A. La Berge (eds.), *Constructing Paris Medicine,* Amsterdam and Atlanta, Rodopi, 1998, 185–219.

206   Alibert, *Monographie des dermatoses*, XXXIX.

207   Ibid., XV: 'La marche que nous allons suivre sera simple; c'est ici de l'histoire naturelle faite avec les maux de l'humanité'.

208   Ibid., 3ff. The particular subspecies is called erythema endemicum (*érythème endémique*).

209   Ibid., 8.

210   Ibid., 15.

211   Ibid.: 'On a consigné dans quelques journaux scientifiques l'histoire d'un fanatique, nommé Matteo Lovat, né dans les montagnes de l'état de Venise, qui fit de funestes tentatives pour clouer l'une de ses mains à une croix qu'il avait fabriquée, et se donner le supplice du Christ'.

212   Goldstein, *Console and Classify*, 121.

médico-psychologique in 1852.[213] In this process, the case was subjected to multiple transformations in its form and content. Depending on the respective interests of the individual authors and the interpretive community they wished
to belong to, certain elements of the narrative were stressed while others were
neglected or eliminated. The more frequently the case was cited, the shorter
the narrative became. In the long run, the alienists reduced the case to a short
example, which, together with numerous other case histories, served to illustrate different aspects of religious madness.

In the second half of the century, Lovat's case continued to be an important
reference for French alienists. The first institutionalisation of their community had been prepared by an important editorial project, the *Annales médico-
psychologiques*, founded in 1843 by the alienists Jules Baillarger, Laurent Cerise
and F.A. Longet in the intellectual legacy of Pinel and Cabanis.[214] This journal
became the platform for various debates about the treatment and the classification of mental diseases that concerned the alienists in the second half of the
nineteenth century, such as, for instance, the debate on hallucinations, but also
that on pellagra or on force feeding.[215] Most of the authors discussed in this
chapter formed part of the *Société médico-psychologique* and contributed many
articles to the *Annales médico-psychologiques*. It is hardly surprising, therefore,
that Lovat's case reappeared in several contributions to this journal.[216] Remarkably, however, authors now increasingly used it as a springboard[217] to discuss

---

213   See for this institution S. Nicolas, 'Les annales médico-psychologiques. Abrégé d'histoire
      sur la fondation de la première revue française de psychiatrie', *Université Paris Descartes,
      BIU Santé*, [website], 2006, http://www.biusante.parisdescartes.fr/histoire/medica/
      annalesmedicopsychologiques.php, (accessed 18 April 2012).

214   J. Baillarger, L.A.P. Cerise, and F.A. Longet (eds.), *Annales médico-psychologiques. Journal
      de l'anatomie, de la physiologie, et de la pathologie du système nerveux, destiné particulière-
      ment à recueillir tous les documents relatifs à la science des rapports du physique et du
      moral, à la pathologie mentale, à la médecine légale des aliénés, et à la clinique des névroses*,
      Paris, Victor Masson, 1843. The névroses was a term used by Philippe Pinel, after William
      Cullen, to classify 'lesions of feelings and movement', see Williams, *Neuroses of the Stom-
      ach*, 58.

215   Nicolas, *Les Annales médico-psychologiques*.

216   This is true for Voisin, Falret, Maury, Boismont and Marchant. Some of their texts were
      in fact published in the *Annales*. See for instance A. Maury, 'Les mystiques extatiques
      et les stigmatisés', in J. Baillarger, L.A.P. Cerise, and J.-J. Moreau (eds.), *Annales médico-
      psychologiques. Journal destiné à récueillir tous les documents relatifs à l'aliénation mentale,
      aux névroses, et à la médecine légale des aliénés, par MM. les docteurs Baillarger, Cerise et
      Moreau*, Paris, Victor Masson, 1855, 181–232. The following articles cited from the *Annales
      médico-psychologiques* are accessible online: http://www2.biusante.parisdescartes.fr/liva
      nc/?fille=c&cotemere=90152, (accessed 11 Jan 2013).

217   Ankeny, *Using Cases to Establish Novel Diagnoses*, 258.

more recent observations and findings, in particular those related to sexual self-mutilation.[218] They briefly referred to Lovat's case only to introduce their analysis of cases of self-mutilation, taking for granted that all the members of the newly founded *Société médico-psychologiques* were familiar with the details of the narrative.

The new focus on Lovat's self-castration rather than on the self-crucifixion signals an increasing interest in this topic. In 1908 Lovat's case was even considered in a book that systematically focused 'on self-mutilation' by presenting a collection of famous cases (*inventaire des faits connus*).[219] Outlining a brief history of the phenomenon of self-castration since ancient times, the author reproduces Lovat's case under the double title 'RUGGIERI-Mutilation sexuelle et crucifiement'.[220] He considers self-mutilation a consequence of a *psychose maniaque* with traits of religious delirium.[221] Calling self-castration a 'sexual self-mutilation',[222] the author argues that 'the important role which the genitals play in human life explains why the concerns regarding the organs of reproduction are frequent with the insane, and also why insane ideas, whatever their nature, motivate their mutilation'.[223]

In addition to this shift in focus, a growing awareness of the publicity and celebrity of Lovat's case is clear in the alienists' rewritings of it from the second half of the century. Authors frequently commented on the high profile of the case. In 1853, Bénédicte-Auguste Morel, chief physician in the mental asylum of Maréville near Nancy, included Lovat in a short list of various voluntary self-mutilations carried out by patients affected by religious delirium.[224] He

---

218   For example, see T. Archambault, 'Lypémanie suicide. Tentative de suicide par section de la verge. – Observation communiquée par M. le docteur Archambault, médecin de la maison royale de Charenton', in J. Baillarger, L.A.P. Cerise, and J.-J. Moreau (eds.), *Annales médico-psychologiques. Journal destiné à récueillir tous les documents relatifs à l'aliénation mentale, aux névroses, et à la médecine légale des aliénés, par MM. les docteurs Baillarger, Cerise et Moreau,* Paris, Victor Masson, 1852.

219   M.M.E.J. Lorthiois, *De l'automutilation. Mutilations et suicides étrangères*, Paris, Vigot Frères, 1908.

220   Ibid., 44f. The source is the *Bibliothèque médicale* and Esquirol's book of 1838.

221   Ibid., 98: '[...] bien souvent la psychose maniaque dépressive est en jeu. Tout naturellement, c'est au cours de la phase dépressive de cette psychose que, de même qu'on observe les boufflées délirantes religieuses, se produisent les automutilations'.

222   Ibid., second chapter entitled 'L'automutilation sexuelle' on 16ff.

223   Ibid., 16: 'Le role important joué par la fonction génitale dans la vie humaine explique pourquoi les préoccupations relatives aux organes de la reproduction sont fréquentes chez les malades et pourquoi aussi les idées délirantes, quelle que soit leur nature, motivent leur mutilation'.

224   B.-A. Morel, *Études cliniques. Traité théorique et pratique des maladies mentales considérées dans leur nature, leur traitement, et dans leur rapport avec la médecine légale des aliénés,*

remarks that 'Mathieu Lovat, this shoemaker of Venice, is one of the most striking examples of self-mutilation. It has been cited by professor Ruggieri, and all
the historians of mental diseases (*aliénation*) have repeated it'.[225] We find a
similar comment in a study on insensitivity in mental diseases and the application of electric therapy published in 1859 by Théodore Auzouy, corresponding
member of the *Société médico-psychologiques*.[226] Talking about the 'existence
of analgesia [i.e. insensitivity to pain, M.B.]' in the majority of melancholics,
and in particular in those affected by 'religious lypémanie and suicidal lypémanie', Auzouy remarks that 'everybody knows the history, told by Marc, of the
shoemaker Mathieu Lovat, who began his long martyrdom with the amputation of the genitals, and by throwing them out of the window [...]'.[227] Auzouy's
summary of Lovat's case is reduced to just a few lines, and he does not refer
to any specific source. Apparently, there was no longer a need to mention any
more details. Within the alienists' interpretive community, Lovat's case had become a standard reference that was passed on as common psychiatric knowledge. But exactly for this reason, it was even the more rewarding to cite the
case, as referring to it was a means to signal commitment and belonging to the
professional community.

9   From Empirical to Doctrinal Knowledge: Lovat's Case in
     Psychiatric Textbooks

As a famous psychiatric case, Lovat's case also entered psychiatric textbooks, a
genre which developed in remarkable ways at the end of the nineteenth century.[228] Because of its cognitive goals, the textbook belongs to the epistemic

---

vol. 2, Paris, Victor Masson et Baillière, 1853, see in particular 163: '§VI. Des troubles de
l'intelligence et des sentiments, dans leur rapport avec lexagération ou la perversion du
sentiment religieux (délire religieux, ses variétés)'.

225   Ibid., 164: 'Mathieu Lovat, ce cordonnier de Venise, est un example de multilation des plus
      frappants. Il a été cité par le professeur Ruggieri, et tous les historiens en aliénation l'ont
      répété'.

226   T. Auzouy, 'Des troubles fonctionnels de la peau et de l'action de l'électricité chez les alié-
      nés', in J. Baillarger, L.A.P. Cerise, and J.-J. Moreau (eds.), *Annales médico-psychologiques.
      Journal destiné à récueillir tous les documents relatifs à l'aliénation mentale, aux névroses,
      et à la médecine légale des aliénés, par MM. les docteurs Baillarger, Cerise et Moreau*, Paris,
      Victor Masson, 1859, 527–563.

227   Ibid., 533: 'On connaît généralement l'histoire, rapporté par Marc, du cordonnier Mathieu
      Lovat, qui commenca son long martyre par s'amputer les parties génitales et les jeter par
      la fenêtre [...]'.

228   Y. Wübben, 'Mikrotom der Klinik. Der Aufstieg des Lehrbuches in der Psychiatrie (um
      1890)', in Y. Wübben and C. Zelle (eds.), *Krankheit schreiben. Aufzeichnungsverfahren in
      Medizin und Literatur*, Göttingen, Wallstein, 2013, 107–133, see also Y. Wübben, 'Einleitung:

genres. In contrast to genres that are directly related to medical practice and therefore transmit empirical knowledge, as the case history or the recipe, the textbook belongs to the doctrinal genres that aim to produce authoritative knowledge and long for standardisation. The framing of Lovat's case in textbooks thus meant that case knowledge was inserted into a doctrinal genre, so that the two epistemic genres interacted. The following examples show the impact this had on the rewriting and the presentation of Lovat's case.

In Gilbert Ballet's textbook on mental pathology, published in four volumes in 1903,[229] Lovat's case appears among the 'constitutional psychoses', under the subcategory 'systematic or partial deliria'.[230] As to 'religious systematic delirium', the author claims that it frequently develops in individuals with 'a weak hereditary constitution', and that education and milieu have a great influence.[231] Here, he briefly comments that 'a famous example of self-crucifixion is that of the Venetian shoemaker Mathieu Lovat, whose case (*histoire*) has been reproduced by Esquirol after Marc'.[232] This framing of Lovat's case shows, firstly, that not only the celebrity of Lovat's case, but also the reference to important psychiatrists who had worked with it, helped the author to display his expertise and his case knowledge in the field. Secondly, it shows that by 1900, psychiatric vocabulary had been elaborated, while the components of understanding of religious madness as a disease had remained essentially the same, except for a new stress on heritable dispositions. All the other aspects

---

Aufzeichnen in Pathologie, Psychiatrie und Literatur', in Y. Wübben and C. Zelle (eds.), *Krankheit schreiben. Aufzeichnungsverfahren in Medizin und Literatur*, Göttingen, Wallstein, 2013, 13–19.

229   G. Ballet (ed.), *Traité de pathologie mentale*, Paris, Octave Doin, 1903. See the introduction on 10: 'Ce livre est un traité de *pathologie mentale:* il vise à présenter, sous la forme didactique et forcément un peu concise qui convient à un traité, les notions principales relatives aux troubles, aux affections, aux maladies de ce que naguère encore appelait l'*Esprit*'. Ballet was a member of the *Société médico-psychologiques* and also of the *Société de psychologie*.

230   Ibid, 483ff.: 'Livre IV, "Psychoses constitutionelles" par F.L. Arnaud. Premiére Partie. Psychoses chez les sujets a prédisposition latente. Chapitre premier. Délires systématisés ou partiels (Paranoia, Verruecktheit des auteurs allemands)'. The definition on 488 reads: 'On désigne, en France, sous le nom de *délires partiels* ou *systematisés*, sous le terme générique de *paranoia*, en Allemagne et en Italie, des états psychopathiques fonctionnels, caractérisés par des idées délirantes permanentes, fixes, méthodiquement liées entre elles, se développant dans un sens déterminé et suivant une évolution logique'.

231   Ibid., 568f.: 'Qu'il y ait ou non hérédité, l'influence de l'*éducation* et du *milieu* paraît avoir une action prépondérante sur l'orientation du délire dans le sens religieux. Dans la plupart des cas, en effet, ce délire atteint des sujets qui, depuis l'enfance, présentaient un gout marqué pour les pratiques de la religion, l'habitude de raisonner sur les dogmes, et souvent une véritable exaltation mystique'.

232   Ibid., 572f.: 'Un example fameux d'auto-crucifiement est celui du cordonnier vénitien Mathieu Lovat, dont l'histoire a été reproduite par Esquirol, d'après Marc'.

mentioned, education, milieu and religious practices, already formed part of Ruggieri's case description from 1806. Ballet's emphasis on 'scientific progress' therefore reveals much more the general vagueness and fugitiveness of psychiatric classifications:

> the classifications change and improve according to the progress of the science: if those adopted in recent textbooks of psychiatry are not without fault, one will readily admit that they show a significant progress compared to those from the beginning of this century: as imperfect as the classification by Morel was, for instance, it is without any doubt much superior to the ones of Pinel and Esquirol.[233]

German psychiatrists, too, used Lovat's case as a standard example in doctrinal genres when constructing *religiöser Wahnsinn* or *religiöse Verrücktheit* as a separate diagnostic category. Consider the successful textbook by Emil Kraepelin (1856–1926), who could be said to have laid the foundations of the classification system of modern psychiatry.[234] In his *Compendium of Psychiatry* published in 1883 'for the use of students and physicians', he developed a classificatory system of the causes and symptoms of mental diseases. In this system, *religiöse Verrücktheit* comes next to the category 'insane delusions of grandeur' (*Größenwahn*).[235] In his description of *religiöse Verrücktheit*, Kraepelin highlights individual disposition, and the development of a whole system of insane thinking (*Wahnsystem*): people who in their youth have demonstrated an affinity for mysticism and exaggerated religious zeal, he explains,

---

233   Ibid., VII: 'Les classifications se modifient et se perfectionnent à mesure que la science progresse: si celles qui sont adoptées dans les traités récents de psychiatrie ne sont pas exemptes de défauts, on n'a pas de peine cependant à reconnaître qu'elles marquent un progrès sensible sur celles du commencement du siècle: tout imparfaite qu'ai été la classification de Morel par example, elle est sans conteste très supérieure à celles de Pinel et d'Esquirol'. On vagueness as a characteristic feature of modern psychiatric diagnoses see G. Keil, L. Keuck, and R. Hauswald (eds.), *Vagueness in Psychiatry*, Oxford, Oxford University Press, 2017.

234   H. Siefert, 'Emil Kraepelin', in Historische Kommission bei der Bayerischen Akademie der Wissenschaften (ed.), *Neue Deutsche Biographie*, vol. 12, Berlin, Duncker & Humblot, 1980, 639–640. With its focus on classifications and statistics, Kraepelin's work contrasts with another branch of psychiatry that developed in late nineteenth-century psychiatry, namely the interpretative approaches of the new psychoanalysis, commonly associated with Sigmund Freud, see Wübben, *Ordnen und Erzählen. Emil Kraepelins Beispielgeschichten*, 382. On Freud's case histories see for instance G. Steinlechner, *Fallgeschichten. Krafft-Ebing, Panizza, Freud, Tausk*, Vienna, WUV Universitätsverlag, 1995.

235   E. Kraepelin, *Compendium der Psychiatrie zum Gebrauche für Studierende und Ärzte*, Leipzig, Ambr. Abel, 1883, 304–306.

are often predisposed for mental diseases, either due to their education or personal disposition (*Anlage*).[236] Instead of developing a sane approach to life, they tend to mystical pondering (*mystische Grübelei*), self-torture (*Selbstquälerei*) and sexual excitability (*sexuelle Erregbarkeit*).[237] Kraepelin consequently describes how some of those affected experience visions, sudden revelations and transfigurations and a belief that they are the messiah. Motivated by imaginary warnings or, like Origen, by the 'insane interpretation of scriptures', they believe that they are fighting against demoniac appeals or that they must hurt themselves. When describing that some of the insane even pull out their eyes, cut off their genitals or crucify themselves, Kraepelin simply puts the name of Lovat in brackets.[238]

In this passing allusion to Lovat's case, the narrative is extremely compressed and reduced to the protagonist's name – the name alone was meant to embody and convey the whole case narrative. This shows not only that by Kraepelin's time, the association of religious madness with Lovat's case had become self-evident for German psychiatrists. The fact that Kraepelin put the name 'Mathieu Lovat' in brackets *after* his general description of the typical behaviour regularly displayed by patients is telling: it demonstrates that the case it not used to deduce knowledge from it, but rather to confirm authoritative knowledge.

---

236 Ibid., 304: 'Sehr ähnlich ist dieser Entstehungsgeschichte des verrückten Grössenwahns die Entwicklung der sog. religiösen Verrücktheit. Der mystische Zug, der überhaupt allen diesen Krankheitsformen gemeinsam ist, tritt hier am stärksten in den Vordergrund. Meist sind die Kranken schon von Jugend auf durch Erziehung oder Anlage (besonders wichtig Epilepsie) in eine bigotte, schwärmerische, religiöse Richtung hineingedrängt und durch die eifrige Lektüre überfrommer Schriften, die Einwirkung fanatischer Geistlicher oder überspannter Freunde genügend für die psychische Erkrankung vorbereitet'.

237 Ibid.: 'Das Interesse für "die Freuden dieser Welt", für eine fruchtbringende Thätigkeit, freie, klare Gedankenbewegung, gesunden Lebensgenuss erlischt, und an seine Stelle tritt die Neigung zu mystischen Grübeleien und skrupulöser Selbstquälerei. Regelmässig gesellt sich dazu eine gewisse sexuelle Erregbarkeit, die sich in Masturbation und schwärmerisch-sinnlicher Ausmalung der religiösen Verhältnisse zum "Seelenbräutigam" und der "Seelenbraut" Luft zu machen pflegt'.

238 Ibid., 305: 'Aus diesen Offenbarungen gehen dann die Kranken als Apostel, Messias, Welterlöser, oder aber als Braut Christi, Jungfrau Maria, Gottesgebärerin u. dergl. hervor. Sie beginnen zu predigen, führen Skandalscenen in der Kirche herbei, warten auf den Bräutigam, der ihnen in der Form irgend eines Mannes erscheint u. s. f. Dazwischen schieben sich zuweilen auch Kämpfe und Versuchungen, in denen sie von Angst gepeinigt mit dem visionären Teufel ringen, Busse thun, sich die schwersten Selbstpeinigungen, Fasten auferlegen und sogar auf Grund hallucinatorischer Mahnungen oder verrückt ausgelegter Bibelstellen, wie weiland Origines, sich gefährliche Verstümmelungen beibringen, sich die Augen ausreissen, die Hoden abschneiden sich kreuzigen (Mathieu Lovat) u. ähnl. Solchen Anfällen folgt dann in der Regel eine um so freudigere und stolzere Erhebung zu himmlischen Würden'.

Lovat is not thought of as an individual patient, but as an ideal type representing a specific mental disease. Accordingly, Kraepelin speaks of 'the' sick as a collective (*die Kranken, der Kranke*) and does not discuss individual cases at length.[239]

Kraepelin's example points to a broader shift in how German psychiatrists worked with cases in their textbooks, as Yvonne Wübben has shown.[240] While authors of earlier psychiatric textbooks followed the ideal of observation and therefore aimed at 'immediacy' in their narrative strategies, which they tried to produce by reporting empirical cases, later textbooks turned away from the programme of casuistry, aiming instead at the construction of systems characterised by narrative 'mediacy'.[241] Wübben emphasises that Kraepelin did not publish case collections and did not 'think in cases' like the psychoanalysts Sigmund Freud or Karl Jaspers.[242] However, she observes that Kraepelin employed literary strategies akin to those of psychological case histories from around 1800, which aimed at an effect of 'narrative immediacy' and extensively relied on the report of empirical observations.[243] She considers Kraepelin's use of narrative techniques – which by around 1900 were regarded as literary devices – to be somewhat inconsistent with the general direction of the psychiatric profession at Kraepelin's time, which called for systematisation, professionalisation and objectivity.[244] She therefore calls Kraepelin's narratives 'literarised exemplary stories' that served to describe the course of diseases over time (*Verlaufsgeschehen*), which formed the basis for his disease classifications.[245] But Kraepelin did not treat all the case histories he cited in his work

---

239   Ibid., 304f.
240   See Y. Wübben, 'Die kranke Stimme. Erzählinstanz und Figurenrede im Psychiatrie-Lehrbuch des 19. Jahrhunderts', in R. Behrens, N. Bischoff, and C. Zelle (eds.), *Der ärztliche Fallbericht. Epistemische Grundlagen und textuelle Strukturen dargestellter Beobachtung*, Wiesbaden, Harrassowitz, 2012, 151–170, 163.
241   Ibid., 164: 'Ist Unmittelbarkeit die Darstellungsstrategie jener Lehrbücher, die Beobachtung zu ihren epistemischen Idealen zählen und sich damit eine Lizenz zum Erzählen gegeben haben, markiert Mittelbarkeit jetzt ein konkurrierendes Programm, das seine Wissenschaftlichkeit auf die Geltung eines Systems gründet und mit den Erzählweisen der Kasuistik bricht'.
242   Wübben, *Ordnen und Erzählen*, 381. See also Y. Wübben, 'Dementia praecox: Emil Kraepelins Lehrbuchfall', in C. Zelle and A. Zein (eds.), *Casus. Von Hoffmanns Erzählungen bis Freuds Novellen. Eine Anthologie der Fachprosagattung 'Fallerzählung'.* Hannover, Wehrhahn, 2015, 207–213.
243   Wübben, *Ordnen und Erzählen*, 388.
244   Ibid., 390.
245   Ibid., 395: 'Kraepelins Lehrbucherzählungen erweisen sich [...] als literarisierte Beispielgeschichten, die ein Verlaufsgeschehen überhaupt erst konturieren, den klinischen Blick lenken und, indem sie die Präsenz erzählerischer Instanzen reduzieren, Unmittelbarkeit erzeugen und Wissen stabilisieren'.

in the same way: in his textbook, we find case narratives in different forms, longer and shorter ones, taken from his own or other physicians' practice, and he used them for different epistemic purposes.[246] The particular way in which Kraepelin appropriated Lovat's case, as a code to be deciphered rather than as a narrative that explains the case, not only reflects the contemporary turn towards a theoretical system of disease. As this chapter shows, it was also due to the history of the case itself. In Kraepelin's time, Lovat's case was so well known to the interpretive community of the German psychiatrists that it sufficed to simply mention his name.

We can see, then, that by the end of the nineteenth century, Lovat's case had undergone a significant shift in terms of the purpose it fulfilled for physicians, from producing and transmitting practical knowledge to confirming doctrinal knowledge. In its original form, the *Storia della crocifissione* transmitted empirical knowledge that Ruggieri had gained from his first-hand observations of Lovat's case. In his narrative, Ruggieri concentrated on the idiosyncratic aspects of the case, and how Lovat's case would fit into a more general disease classification was only a secondary concern. In contrast, Kraepelin's interest at the end of the nineteenth century was the very opposite. Sketching a general clinical picture of *religiöse Verrücktheit* in his textbook, the brief reference to Lovat's name served to confirm his general description of this disease. The transformation of Lovat's case from empirical to doctrinal knowledge in the history of psychiatry shows how nineteenth-century psychiatric knowledge was constructed on the basis of case material, that is narrative knowledge, that circulated from author to author, to finally establish itself in certain contexts. Michael Hagner has suggested that there are periods of 'diffusion' and periods of 'settlement' in the constitution of case knowledge. While in the period of diffusion, the discourse broadens, in the period of settlement it is reduced, amputated and integrated into a 'matrix'. Important elements can get lost in this process: 'by being canonised, knowledge dissociates itself from the original events and is turned into a general stipulation, which has enough profile to be recognised and identified, but can still be adjusted in various ways, so that it can be applied to other cases as well'.[247] Although the media channels

---

246   Ibid., 381–395.
247   Hagner, *Der Hauslehrer*, 216f.: 'Damit sich Wissen konstituiert [...] bedarf es der Phasen der Ausbreitung und der Setzung. Die Ausbreitung wird durch einen Skandal [...] erheblich befördert: die Setzung hingegen erscheint als Beruhigung, als Zurechtstutzen der diskursiven Aussprossungen und Einordnung in eine übersichtliche Matrix. Dieser Vorgang hat erhebliche Konsequenzen, denn er impliziert zum einen die aktive Produktion von Unwissen, das heißt des Weglassens verschiedener Elemente, Aspekte, Verwicklungen und Komplexitäten, die nicht in die Matrix passen; zum anderen garantiert er nicht, daß

necessary for the successful distribution of a case[248] were different in the case Hagner describes from those involved in Lovat's case, Hagner's observation fits with the development described in this chapter: toward the end of the century, the knowledge transmitted by Lovat's case experienced such a settlement in that it was archived as a doctrinal example in important textbooks of French and German psychiatry.

---

am Ende eine gereinigte, wahrere Version der Geschichte herauskommt. Indem das Wissen kanonisch wird, entfernt es sich vom ursprünglichen Geschehen und wird zu einer allgemeinen Klausel, die scharf genug konturiert ist, damit sie identifizierbar bleibt, und gleichzeitig eine hinreichende Modulationsfähigkeit aufweist, damit andere Fälle auf sie bezogen werden können'.

248   See ibid., 153ff.

CHAPTER 6

Professional Readings: Suicide

A third reading on Lovat's case that contemporaries established in the course of the nineteenth century was that Lovat's self-crucifixion was an extraordinary suicide. As we saw in the first chapter, Lovat's case had already been registered in 1805 as a 'surprising suicide' by the Venetian authorities.[1] In the *Storia della crocifissione*, Ruggieri had, however, questioned if Lovat should be considered a suicide. In his eyes, Lovat's longing for pain contradicted the suicides' usual desire for a rapid and painless death. Ruggieri emphasised that Lovat's primary aim, when crucifying himself, was not to die but to become a martyr. And in fact, thanks to immediate medical assistance, Lovat did not die as a result of his self-crucifixion, but from an undesignated 'disease of the chest' several months later. As this chapter will show, however, several professionals in nineteenth-century Europe – mainly theologians, forensic doctors, and psychiatrists – understood and classified Lovat's self-crucifixion as a suicide attempt. The reason why they took a special interest in Lovat's case was that the act of suicide had become an important research object in their respective scientific fields. The professional debates on suicide were in many ways connected with the medical critique of enthusiasm as well as with the rise of psychiatry. However, with important differences in the respective national contexts, suicide became a specialist debate and a field of knowledge per se. Within the international suicide debate, Lovat's case thus came to be read and framed in ways that were distinct from the two interpretive communities described so far. Moreover, suicide represented not only an important topic in professional debates, but one that was also dealt with extensively in popular publications that addressed a wider lay readership. Tracing how and why Lovat's case was read as a suicide case in nineteenth-century Europe, this chapter argues that the notion of Lovat as a suicide helped to popularise the case narrative, making it particularly appealing to a broader readership.

Long an important research subject for sociologists, suicide has become a topic of historical scholarship since the 1980s. While historians of modern European societies tend to put a strong focus on the relation between suicide

---

1   ASV, Direzione Generale Polizia, protocolli degli esibiti, b. 18, numero dell'esibito 4684, 19 luglio 1805: 'Il Reverendo Comando di Polizia di Canal Regio subbordina il proprio Rapporto col sopraluoco praticato in questa mattina dal suo officio in punto di sorprendente suicidio da se tentato di certo Matteo Casal di Soldo'.

© KONINKLIJKE BRILL NV, LEIDEN, 2019 | DOI:10.1163/9789004353602_008

rates, industrialisation and modernisation, as suggested by the important study of Durkheim,[2] early modernists have focused mainly on the shift 'from sin to insanity'.[3] They have shown what the increasing secularisation and medicalisation of suicide since the seventeenth century can tell us about changing cultural, social and moral attitudes and values in different societies. The overall narrative suggests that by the end of the eighteenth century, the debate on suicide was to a great extent secularised.[4] During the early modern period, it had been largely dominated by theological arguments, but in a long and complex process, the demonisation and criminalisation of suicide was largely replaced by medical explanations. As an effect, there was a 'shift from severity to tolerance'[5] in the treatment of suicide. At least amongst the Enlightened elite in Europe, it became a common opinion that suicides should not be penalised but rather be encountered with pity. In relation with a general spread of medical explanations in various contexts, suicide increasingly came to be equated with insanity. Physicians spread the notion that committing suicide was itself an insane act.[6] By the nineteenth century, therefore, the previous criminalising and moralising attitudes toward suicides had given place to more tolerant

2   E. Durkheim, *Le suicide: Étude de sociologie,* Paris, Félix Alcan, 1897; M. Barbagli, *Farewell to the World. A History of Suicide,* Cambridge, UK, Polity Press, 2015; A. Bähr and H. Medick (eds.), *Sterben von eigener Hand: Selbsttötung als kulturelle Praxis,* Cologne, Böhlau, 2005; J.C. Weaver, *A Sadly Troubled History: The Meanings of Suicide in the Modern Age,* Montréal and Kingston, McGill-Queen's University Press, 2009. M.T. Brancaccio, E.J. Engstrom, and D. Lederer, 'The Politics of Suicide: Historical Perspectives on Suicidology before Durkheim. An Introduction', *Journal of Social History,* vol. 46, no. 3, 2013, 607–619.

3   J.R. Watt (ed.), *From Sin to Insanity: Suicide in Early Modern Europe,* Ithaca, Cornell University Press, 2004.

4   For a general history on suicide in Western culture see Minois, *History of Suicide* in particular the chapter on 'The Elite. From Philosophical Suicide to Romantic Suicide', 248–278. On suicide in the early modern German speaking countries see for instance V. Lind, *Selbstmord in der frühen Neuzeit. Diskurs, Lebenswelt und kultureller Wandel,* Göttingen, Vandenhoeck & Ruprecht, 1999; M. Schär, *Seelennöte der Untertanen. Selbstmord, Melancholie und Religion im Alten Zürich, 1500–1800,* Zurich, Chronos, 1985; G. Signori (ed.), *Trauer, Verzweiflung und Anfechtung. Selbstmord und Selbstmordversuche in mittelalterlichen und frühneuzeitlichen Gesellschaften,* Tübingen, edition diskord, 1994; J. Schreiner, *Jenseits vom Glück. Suizid, Melancholie und Hypochondrie in deutschsprachigen Texten des späten 18. Jahrhunderts,* Munich, R. Oldenbourg, 2003. With a focus on England see the groundbreaking works by M. MacDonald, 'The Medicalization of Suicide in England: Laymen, Physicians, and Cultural Change, 1500–1870', *The Milbank Quarterly,* vol. 67, Supplement 1, *Framing Disease: The Creation and Negotiation of Explanatory Schemes,* 1989, 69–91 and MacDonald and Murphy, *Sleepless Souls.*

5   MacDonald, *The Medicalization of Suicide in England,* 74.

6   MacDonald and Murphy, *Sleepless Souls,* 201.

views and to the rise of verdicts of insanity. As John Weaver and David Wright put it, '(s)uicidality became a pathological symptom of ill individuals, something to be identified, classified, institutionalised, and prevented'.[7]

This notion of a linear and comprehensive process of the medicalisation of suicide has, however, been challenged by calls for more nuanced descriptions of what exactly was 'medicalised' in specific historical contexts. Historians of suicide have emphasised that '[...] the process of medicalisation was patchy and uneven [...]', and that '[t]he competition of discourses – religious and lay, medical and popular, cultural and "scientific" – remains an important aspect of the history of suicide'.[8] So while at the level of language, medical terms clearly dominated nineteenth-century debates on suicide, competing views of and attitudes to suicide continued to co-exist for a longer time.[9] As historian Jeff Watt has observed with view to London, 'In the early 1800s, both the popular press and learned opinion were torn between seeing suicide as a product of sickness or of sin, as acts of mental anguish or opprobrious vice. These findings show that even by the nineteenth century, one of Europe's most "modern" societies was still quite ambivalent about voluntary self-destruction [...]'.[10]

The occurrence of suicide, its public discussion as well as the societal attitude towards individual cases varied remarkably from place to place. While in Britain, for instance, suicide came to be a subject of vivid intellectual and popular debates, in Italy it was rarely a public issue before the nineteenth century, partly because of the prevalence of a distinct morality shaped by Roman Catholicism in the Italian States. As was the case for other emerging nations in Europe, the culture of death was to play a role in the construction of Italian nationality.[11]

Initially, the emerging science of suicide put a strong focus on individual case studies. Over the course of the nineteenth century, however, social scientists began to systematically collect and produce data in order to establish

---

7   D. Wright and J.C. Weaver, 'Introduction', in J.C. Weaver and D. Wright (eds.), *Histories of Suicide. International Perspectives on Self-Destruction in the Modern World*, Toronto, University of Toronto Press, 2009, 3–18, 4.

8   Ibid., 11f.

9   Ibid.

10   Watt, *From Sin to Insanity*, 8.

11   On suicide in England see MacDonald and Murphy, *Sleepless Souls*; MacDonald, *The Medicalization of Suicide in England*. On suicide in Italy see P.L. Bernardi, 'Introduction: A Culture of Death: Suicide in Italy in the Long Nineteenth Century 1798–1915', in P.L. Bernardi and A. Virga (eds.), *Voglio morire! Suicide in Italian Literature, Culture and Society 1789–1919*, Cambridge, UK, Cambridge Scholars Publishing, 2013, 1–26, 4. On the construction of nationality and related cults, see L. Riall, 'Martyr Cults in Nineteenth-Century Italy', *Journal of Modern History*, vol. 82, no. 2, 2010, 255–287.

suicide statistics for their respective nations.[12] Tracing how Lovat's case was employed as an individual suicide case in various debates allows one to explore the role of individual case histories in some of the competing discourses on suicide, and sheds light on the interdisciplinary and international construction of suicide as an object of scientific research. This chapter also demonstrates that despite the prevalence of a medical perspective on the topic, religion remained in many ways a crucial factor in the nineteenth-century debates of suicide.

1   Lovat's Case in the Construction of a *délire-suicide* in France

In the various readings of Lovat's case as an extraordinary suicide case, the general influence of a psychiatric perspective on suicide is very strong. We can see that most clearly when reconsidering some French publications we have already examined in the previous chapter on madness. Discussing Lovat's case as one of religious madness, several French alienists also classified him as a suicide caused by insanity. Most influential in this respect was Esquirol's article on suicide, published in the *Dictionnaire des sciences médicales* in 1821.[13] Esquirol's intention was not to study the legal aspects of suicide, but to conceptualise suicide as 'one of the most important objects of clinical medicine'.[14] Among a broad spectrum of individual, social, environmental and political causes, Esquirol considers Christian belief as a causal factor of self-murder, writing that

> in this age, there are a lot of factors producing suicides. Just as many superstitious monomanias (*les monomanies superstitieuses*) are predominant in times of ignorance in which religious ideas prevail we then find magicians, sorceries, possessed, etc., suicide predominates when excesses of civilisation threaten the empires.[15]

---

12   Wright and Weaver, *Introduction*, 5.
13   Esquirol, *Suicide*.
14   Ibid., 213: 'Il n'est point de mon sujet de traiter du suicide sous le rapport légal, par conséquent de sa criminalité; je dois me borner à faire connaître le suicide comme un des objets les plus importants de la médecine clinique'.
15   Ibid., 276: 'En parlant des causes particulières du suicide, j'ai fait sentir que l'age présent était fécond en causes propres à produire les suicides; de même que, dans les temps d'ignorance, dans les temps où les idées religieuses sont dominantes, règnent les monomanies superstitieuses, alors on voit des magiciens, des sorciers, des possédés, etc.; de même le suicide règne lorsque les excès de la civilisation menacent les empires'.

For Esquirol, *monomanie* was a cause of suicide, as '[...] every kind of mono-mania can lead to self-murder, be it that the monomaniac responds to hallu-cinations, be it that he becomes a victim of an insane passion'.[16] In his article, Esquirol frames Lovat's case as a telling example of suicide caused by *lypémanie*, his new term for melancholy.[17] Under the column 'suicide caused by the pas-sions', he presents Lovat's case between two other case narratives of so-called monomaniacs who follow inner voices to commit suicide. The first example is a man of a 'biblio-sanguine temperament' who falls down from a horse and consequently suffers from 'furious delirium' and 'aberrations in his ideas'.[18] This man quits his job to dedicate himself fully to his great project, which is to unify all peoples of the world. In order to receive public attention, he then jumps from a bridge in Paris and throws himself on crossroads, convinced he is invulnerable. Admitted to the mental asylum, he continues thinking about his project. As Esquirol emphasises, 'for the rest, M.*** is reasonable when he talks about things which have nothing to do with his project'.[19] The other case Esquirol cites is that of a state official who, after a national uprising, feels so responsible and guilty that he cuts his throat with a razor, following an inner order to commit suicide.[20] Hence, the common feature of the three case nar-ratives, that of Lovat included, is that all three protagonists were driven by one or the other *idée fixe*, leading them to their suicide attempts, while they were able to reason on other subjects. With the comparison and juxtaposition of the three cases, Esquirol thus sought to support and illustrate his general view that in many cases, suicide was nothing more than the effect of a partial delirium.

Following Esquirol's presentation of Lovat's case in his article on suicide, many of the alienists read Lovat's case from that perspective, although they focused on different aspects. The alienist Jean-Pierre Falret included Lovat's case in his book *De l'hypochondrie et du suicide*, where he put a strong focus on Lovat's presumed voluntary fasting. Ultimately, however, Falret too un-derstood Lovat as a suicide when considering the case under the broader category of a 'suicidal delirium' (*délire-suicide*)[21] and presenting it under the

---

16   Ibid., 221: 'Toute monomanie peut conduire au meurtre de soi-même, soit que le mono-maniaque obéisse à des hallucinations, soit qu'il agisse comme victime d'une passion délirante'.

17   Ibid., 223f.: 'M. le docteur Marc a fait connaître l'observation suivante, publiée par le docteur Ruggièri, pharmacien à Venise. Elle prouve toute l'influence de la lypémanie sur la détermination au meurtre de soi-même'.

18   See ibid., 221–224.

19   Ibid., 222: 'D'ailleurs, M.*** est raisonnable quand il parle des choses étrangères à son projet'.

20   Ibid., 224.

21   Falret, *De l'hypochondrie et du suicide*, 289.

headline 'ascetic melancholy followed by suicide'.[22] For Falret, it was clear that Lovat's final aim was to kill himself by means of voluntary fasting, and by crucifying himself. Another example is psychiatrist Gerard Marchant, who in his *Recherches sur les aliénés* wrote that 'mystical ideas are often followed by suicide. Lovat, a shoemaker in Venice who was obsessed by ideas of this kind, convinced himself that he had to die on the cross [...]'.[23] In many specialist publications on the relation between mental illness and suicide, the French alienists thus established an understanding of Lovat as an exemplary suicide who tried to kill himself because he suffered from a specific mental disease which they called, in alternative terms, religious madness.

Transmitting Lovat's case as a famous suicide in important French psychiatric publications, several alienists regarded not only Lovat's attempt at self-crucifixion, but also his self-mutilation as a suicidal act. In 1852, an article entitled 'lypémanie suicide' was published in the *Annales médico-psychologiques*.[24] Under the category 'Repertory of inedited observations', the author reports on an attempt at suicide, which was carried out through amputation of the genitals. In a short introduction to the case narrative, he writes that 'because of its bizarreness and the circumstances which have preceded and accompanied its execution, it seems to me that this observation can be ranked next to the one of this shoemaker from Venice, Matthieu Lovat, which Esquirol cites after the physician Ruggieri'.[25] By means of the following comparative case, the author puts his focus on the fact that Lovat had amputated his genitals. Thanks to this and similar publications, the alienists considered Lovat's case still worth citing in their specialist studies on suicide at the end of the century. In his book on 'suicides and strange crimes', published in 1899, Jacques-Joseph Moreau de Tours, a member of the Esquirol circle who had worked in the Parisian asylums Charenton and Bicêtre,[26] referred to it as one of the 'most famous cases' of religious delirium followed by suicide.[27]

---

22   Ibid., 330–333: 'Observation quatorzième. Mélancolie ascétique suivie de suicide'.

23   Marchant, *Recherches sur les aliénés*, 52: 'Les idées mystiquent provoquent quelquefois le suicide. Lovat, cordonnier à Venise, dominé par des idées de cette nature, après s'être plusieurs fois mutilé, se persuada qu'il devait mourir sur la croix. [...]'.

24   Archambault, *Lypémanie suicide*.

25   Ibid., 146: 'Lypémanie suicide. Tentative de suicide par section de la verge. – Observation communiquée par M. le docteur Archambault, médecin de la maison royale de Charenton. Elle m'a semblé par sa bizarrerie et les circonstances qui ont précédé ou accompagné son éxecution, pouvoir se placer auprès de celle de ce cordonnier de Venise, Matthieu Lovat, que cite Esquirol, d'après le médecin Ruggieri'.

26   On Moreau de Tours see the register in Goldstein, *Console and Classify*, 390f. and 266.

27   J.-J. Moreau, *Suicides et crimes étranges*, Paris, Société d'éditions scientifiques, 1899. Lovat's case is on 22–24 and begins with: 'Mais le genre de délire qui conduit le plus souvent à des crimes étranges, est, sans contredit, le délire religieux. Là les faits abondent et il suffirat

2   Lovat's Case in the Italian Suicide Debate

The French alienists set the tone as regards psychiatric discussions in nineteenth-century Western Europe. Many physicians specialising in mental diseases in Italy, Germany and Britain were inspired by the works of the French alienists, and borrowed the case histories they came across when reading French publications, employing them in their own studies. The ways in which Lovat's case circulated between psychiatric authors from different countries mirrors this broader tendency, as the following two examples from the Italian context show. The Italian forensic doctor Antonio Fossati included Lovat's case in his dissertation *Del suicidio nei suoi rapporti colla medicina legale, colla filosofia, colla storia* ('On Suicide in its Relations with Legal Medicine, Philosophy, and History'), which he published in Milan in 1831.[28] Fossati used Lovat's case primarily to reflect on the problem of insensitivity to pain in suicides, an aspect which Ruggieri, as we have seen, had already emphasised in the *Storia della crocifissione*. Essentially, Fossati argues that if the mental faculties are fixed on one point only, all the other organs no longer react to any other stimuli. Therefore, if one had the fixed idea of dying, all reactions of the body would align themselves with this desire. According to the author, this phenomenon was most frequently met with suicides relating to erotomania, theomania, and demonomania. Fossati then remarks, 'I could not give you a better example than that provided by doctor Ruggieri which happened to a certain shoemaker Matteo Lovati [sic!] in Venice [...]'.[29] As the following narrative reveals, Fossati

---

d'en rappeler quelques-un des plus célèbres. Mathieu Lovat, cordonnier à Venise [...]'. The source is the *Bibliothèque médicale*.

28   A. Fossati, *Del suicidio nei suoi rapporti colla medicina legale, colla filosofia, colla storia. Dissertazione inaugurale cui per conseguire la lauree dottorale in medicina nell'I.R. università di Pavia nel mese di settembre MDCCCXXXI*, Milan, Presso Luigi Nervetti, 1831. On this study see E. Bianco, 'Suicidi di primo ottocento: Riflessioni sulla liceità della morte volontaria nell'Italia preunitaria', in P.L. Bernardi and A. Virga (eds.), *Voglio morire! Suicide in Italian Literature, Culture and Society 1789–1919*, Cambridge, UK, Cambridge Scholars Publishing, 2013, 85–114.

29   Ibid., 83f.: 'Occupate e concentrate le mentali facoltà su di un solo punto, ed a quello fissamente aderenti, inerte si rende la vitale efficacia per gli altri, di modo che non agisce verso gli stimolo che la eccitano. [...] onde ne avviene che fissa l'immaginazione nella idea di morire, imprime alla volontà le opportune condizioni onde regolate vengano le corporee azioni al prefisso scopo. [...] Un tale stato di inerzia delle estremità periferiche de'nervi e di soverchio eccitamento del centro, riscontrasi facilmente ne' suicidi per Erotomania (amor furioso), Theomania (mania religiosa con liete speranze) e Demonomania (mania religiosa con spaventi e terrori). Non saprei a questo proposito citare miglior esempio di quello riportato dal Dotto Ruggieri ed accaduto in Venezia, a certo Matteo Lovati calzolajo'.

had literally copied Lovat's case from Esquirol's article on suicide.[30] In order to frame the case according to his interest in physical insensitivity, he compared it with other case narratives about individuals who harmed themselves in various ways and were thereby apparently resistant to pain. Fossati's presentation of Lovat's case concludes with the rhetorical question of whether Lovat 'could have accomplished his idea if his body had been susceptible to pain? [...]'.[31] On the whole, Fossati's study demonstrates that his ideas were strongly modelled on existing French works on legal medicine and psychiatry. Throughout his book, he cites well-known French physicians, such as Esquirol, Falret or Fodéré who were leading figures in the psychiatric discourse. Fossati was eager to apply the findings of the French alienists to Italian suicide cases and statistics, as a table providing statistics about Italian suicides at the end of his book shows.[32]

Another important promoter of Lovat's case in the Italian suicide debate was the physician and writer Mosè Giuseppe Levi.[33] Between 1830 and 1840, Levi translated and edited an important contemporary French medical dictionary that he published in Venice with annotations under the title *Dizionario classico di medicina interna ed esterna*.[34] In the volume published in 1839, Levi reprinted a full copy of Ruggieri's second Italian edition of the *Storia della crocifissione* from 1814 in the final part of a long article on suicide.[35] This article

---

30   Esquirol, *Suicide*.

31   Fossati, *Del suicidio nei suoi rapporti colla medicina legale*, 85: 'Avrebbe egli potuto compiere il suo disegno se sensibile fosse stato il suo corpo all'impressione del dolore? Io pure conobbi non è gran tempo uno sciagurato giovane risoluto di uccidersi, cui fallito un colpo di pistola diretto contro la testa [...] Al qual fatto altri molti aggiungere ne potrei di individui che lenta e tormentosa per sivariate circostanze si procacciaron morte; ma solo mi limito al fatto marcato nelle tavole, 10 giugno 1829, ove scorgesi un individuo che si recò 64 ferite di propria mano, prima di gettarsi in un pozzo, ove poi trovò morte'.

32   Ibid., 137ff.: 'Prospetto dei suicidj e degli attentati accaduti in Milano dal I. Gennajo 1821 a tutto Agosto 1831'.

33   Levi was the author of an important encyclopaedia on eighteenth- and nineteenth-century Venetian physicians and surgeons. Levi, *Ricordo intorno agli incliti medici chirughi e farmacisti che praticarono loro arte in Venezia*.

34   M.G. Levi (ed.), *Dizionario classico di medicina interna ed esterna. Prima tradizione italiana di M. Giuseppe Levi*, Venice, G. Antonelli, 1831–1846. The French original is: N.-P. Adelon *et al.* (eds.), *Dictionnaire de médecine ou répertoire général des sciences médicales considérées sous le rapport théorique et pratique, par MM. Adelon, Béclard, Bérard, Biett et al.*, Paris, Béchet Jeune et Labé, 1832–1846. This dictionary was preceded by the *Dictionnaire de médecine* by the same editors: N.-P. Adelon *et al.* (eds.), *Dictionnaire de médecine par MM. Adelon, Béclard, Biett et al.*, Paris, Béchet Jeune, 1821–1828.

35   M.G. Levi, 'Suicidio', in M.G. Levi (ed.), *Dizionario classico di medicina interna ed esterna. Prima tradizione italiana di M. Giuseppe Levi*, Venice, G. Antonelli, 1839, 477–562, the 'Storia della Crocifissione di Mattio Lovat' is on 554–562.

essentially consists of a compilation of different contributions on suicide written by French authors, and many comments added by Levi himself. Tellingly, Levi refers to Étienne Georget, a famous French specialist in legal medicine who prominently fought for the position of physicians in the courtroom. According to Jan Goldstein, 'Georget proposed, in brief, that monomania form the basis of broadened insanity defence in criminal cases, and concomitantly that the new *médecin des aliénés* be given a central place in the deliberations of the courtroom'.[36] Levi complained that Georget's discussion of Lovat's case was vague and full of omissions. In particular, he claimed that Georget had wrongly called Ruggieri a 'pharmacist'. In order to rectify the authority of his 'beloved friend and teacher Ruggieri' as well as of 'this unique history in the annals of surgery', Levi therefore reproduced the full original text of the *Storia della crocifissione*, including Lovat's letter that Ruggieri had added in the second edition only.[37] It seems that Levi was very fond of Ruggieri's works: besides the *Storia della crocifissione*, he included several other contributions by and on Ruggieri in different volumes of the *Dizionario classico di medicina*.[38] Levi's inclusion of the *Storia della crocifissione* in the *Dizionario classico di medicina* is revealing for several reasons. Firstly, his translation demonstrates that Italian physicians were strongly influenced by the French alienists and

---

36   Goldstein, *Console and Classify*, 162.

37   M.G. Levi, *Suicido*, 479: '[...] eppur in questo articolo, cerchiamo invano il medico psicologico, il medico moralista, il medico anatomico, il medico pratico; che più un informissimo sunto di certo grandissimo omicidio accaduto in Venezia già parecchi anni, vi è colà così sgarbatamente accennato, che, fra le altre storpiature, l'autore della descrizione di esso, mio amatissimo amico e maestro Cesare Ruggieri, vi è detto *farmacista*, ragioni per le quali immettemmo tradurlo e preferimmo riportare per intero la storia del fatto come unica negli annali chirurgici, e c'ingegneremo pure riprodurre qui vari altri scritti di alcuni incliti autori, onde riparare alle gravi immissioni di Georget'.

38   C. Ruggieri, 'Storia ragionata di una donna avente gran parte del corpo coperta di pelle e pelo nero', in M.G. Levi (ed.), *Dizionario classico di medicina interna ed esterna. Prima tradizione Italiana di M. Giuseppe Levi*, Venice, G. Antonelli, 1837; C. Ruggieri, 'Del processo litotomico di lecat seguito dal dottor Francesco Pajola', in M.G. Levi (ed.), *Dizionario classico di medicina interna ed esterna. Prima tradizione italiana di M. Giuseppe Levi*, Venice, G. Antonelli, 1835, 318–320.; C. Ruggieri, 'Delle variazioni riguardanti la esecuzione del taglio nell'apparecchio laterale fatto da più accreditati autori italiani', in M.G. Levi (ed.), *Dizionario classico di medicina interna ed esterna. Prima tradizione italiana di M. Giuseppe Levi*, Venice, G. Antonelli, 1835, 686–688; C. Ruggieri, 'Taglio laterale eseguito alla parte destra del perineo', in M.G. Levi (ed.), *Dizionario classico di medicina interna ed esterna. Prima tradizione italiana di M. Giuseppe Levi*, Venice, G. Antonelli, 1835, 699–701; C. Ruggieri, 'Dei polipi dell'ano', in M.G. Levi (ed.), *Dizionario classico di medicina interna ed esterna. Prima tradizione italiana di M. Giuseppe Levi*, Venice, G. Antonelli, 1837, 228–231; M.G. Levi, 'Ruggieri Cesare, sua vita', in M.G. Levi (ed.), *Dizionario classico di medicina interna ed esterna. Prima tradizione italiana di M. Giuseppe Levi*, Venice, G. Antonelli, 1838, 520–523.

their growing body of psychiatric knowledge. Secondly, it shows that for Italian physicians, Ruggieri's case history was not ephemeral but was part of standard contemporary medical knowledge, in particular in relation to the growing international corpus of suicide cases. And thirdly, Levi's promotion of Lovat's case sheds light on the complex trajectories of Lovat's case between French and Italian authors. Levi's reference to Georget suggests that Italian physicians came across Lovat's case not by reading one of Ruggieri's original Italian editions of the *Storia della crocifissione*, but by consuming foreign publications. More often than not, the primary attention of Italian readers to Lovat's case was indeed triggered by French publications and Lovat's case had made a detour via France before Italian authors appropriated it in their works. It is striking that even Italian physicians would refer to the French booklet when citing Lovat's case, rather than to the first Italian edition of the *Storia della crocifissione* contained in Carlo Amoretti's miscellanea.[39] Last but not least, Levi's reproduction of Lovat's case is interesting because it suggests that for local authors who knew Lovat's case and its first author from its original Venetian context, it was important to correct the minor changes and misunderstandings that foreign authors had transmitted in their readings of the case. Italian authors thus claimed a certain interpretive authority over 'their' case. Generally speaking, however, the circulation of Lovat's case in the Italian debate on suicide was less pronounced and, in quantitative terms, did not reach the extent it had in France, Germany and Britain. At least, it appears that Lovat's case did not become a standard reference in important Italian publications on suicide.[40] One reason probably lies in the fact that in the first half of the nineteenth century, studies on suicide were still comparatively rare in the Italian States. As a result of a relatively reluctant attitude to this topic, Italian publications on suicide began to be common only in the second half of the nineteenth century.[41]

Interestingly, Lovat's case nevertheless went down in Italian history as a famous suicide case, thanks to its late inclusion in a huge editorial project of a national history of Italy in the nineteenth century, published by Alfredo Comandini between 1907 and 1942: *L'Italia nei cento anni del secolo XIX (1801–1900)*

---

39   For instance, Moschini refers to the French version of the *Storia della crocifissione*, see G. Moschini, *Della letteratura veneziana del secolo XVIII fino ai giorni nostri*, vol. 4, Venice, Dalla Stamperia Palese, 1808, 35.

40   For instance, the case is not cited in E. Caluci, *L'omicidio-suicidio. Cenni critici*, Venice, Fontana, 1884; Anonymous, *Sopra il suicidio. Saggio filosofico, pubblicato con annotazioni da G.V.*, Venice, Nella tipografia Picotti, 1824.

41   P.L. Bernardi and A. Virga (eds.), *Voglio morire! Suicide in Italian Literature, Culture and Society 1789–1919*, Cambridge, UK, Cambridge Scholars Publishing, 2013, XI.

giorno per giorno illustrata.[42] Due to the specific nature of this publication, Lovat's case was turned into an event of Italian national history. Comandini was a political journalist, editor of several journals and an advocate of the Italian national movement.[43] His concern was to illustrate the process of Italian unification in an encyclopaedic format, reporting on the political, societal and cultural events day by day that he considered important for the rise of Italy as a nation, Italian's national 'Resurrection', the *Risorgimento*. In order to sketch his broad historical and iconographical panorama, he used various nineteenth-century print media from his own library and beyond.[44] His main sources were periodicals and newspapers from which he took the succession of events, but also a great variety of visual prints, representing revolutionary scenes, monuments, coins, medals or portraits of heroes and martyrs.[45]

Given the historiographical genre of Comandini's work, it is surprising to find Lovat's case mentioned among the several thousand day-by-day accounts of political events. In the first volume, covering the early years of the nineteenth century, we find the following note for the nineteenth of July 1805: 'Great tumult in Venice due to the fact that a certain Matteo Lovat, a day labourer born in the region of Belluno, after he had emasculated himself voluntarily in 1802, succeeded in Venice in nailing himself to a cross, crowned with thorns, his feet and hands pierced with nails. The physician Ruggieri defined him *pellagroso*'.[46] And among the events registered for 1806, the entry for 8 April reads: 'Dies in Venice, much commented-on by the public, Matteo Lovat from Belluno, who,

---

42   A. Comandini, *L'Italia nei cento anni del secolo XIX (1801–1900) giorno per giorno illustrata*, vol. 1, Milan, Antonio Vallardi, 1900–1901.

43   D. Savoia, 'Dalla parte di Alfredo Comandini. Note per una biografia', in G. Benassati and D. Savoia (eds.), *L'Italia nei cento anni. Libri e stampe della biblioteca di Alfredo Comandini*, Bologna, grafis, 1998, 1–9.

44   G. Benassati and D. Savoia (eds.), *L'Italia nei cento anni. Libri e stampe della biblioteca di Alfredo Comandini*, Bologna, grafis, 1998, 29: '[…] un grande e complesso mosaico storico-iconografico sul Risorgimento italiano elaborato a partire da molteplici fonti, molte delle quail presenti nella biblioteca dell'Autore'.

45   Ibid.: 'Il susseguirsi degli avvenimenti che gradatamente, o convulsamente, condussero all'indipendenza ed all'unificazione dello Stato è definito da un succedersi ordinato di notizie illustrate a partire da dipinti, stampe, monete e monumenti ove sono raffigurati moti rivoluzionari, celebri battaglie, apparati effimeri e ritratti; icone attraverso cui avviene il processo di eroicizzazione di uomini ed eventi che, insieme, danno vita alla rappresentazione di ciò che è comunemente definito il mito del Risorgimento'.

46   Comandini, *L'Italia nei cento anni del secolo XIX (1801–1900)*, 148: 'Luglio 1805, 19. Grande baccano a Venezia per il fatto che certo Matteo Lovat, bracciante, nativo del bellunese, dopo essersi nel 1802 volontariamente evirato è riuscito in Venezia a conficcarsi su di una croce coronato di spine, coi piedi e le mani trafittisi da se con chiodi. Il medico Ruggeri [sic!] definiscelo pellagroso'.

on the nineteenth of July in 1805, carried out the self-crucifixion'.[47] Probably, a copy of Ruggieri's case history was on hand in Comandini's library, or he had read about Lovat's case in some other publication. In any case, he transformed the narrative into a factual report, in order to include it in his *L'Italia nei cento anni del secolo* as an extraordinary historical event.

This framing of Lovat's crucifixion attempt suggests a specific reading of Lovat's case: Lovat as an early hero or martyr of the political upheavals in early nineteenth-century Italy, or, more specific, of Napoleonic Italy. To be sure, there is not enough evidence to assert that Comandini explicitly understood Lovat's case in this way. However, the specific framing could inspire his readers for such a reading. Comandini's panorama of historical events recalls the major events happening before and after Lovat's self-crucifixion: In May 1805, Napoleon crowned himself in the Milan dome, thereby establishing his *Regno d'Italia*.[48] But it was only at the end of December in 1805, that Venice, together with Dalmatia and Istria, was annexed to the *Regno d'Italia* as well, as a result of the peace of Pressburg.[49] For the year 1806, Comandini recalls the great impact that this important change had on Venetia and the Italian Kingdom in general. Apart from listing political ceremonies and celebrations that took place in Venice during this year,[50] he also notes important political and administrative events, such as the introduction of a new currency and the application of the Napoleonic *code civil* in April 1806.[51] Encountering Lovat's case among these local, national and international political events, the reader inevitably establishes possible relations between these political macro-events, and Lovat's self-crucifixion. Through this perspective, Lovat's self-crucifixion appears as a form of social protest: in the very year of 1805, only several weeks after Napoleon had crowned himself King of Italy in Milan, Lovat committed

---

47   Ibid., 183: 'Aprile 1806, 8. Muore in Venezia, fra i commenti del popolino, il bellunese Matteo Lovat che il 19 luglio 1805 fece l'autocrocifissione'.

48   Ibid., 132: year 1805, May 26: 'Napoleone Bonaparte cingesi il capo, nel duomo di Milano, con la corona ferrea, in mezzo a pompa solenne e pronunziando le famose parole: Dio me l'ha data, guai a chi la toccherà'.

49   Ibid., 159: year 1805, December 26: 'Alle 5 del mattino a Presburgo è segnata fra Talleyrand, per Napoleone, e il principe di Lichtenstein, per Francesco I. la pace onde la città di Venezia e tutti gli stati veneti sono uniti al regno d'Italia'.

50   See for instance ibid., 165: year 1806, February 3: 'Solenne ingresso del vice-re Eugenio e della vice-regina Amalia di Baviera in Venezia'.; February 6: 'Grande cerimonia e rivista militare in piazza S. Marco a Venezia passata dal vice-re, e corso di peone, bissino e gondole sul Canal grande'.

51   Ibid., 180: year 1806, March 21: 'Decreto di Napoleone dalle Tuileries ordinante la coniazione di monete d'oro d'argento, di rame, a sistema decimale per il regno d'Italia'.; ibid., Aprile 1: 'È posto in attività in tutto il Regno il codice civile Napoleone'.

a suicide attempt that was deeply charged with Christian symbols. In the light of the violent secularisation policies to which Venice was going to be subjected about one year later – in the summer of 1806, Napoleon secularised about 24 Venetian churches and 60 monasteries[52] – one could therefore be tempted to interpret Lovat's crucifixion attempt as an anticipated martyr-like revolt against Napoleon, the Antichrist.[53]

Historian Lucy Riall has shown how nineteenth-century Italy saw a 'revival of the martyr as a collective symbol and tool of propaganda [...]'.[54] In public discourse, Catholic and nationalist martyr cults were closely interrelated. On the one hand, the general Catholic revival in the Restoration period saw a rise of Catholic martyr cults. On the other hand, there was the national discourse that saw a clear 'transposition of religious vocabularies on to the nation', and attributed the nation a certain 'divine quality'.[55] As Riall states, '[...] Italian nationalism was neither a secular doctrine nor a new religion that sought to replace the Christian God with the divinity of the nation. Instead, it was the expression of a romantic culture acting within a symbolic environment that was conspicuously Catholic'.[56] In this context, self-sacrifice and the dying volunteer were figures – both real and rhetorical – that served to enhance the sense of a nation. In Riall's words, 'Italy required martyrs to be symbols of national belonging. As part of a collective tradition martyrs served to create the sense, otherwise largely lacking, of a unified national past'.[57] This historical background provides us with an explanation as to why Comandini believed it relevant to include Lovat's case in his *L'Italia nei cento anni del secolo XIX*. Representing the figure of the Christian martyr in the midst of the Napoleonic upheavals, Lovat was, in Comandini's retrospective view, illustrative of the Zeitgeist that he sought to convey with his work.

3   Lovat's Case in the British Suicide Debate

Like the Italian physicians, British medical writers were inspired by reading the publications of the French alienists, and appropriated the suicide cases

---

52   On Napoleon in Venice see for instance Zorzi, *Napoleone a Venezia* and A. Zorzi, *Venezia scomparsa*, Milan, Mondadori, 1972.

53   As Matthias Pohlig has shown, several contemporary writers demonised the figure of Napoleon and associated it with the Antichrist, see Pohlig, *Individuum und Sattelzeit*, 274.

54   Riall, *Martyr Cults in Nineteenth-Century Italy*, 256.

55   Ibid., 259.

56   Ibid., 286.

57   Ibid., 273.

reported by foreign physicians for their own purposes. In 1840, the physician and specialist in insanity Forbes Winslow (1810–1874), president of the Medical Society of London,[58] published *The Anatomy of Suicide*, which, according to the author's own contention, provided the first systematic study in Britain considering suicide 'in reference to its pathological and physiological character'.[59] An early adherent of phrenology, Winslow considered mental disorder to be primarily an organic disturbance, but nevertheless emphasised 'psychology and philosophical inquiry in relation to mental disorder'.[60] He aimed to show that suicides were victims of mental diseases rather than criminals.[61] Winslow's ideas about mental diseases were clearly influenced by the French alienists, in particular by Pinel, Esquirol and Fodéré, to whom he explicitly refers in his foreword.

Winslow presents Lovat's case in the last part of his study where he discusses 'singular cases of suicide'.[62] The introduction to this chapter reveals the author's eagerness to find the true causes of suicidal actions. At the same time, it reveals the difficulty of explaining suicide in general terms, and in particular on the basis of accounts written by others:

> In investigating, as we have endeavoured to do, the motives that have led to this heinous offence [the suicide, M.B.] we have in many cases been unsuccessful in tracing the act to any definite principle. Either no reasons have been assigned, or the accounts of the cases transmitted to us have been imperfect. These individuals stand apart from the rest of the world, and exhibit an anomaly in the last act of life totally irreconcilable to all acknowledged principles of reason and human action.[63]

Eliminating the last part of Ruggieri's original case history, Winslow laconically comments: 'In the course of a short time Lovat was completely restored to bodily health, but his mind retained the same melancholy caste until his death, although he never had another opportunity of putting his sanguinary project into execution'.[64] As Barbara Gates has rightly remarked in her study

---

58   A. King and J. Plunkett (eds.), *Victorian Print Media. A Reader*, Oxford, Oxford University Press, 2005, 58. On Winslow see J. Andrews, 'Winslow, Forbes Benignus (1810–1874)', *Oxford Dictionary of National Biography*, 2004, http://www.oxforddnb.com/view/article/29752, (accessed 20 July 2017).

59   F. Winslow, *The Anatomy of Suicide*, London, Henry Renshaw, 1840, VI.

60   See Andrews, *Winslow, Forbes Benignus*.

61   Winslow, *The Anatomy of Suicide*, V.

62   Ibid., 329–333.

63   Ibid., 283.

64   Ibid., 333.

of Victorian suicides, for Winslow, 'Lovat's attempt seemed like a sick echo of Christianity, but certainly no self-sacrifice for the sake of others'.[65] By applying an attribute which, as we shall see, was specific to the British scientific and popular debates on social deviance, Winslow finally describes suicides as 'eccentric' characters who are just very consistent in their eccentric deeds: 'Eccentric in their lives, they have been desirous of manifesting the ruling passions strong in death'.[66] Apparently, Winslow considered Lovat's case as the most telling one of his whole collection. He produced a new engraving of Ruggieri's original illustration, showing Lovat hanging on the wooden cross out of the window, and used it as frontispiece to his book (see illustration 8).

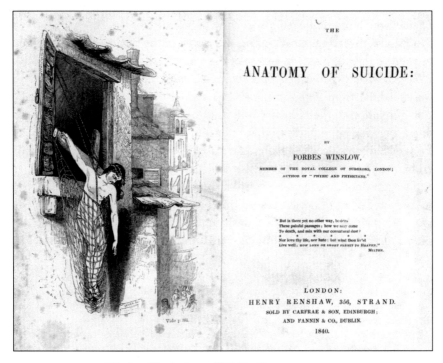

ILLUSTRATION 8   Winslow, *The Anatomy of Suicide*, 1840.

---

65   B.T. Gates, *Victorian Suicides. Mad Crimes and Sad Histories*, Princeton, Princeton University Press, 2013. Available from: http://www.victorianweb.org/books/suicide/04.html, (accessed 1 June 2017).

66   Winslow, *The Anatomy of Suicide*, 283. One has to be aware that in general, 'science' and 'eccentricity' should not be considered as separated and contradicting discourses in nineteenth century Britain, see V. Carroll, *Science and Eccentricity: Collecting, Writing and Performing Science for Early Nineteenth Century Audiences*, London, Pickering & Chatto, 2008.

Probably due to a mistake in the process of reproduction, the illustration is represented in the wrong way: Lovat's left arm hangs down whereas according to the original narrative and the original illustration, it was the right. Winslow adjusted his narrative of Lovat's case accordingly.[67]

Winslow's *Anatomy of Suicide* proved important not only for the further transmission of Lovat's case in Britain but in turn became also the source for some French authors writing on Lovat's case as a suicide case. Brière de Boismont, who had not referred to Lovat's case in his study of pellagra, did include it in his later study on suicide. Tellingly, Brière's source was not the *Bibliothèque médicale* or any other French contribution, but Winslow's study. In *Du suicide et de la folie suicide*, Brière lists Lovat's case in a series of cases that served him as examples for suicide as a result of melancholy and compares it with the case of a man who burned himself in an access of insanity.[68]

In Britain, several medical authors interested in the rising field of psychology would convey Winslow's version of the narrative. It appeared, for instance, in *The Journal of Psychological Medicine and Mental Pathology,* which Winslow himself edited from 1848 onwards.[69] '[D]evoted to the discussion of questions in relation to the Human Mind in its abnormal condition', the journal aimed at 'giving an impetus to that branch of the science of medicine which is termed Psychological'.[70] As Jonathan Andrews states, '[t]hrough this journal and his prolific publications, Winslow contributed perhaps more than anyone to the dissemination of psychological medicine as a term and concept'.[71] The author who discussed Lovat's case in this journal, a certain R. Horne, included it in his 'Analysis of crime' that dealt with 'Misdirected strength, and the criminal actions which result from it'. For Horne, Lovat's self-crucifixion was a

---

67   Ibid., 332: 'He then, by way of finishing, nailed his right hand to the arm of the cross, but could not succeed in fixing his left, although the nail by which it was to have been fixed was driven through it, and half of it came out of the other side'.

68   A. Brièrre de Boismont, *Du suicide et de la folie suicide: considérés dans leurs rapports avec la statistique, la médecine et la philosophie*, Paris and New York, Baillière, 1856, 560: 'Le fait observé par M. Madin peut être rapproché de celui de Mathieu Lovat, ce cordonnier de Venise qui s'était lui-même crucifié, après c'être couronné d'épines, amputés les parties génitales et fait au flanc une large plaie avec un tranchet. Ce malheureux, qui ne succomba point à ses blessures, ne souffrait pas dans les redoublements de son délire, mais seulement dans les intervalles lucides'.

69   M. Shepherd, 'Psychiatric Journals and the Evolution of Psychological Medicine', in W.F. Bynum, S. Lock and R. Porter (eds.), *Medical Journals and Medical Knowledge. Historical Essays*, London and New York, Routledge, 1992, 188–206, 193.

70   F. Winslow (ed.), *The Journal of Psychological Medicine and Mental Pathology*, vol. 1, London, John Churchill, 1848, 111f.

71   See Andrews, *Winslow, Forbes Benignus.*

'martyrdom' caused by pathologic fanaticism. Interestingly, Horne speculates about the strong influence of Catholic visual culture that may have inspired Lovat:

> [...] influenced no doubt by fanaticism, his imagination being constantly fed by the various images and pictures in the Roman-catholic churches, chapels, and streets, he conceived the idea of imitating in his own person, the last mortal scene of the Saviour. Totally overlooking the grand fact of self-devotion for a mighty and disinterested object, and that the most distant resemblance would still demand a great cause and purpose, he saw the resemblance only in the external form – such as his imagination was familiar with – and accordingly he conceived and executed, with infinite ingenuity and unsurpassable resolution, the apparently impossible feat of crucifixing himself.[72]

Like many other medical authors, Horne thus used Lovat's case to illustrate more general claims in the context of a general pathology of suicide and religion. Unusually, however, his comment contains an implicit confessional demarcation. The author describes Catholicism as an intrinsically 'visual confession' that relies on liturgical formalities and a literal understanding of belief – the 'external form' – rather than on its internal meaning. According to Horne, the Catholic Lovat took this tendency to extremes in that he became obsessed by the idea of imitating Christ, at least through his outward appearance. Remarkably, this is the only British commentator to display a certain resentment against Italian Catholicism by blaming the effect of the Catholic visual culture for having conditioned Lovat's fanaticism.

Like Italian physicians who encountered Lovat's case when reading French publications, several British authors came to know Lovat's case by reading English translations of French publications.[73] As most of the French authors

---

72   R. Horne, 'Analysis of Crime. Being an Attempt to Distinguish Its Chief Causes, in Answer to the Statistical Deductions of M. Guerry, and the Rev. Whitworth Bussell; the Former Finding that Popular Education Did Not Prevent Crime – the Latter That It Was the Cause of Crime', in F. Winslow (ed.), *The Journal of Psychological Medicine and Mental Pathology*, vol. 3, London, John Churchill, 1850, 94–123, 112f.

73   For instance, this is the case for a text by the French alienist Théodore Auzouy already mentioned in the chapter on France. His article 'On Lesions of the Cutaneous Sensibility among the Insane', in which Lovat is cited as an example of the absence of physical sensitivity in monomania, appeared in the *Journal of Psychological Medicine and Mental Pathology*: T. Auzouy, 'Art. IV. – On Lesions of the Cutaneous Sensibility among the Insane', in F. Winslow (ed.), *The Journal of Psychological Medicine and Mental Pathology*, vol. 13, London, John Churchill, 1860, 68–82.

had done, English specialists in mental diseases therefore generally ignored Ruggieri's original reference to pellagra as a possible cause of Lovat's mental disorder. Tellingly, already in the English translation published in 1814 in the *Pamphleteer*, the term pellagra had been replaced with 'leprosy', indicating that the British readership at that time was not familiar with the Italian local debate on pellagra. Nevertheless, pellagra was rewritten into Lovat's case much later at least in one British contribution. In *The Journal of Mental Science* published in 1861, we find an article on 'Endemic Degeneration' by William Browne, Commissioner in Lunacy for Scotland.[74] He describes pellagra as a new hereditary disease in Europe, especially in Italy, affecting in particular poor farmers. He briefly mentions that '[t]he celebrated M. Lovat, who attempted to destroy himself by crucifixion, was a pellagrin [...]'.[75]

Broadly speaking, however, Lovat's circulated within the emerging sciences of psychology and mental pathology in Britain as an extraordinary case of suicidal insanity. What distinguishes the British discussions of Lovat's case from those in the other countries is, however, that in Britain the boundaries between scientific and popular debates were particularly blurred when it came to questions of mental disorder and suicide. Historians of science popularisation in Britain have shown that the human mind and mental conditions were topics that were discussed in a broad range of print media, professional and lay, and adapted for different audiences:

> [m]ost nineteenth-century writers were prepared to include discussions of the nature of mind within their definitions of "science"; indeed, during the middle decades of the century the main contributors to the "science of mind" published extensively in the general periodical press. It is here that the historian can find the changing meanings of the term "science" and the early stages in the emergence of psychology as a separate subject.[76]

As described by Rick Rylance, the field of psychology in Britain included authors from various disciplines and, for a long time, remained rather eclectic, generalist and controversial, which made it appealing for a general

---

74   W.A.F. Browne, 'Endemic Degeneration. By W.A.F. Browne, Commissioner in Luncay for Scotland', in J.C. Bucknill (ed.), *The Journal of Mental Science. Published by Authority of the Association of Medical Officers of Asylums and Hospitals for the Insane*, vol. 7, London, John Churchill, 1861, 61–76.

75   Ibid., 68.

76   Henson *et al.*, *Introduction*, XVIII.

readership.[77] Several Victorian periodicals contributed to the distribution of 'psychological knowledge' into a wider reading public and therefore played an important role in the construction of psychology as a modern discipline.[78] In this context of the rising psychological and psychiatric sciences in Britain, suicide played an important role. If this, as we have seen before, was also the case in France, specific to Britain was the public dimension of the suicide debate from the eighteenth century onwards. Historian of suicide George Minois has therefore argued that,

> [t]he English attitude was diametrically opposed to the French one. Suicide was news in England. It was given full coverage in the newspapers, and it received abundant commentary, a habit that did much to secularize and normalize suicide. The extraordinary growth of the press helped create more open, more liberal ways of thinking that were very different from the ones that predominated on the Continent.[79]

Similarly, Michael MacDonald has observed that '[t]he press made suicide a much more public event than it had been before; the newspapers in particular became the principal means of learning about such deaths', and '[t]he ways in which suicide was depicted in the press helped to foster a more secular and tolerant view of the act'.[80] As MacDonald's works show, reports on suicides could be found everywhere and in various forms in London newspapers among other 'casualties'.[81] This explains the prominent reproduction of Lovat's case in *The Pamphleteer* and other magazines.

British physicians, although they clearly fostered medical explanations of suicide, frequently tried to benefit from the sensational dimension of suicide cases when addressing a broader readership. *Bentley's Miscellany*, a literary magazine issued by the London printer Richard Bentley from 1837 onwards and edited, among others, by Charles Dickens, provides a good example in this regard.[82] In an American copy of *Bentley's Miscellany* that was launched

---

77   R. Rylance, '"The Disturbing Anarchy of Investigation": Psychological Debate and the Victorian Periodical', in L. Henson *et al.* (eds.), *Culture and Science in the Nineteenth-Century Media*, London, British Library, 2009, 239 and 241.
78   Ibid., 249.
79   Minois, *History of Suicide*, 293.
80   MacDonald and Murphy, *Sleepless Souls,* see the chapter 'The Medium and the Message', 301–337, especially 302f.
81   Ibid., 305f.
82   C. Dickens, W.H. Ainsworth, and A. Smith (eds.), *Bentley's Miscellany*, vol. 1, London, Richard Bentley, 1837.

in New York in 1839, the British army surgeon John Gideon Millingen featured Lovat's case in an article called 'Remarkable suicides'.[83] Millingen was also the author of a book called *Curiosities of Medical Experience* that had been published in the same year with Bentley in London.[84] As the title suggests, he was eager to communicate news from the realm of medical science to a lay audience. Accordingly, his brief summary of Lovat's case ends with the somewhat didactic comment: 'Had this man died, the verdict should certainly have been insanity, brought on by religious delusions'.[85] This example demonstrates that medical British authors readily published medical case histories in publications that they themselves explicitly saw as non-scientific. Adapting authentic case histories from the realm of science for a literary readership was a trend that was also prevalent in the German context.

The boundaries between the British and the American bookmarket were also fluid. This is signalled most clearly by *The Popular Science Monthly*, an American periodical that was founded in 1872 with the explicit intention of communicating scientific knowledge to a lay public.[86] This publication, as already *Bentley's Miscellany*, indicates that Lovat's case easily travelled from Britain to America to continue its journey overseas. The article by a certain Charles W. Pilgrim not only demonstrates that Lovat's case, by the last quarter of the century, had become a canonical example of an extraordinary suicide in both British and American publications, it also demonstrates that English-speaking authors had started to reflect on the history of Lovat's case itself. In his 'Study of Suicide', Pilgrim wrote that '[a]nother very deliberate attempt, probably the most extraordinary ever known, was that made by an Italian shoemaker, named Matthew Lovat. This case was originally reported by Dr. Bergierre [sic!], afterward enlarged upon by Dr. Winslow in his "Anatomy of Suicide", and has since been frequently quoted by various writers'.[87] Here again, the reference to medical authorities who had worked on the case before allows the author to confirm the importance of the case as well as to signal his membership of a specific interpretive community.

83 C. Dickens, W.H. Ainsworth, and A. Smith (eds.), *Bentley's Miscellany*, vol. 4, New York, Jemima M. Mason, 1839.

84 J.G. Millingen, *Curiosities of Medical Experience*, London, Richard Bentley, 1839.

85 J.G. Millingen, '*Remarkable Suicides* by Dr. Millingen, the Author of "Curiosities of Medical Experience"', in C. Dickens, W.H. Ainsworth, and A. Smith (eds.), *Bentley's Miscellany*, vol. 4, New York, Jemima M. Mason, 1839, 516–528, 523.

86 W.J. Youmans (ed.), *The Popular Science Monthly*, vol. 1, New York, D. Appleton and Company, 1872.

87 C.W. Pilgrim, 'A Study of Suicide', in W.J. Youmans (ed.), *The Popular Science Monthly*, vol. 35, New York, D. Appleton and Company, 1889, 303–313, 308f.

Both the eagerness of British authors to popularise science for a broader readership and the British readership's demand for scientific information meant that a more popular appropriation of Lovat's case dominated in the British context. In particular, the notion of Lovat as an 'eccentric', as already suggested by Winslow, played an important role in a contemporary literary genre that was very successful on the British book market, the so-called 'eccentric biographies' examined in the following chapter. Rather than discussing deviant behaviour as a mental disease threatening individuals and society, this genre promoted a popular and positive recognition of social deviance under the label of 'eccentricity'.

4   Lovat's Case in the Making of *gerichtliche Medizin* in Germany

Lovat's case also became a prominent example in German medical publications on suicide. In the German-speaking world, the debate on suicide was, at least in the first half of the century, closely connected with the medical critique of religious enthusiasm. German authors increasingly regarded religious melancholy and zeal as pathological symptoms of mental disorder. Insanity, in turn, was regarded the cause of suicide. Consider an influential study on suicide entitled *Über den Selbstmord, seine Ursachen, Arten, medicinisch-gerichtliche Untersuchung und die Mittel gegen denselben*, which Friedrich Benjamin Osiander (1759–1822), professor of medicine in Göttingen, published in 1813, and in which he presented Lovat's case.[88] Offering a systematic discussion of suicide in its theological, moral, philosophical, juridical, administrative, and medical aspects, Osiander directs his book at state officials such as policemen and lawers, physicians and surgeons specialising in legal medicine, as well as psychologists and school teachers. As Vera Lind has rightly remarked, Osiander was more interested in discussing state measures to prevent suicide than in proposing individual therapies.[89] His study therefore explores the presence and significance of suicide on both the individual and the social scale, considering Europe (especially Germany and Britain), but including also other parts of the world. Essentially, Osiander identifies suicide as the final point of an illness, because, as he argues, 'a sane man does not throw away his life, thus the irrationality of the act in itself confirms his madness'.[90] Accordingly, he

---

88   F.B. Osiander, *Über den Selbstmord, seine Ursachen, Arten, medicinisch-gerichtliche Untersuchung und die Mittel gegen denselben: Eine Schrift sowohl für Policei- und Justiz-Beamte, als für gerichtliche Aerzte und Wundärzte, für Psychologen und Volkslehrer*, Hannover, Hahn, 1813.

89   Lind, *Selbstmord in der frühen Neuzeit*, 95–97.

90   Osiander, *Über den Selbstmord*, 11.

considers suicide as an expression of a contemporary social aberration, a lack of enlightenment and false ideas about religion. By giving numerous examples of suicides of different nations and from different times, Osiander classifies various causes and methods of suicide.

One of the 'causes' of suicide Osiander identifies in his study is enthusiasm (*Schwärmerei*), which he describes as a medical problem.[91] According to Osiander, the false desire for God, the longing for beatitude and salvation could in many cases lead to the most terrible consequence of murder and suicide.[92] To illustrate his argument, Osiander reminds the reader of the frequency of self-murder in the history of monastic life and he also mentions cases in which people killed someone else just in order to receive the death penalty. Osiander concludes that mysticism in general leads to eccentrics.[93] He puts enthusiasm on the same level with mania, melancholy and hypochondria, which shows that for him, it was a medical term.[94] Lovat's case is presented in a subchapter on 'different ways to commit suicide'.[95] Firstly, Osiander calls self-crucifixion the 'most seldom, most curious, most sophisticated and most artful' way of suicide. He then introduces Lovat's case by recalling that the idea of restraining desires and passions was inherent in Christendom since its inception. In Osiander's view, Lovat outdid all precedent attempts in his radical attack on his own desires.[96] It is clear that in his narrative of Lovat's case, Osiander adopts several of the comments Schlegel had made in his German translation of it. Like Schlegel, he believes in a causal relation between Lovat's trade and his mental disorder, stating that 'he chose shoemaking as a trade, which before and after Jacob Böhm [sic!] created various enthusiasts [*Schwärmer*], and which also made poor Lovat into an enthusiast and a fool'.[97] Shoemakers tended to be enthusiasts, which in turn was linked to madness and suicide. Again, the critique of enthusiasm is directly connected with insanity and suicide, and combined with a critique of workers' diseases. Osiander's reference to the Protestant natural philosopher and mystic Jakob Böhme (1575–1624) is telling. Because of his writings, orthodox Lutherans considered Böhme a heretic.[98] So there is again a notion of heresy associated with Lovat's case – as

---

91   Ibid., 65–68.
92   Ibid., 65.
93   Ibid., 343.
94   Ibid., 66.
95   Ibid., 90.
96   Ibid.
97   Ibid., 191: '[...] er wählte daher das Schuhmacherhandwerk, das vor und nach Jacob Böhm [sic!], dem schwärmerischen Schuster in Görlitz, manchen Schwärmer erzeugte, und auch den armen Lovat zum Schwärmer und Narren machte'.
98   F.W. Bautz, 'Böhme, Jacob, Mystiker und Naturphilosoph', in F.W. Bautz (ed.), *Biographisch-Bibliographisches Kirchenlexikon*, vol. 1, Hamm, Traugott Bautz, 1990, 661–665.

we have seen before, Origen was another important figure traditionally associated with heresy and linked to Lovat's self-castration. In his conclusion, Osiander contrasts religious enthusiasm and 'reasonable' religion. He puts forward his view that in all ages, religious enthusiasm has brought about voluntary suffering and defiance of death, but the 'cold religion of reason has never risked its life in order to confirm its dogma'.[99] As this comments suggest, physicians frequently associated enthusiasm with uncontrolled and 'warm' passions, as opposed to an enlightened, reasonable religion which, by contrast, they associated with cold blood.[100] Similarly, in his study on suicide from the standpoint of psychology, the German physician Carl August Diez refers several times to Lovat's case to illustrate characteristic traits and behaviour of suicides caused by religious enthusiasm. According to Diez, enthusiasts frequently display an aversion to their sexual organs and this is why they tend to self-destructive acts such as self-mutilation and ultimately suicide.[101]

As these examples show, religious enthusiasm was important in the German suicide debate because it was considered one of the many psychological causes of suicide and a characteristic trait of many suicides. Osiander's book was broadly received in the German-speaking debate on suicide, not only by physicians but also by theologians, who were likewise concerned with dealing with suicide. In 1837 Ferdinand Friedrich Zyro, professor of theology in Bern, published a study on suicide entitled *Wissenschaftlich-praktische Beurtheilung des Selbstmords nach allen seinen Beziehungen als Lebensspiegel für unsere Zeit*.[102] Inspired by Osiander's book, Zyro reviewed Lovat's case in his second chapter on 'the sources and causes of suicide'.[103] The author lists 21 different causes of suicide, ranging from madness, illness, masturbation, crapulence, loneliness, desperation, misfortune and a broken heart up to excessive intellectual effort.

---

99   Osiander, *Über den Selbstmord*, 195: 'Dergleichen Verweise von Todesverachtung und selbstgewählten Leiden hat die religiöse Schwärmerei in allen Zeitaltern aufgestellt; aber nie hat die kalte Vernunft-Religion zu Begründung ihrer Lehre sich selbst in Lebensgefahr gewagt'.

100   For another example see for instance J.H. Hoffbauer, 'Welches sind die Ursachen der in neuerer Zeit so sehr überhand nehmenden Selbstmorde und welche Mittel sind zu deren Verhütung anzuwenden?', in A. Erlenmeyr *et al.* (eds.), *Archiv der Deutschen Gesellschaft für Psychiatrie und gerichtliche Psychologie*, vol. 2, Neuwied, J.H. Heuser, 1859, 1–138, 15: 'Die Seele des Selbstmörders kurz vor und während der That ist verstimmt, und tödtet sich nie ein Mensch mit kaltem Blute'.

101   C.A. Diez, *Der Selbstmord, seine Ursachen und Arten vom Standpunkte der Psychologie und der Erfahrung*, Tübingen, In der Laubb'schen Buchhandlung, 1838, 53, 67f., 165, and 296.

102   F.F. Zyro, *Wissenschaftlich-praktische Beurtheilung des Selbstmords nach allen seinen Beziehungen als Lebensspiegel für unsere Zeit*, Bern, Chur and Leipzig, J.F.J. Dalp, 1837.

103   Ibid., 122–145.

Enthusiasm, 'whether of political, religious or romantic nature' also forms part of the list.[104] Surprisingly, however, we find Lovat's case not in this category, but classified among the eighth cause, which is a sedentary way of life.[105] Like Schlegel in his German translation and Hoffbauer in his essay, Zyro promotes the medical view that too much sitting, as required by several trades, brings about hypochondria and melancholy. He presumes that this is the reason why shoemakers are often enthusiasts, and he cites Lovat's self-mutilation and attempted self-crucifixion as an outstanding example:

> A sedentary lifestyle and a lack of necessary physical work, while eating and drinking abundantly, easily produces disorder in the digestive system, inducing hypchondria and melancholy. This is why we frequently find shoemakers and tailors who dedicate themselves to exaggerated views of life and enthusiastic feelings. Such as has been the case with Matthias Lovat of Belluno in Venetia, a shoemaker, who in 1802 cut off his testicles with a shoemaker's knife, and crucified himself in the most painful way in 1806.[106]

Zyro concludes that suicide does not fit into the categories of other crimes since it is an action of a very different nature, namely one that deserves pity and absolution because at its origin, it is a 'real illness' or a 'sick mood'.[107] Zyro's extensive use of medical opinions shows quite plainly to what extent the medical critique of enthusiasm was adopted even by theologians in the German suicide debate.

As a famous suicide case, the narrative of Lovat's self-crucifixion also featured prominently in professional discussions about the introduction of a legal medicine in the German states. Since the eighteenth century, physicians

---

104   Ibid., 140–143.
105   Ibid., 129.
106   Ibid.: 'Sitzende Lebensart und Mangel an der nöthigen Bewegung, bei gut essen und trinken, erzeugt leicht Unordnung in dem Verdauungsgeschäft, woraus Hypochondrie und Schwermuth hervorgeht. Daher auch kömmt es, daß man so oft Schuster und Schneider findet, welche sich überspannten Lebensansichten und schwärmerischen Gefühlen hingeben. So vor Allen Matthias Lovat von Belluno im Venetianischen, ein Schuster, der sich i. J. 1802 mit seinem Schustermesser die pudenda wegschnitt, und i. J. 1806 sich auf die martervollste Weise selber kreuzigte'.
107   Ibid., 152: 'Und so ist denn offenbar / daß wir den Selbstmord nicht in die Kategorie der übrigen Verbrechen stellen können/ sondern daß er eine Uebelthat ganz eigener Art ist/ die um so eher unser Mitleid und unsere Entschuldigung verdient/ als sie aus einer wirklichen Krankheit oder krankhaften Stimmung hervorgegangen ist'.

had tried to promote their competence in the domain of law, and to establish a specialised medical discipline, called in German *Gerichtliche Medizin*.[108] Shortly after its publication in 1807, Schlegel's translation of Ruggieri case history had been advertised in several German publications as an interesting suicide case to consider within this specialist debate. For instance, it was discussed with a short summary in the *Jahrbuch der Staatsarzneykunde* under the category *Gerichtliche Medizin*[109] as well as in the *Kritische Jahrbücher der Staatsarzneykunde für das 19. Jahrhundert*, which announced Lovat's case under the same category.[110] In the *Annalen der Staats-Arzneikunde* published in 1840, Lovat's case was cited next to that of Margarethe Peter in an article providing 'instruction for forensic doctors, when they examine and evaluate diseases of suicides'.[111] These and other medico-legal publications on suicide demonstrate the growing desire of German physicians to put suicide on a scientific basis as an object of legal medicine. In systematic studies on suicide, they tried to register and categorise different ways of commiting suicide. Self-crucifixion is categorised as an an extreme and very rare form of suicide, and Lovat is frequently cited as the most prominent example. The author of the article published in the *Annalen der Staats-Arzneikunde* for instance writes, 'Self-crucifixion happens very rarely; and if it does, one must ask if it was really intended as a self-murder. The first elaborated history of a self-crucifixion is about a Venetian, Lovat. This was a hypochondriac, fanatic shoemaker who suffered from pellagra and had already cut off his genitals [...]'.[112]

---

108 On the involvement of physicians in eighteenth- and nineteenth-century law see I. Müller *et al.*, 'Protokolle des Unsichtbaren: Visa reperta in der gerichtsmedizinischen Praxis des 18. und 19. Jahrhunderts', in R. Behrens, N. Bischoff, and C. Zelle (eds.), *Der ärztliche Fallbericht. Epistemische Grundlagen und textuelle Strukturen dargestellter Beobachtung*, Wiesbaden, Harrassowitz, 2012, 36–62; Lorenz, *'Er ließe doch nicht nach biß er was angefangen'*. See also the classic study by E. Fischer-Homberger, *Medizin vor Gericht: Gerichtsmedizin von der Renaissance bis zur Aufklärung. Mit 70 illustrierenden Fallbeispielen, zusammengestellt von Cécile Ernst*, Bern, Hans Huber, 1983.

109 J.H. Kopp (ed.), *Jahrbuch der Staatsarzneykunde*, vol. 1, Frankfurt, Bei Johann Christian Hermann, 1808, 449f.

110 C. Knape and A.F. Hecker, *Kritische Jahrbücher der Staatsarzneikunde für das 19. Jahrhundert*, Berlin, Bei Friedrich Maurer, 1809, Lovat's case is on 318–320.

111 F.C.K. Krügelstein, 'Agende zum Gebrauch für Gerichtsärzte bei Untersuchung und Begutachtung der Krankheit der Selbstmörder. Nach eignen und fremden Beobachtungen und Erfahrungen bearbeitet', *Annalen der Staats-Arzneikunde*, vol. 5, no. 1, 1840, 673–775, 727.

112 Ibid.: 'Die Selbstkreuzigung kommt nur selten vor und dann ist noch die Frage, ob sie wirklich eine Selbsttötung zur Absicht hatte. Die erste ausführliche Geschichte einer Selbstkreuzigung ist von einem Venetianer Lovat. Dieser war ein hypochondrischer fanatischer Schuhmacher, der am Pellagra litt und sich schon die Schamtheile abgeschnitten hatte [...]'.

By the middle of the century, German legal medicine had become an established medical discipline that affirmed its authority through specialised publications. In this context, Lovat's case continued to circulate. While medical journals from the beginning of the century had reported on Lovat's self-crucifixion as a singular and remarkable case of suicide without placing it in a wider context, now the case represented a specific type of suicide caused by insanity. For instance, in a German textbook for legal medicine published in 1850, the author considers the specific way that individuals choose for their suicide attempts as an indicator for their pathological condition:

> the choice of the manner of death sometimes reveals the mental disturbance of the individual; if the manner of death is very painful, cruel, or bizarre, like, for instance the self-crucifixion of the shoemaker Lovat, then this confirms a mental disturbance.[113]

As these examples show, in the professionalising field of legal medicine in Germany, the case narrative of Lovat's self-crucifixion became doctrinal knowledge. It was gradually reduced to a short reference that allowed authors to confirm their theories about the presumed causal nexus between suicide and insanity. The same happened in the neighbouring field of German psychiatry, which also focused on suicide as an object of psychiatry. In the *Archiv der Deutschen Gesellschaft für Psychiatrie und gerichtliche Psychologie*, a journal edited by the director of a private asylum near Koblenz, Lovat is mentioned in 1859 in a list of other prominent and historical examples of suicides in a chapter on 'means and ways of committing suicide'. Even if he had not died as a result of his crucifixion attempt, he even ranks here with the legendary suicides of Cleopatra, Porcia and Dido.[114] Signalling the integration of Lovat's case into the body of common psychiatric knowledge about suicides, Wilhelm Griesinger,

---

113   B. Brach, *Lehrbuch der gerichtlichen Medizin*, Cologne, Franz Carl Eisen, 1850, 593f.: 'Auch die Wahl der Todesart gibt mitunter Aufschluss über das physische Gestörtsein des Individuums; ist die Todesart eine sehr schmerzhafte, grausame, oder eine sehr seltsame, wie z.B. die Selbstkreuzigung des Schusters Lovat, so spricht dies für psychische Störung'.

114   Hoffbauer, *Welches sind die Ursachen der in neuerer Zeit so sehr überhand nehmenden Selbstmorde*, 15: 'Der freiwillige Tod einer wollüstigen Cleopatra durch den Biss einer giftigen Natter, – der Selbstmord einer heldenmüthigen Poreia durch das Verschlucken glühender Kohlen, – die Entleibung einer gekränkten Dido durch den Scheiterhaufen, und die des venetianischen Schusters Mathieu Lovat durch eigenhändige Kreuzigung sind bekannt. Und haben sich nicht auch Viele mit eigenen Händen und Zähnen zerfleischt, bis der schmachvollste Tod sie erlöste'. We find such a listing of Lovat's case among other legendary suicides already in 1842 in a book on suicide by J.H. Hoffbauer, *Über den Selbstmord, seine Arten und Ursachen*, Lemgo, Verlag der Meyerschen Hofbuchhandlung, 1842, 77.

professor of psychiatry in Zurich, cited Lovat's case in a similar brief way in his textbook *Die Pathologie und Therapie der psychischen Krankheiten* ('Pathology and Therapy of Psychic Diseases'), published in 1861. Reflecting on suicide attempts caused by insanity, Griesinger simply states in a footnote: 'Compare the case of Matthieu Lovat who crucified himself etc.'[115]

Suicide was, however, not only an important topic in professional circles, it also provoked public debates. In the German context, the literary presentation of suicide cases had stimulated an intensive discussion of the topic in nineteenth-century popular print media as well as in literature. Famous examples are Goethe's novel *Die Leiden des jungen Werther* (1774) and the *Biographien der Selbstmörder* (1785–1789) published by the German writer Christian Heinrich Spieß, author of many other works of light fiction.[116] While the story of *Werther* appeared in the genre of an epistolary novel, Spieß's book presented a collection of suicide cases oscillating between authenticity and fiction. Thanks to these and other works, suicide, traditionally a taboo, became a vogue topic with German writers and editors who sought to educate and entertain a broader readership. Journals that explicitly aimed at 'literary entertainment' regularly featured case histories about suicides. In 1845, for instance, the *Blätter für literarische Unterhaltung* ('Journal for Literary Entertainment') included Lovat's case in a long article on the history and the moral implications of suicide, as a famous example of self-murder caused by *Schwärmerei*.[117] Among many other case narratives that reported on murders, criminals and suicides, the narrative of Lovat's self-crucifixion allowed the editors of such journals to attract a broader educated readership, and to satisfy a growing anthropological interest in human nature.

The previous chapters have shown how the narrative of Lovat's self-crucifixion attempt attracted the interest of different professionals which formed different 'interpretive communities' of Lovat's case. The boundaries between these disciplinary debates were extremely fluid in early nineteenth-century Europe, and much depended on the specific medium and interpretive

---

115   W. Griesinger, *Die Pathologie und Therapie der psychischen Krankheiten*, Stuttgart, A. Krabbe, 1861, 258: 'Vgl. [...] den Fall des Matthieu Lovat, der sich selbst kreuzigte etc'.

116   C.H. Spieß, *Biographien der Selbstmörder*, ed. A. Košenina, Göttingen, Wallstein, 2005. Spieß also published the *Biographien der Wahnsinnigen*, Leipzig, Voß , 1796. On Spieß see Pethes, *Zöglinge der Natur*, 278.

117   K. Hohnbaum, 'Der Selbstmord', in *Blätter für literarische Unterhaltung, Erster Band*, Leipzig, F.A. Brockhaus, 1845. The article 'On suicide' begins with no. 113, 23 April 1845, 453–455: 'Der Selbstmord. Die Liebe zum Leben hat der Mensch mit allen übrigen Geschöpfen der Erde gemein [...]'. Lovat is mentioned in no. 114, 24 April 1845, 458 ('Überspannung der Gefühle und Schwärmerei').

framework in which Lovat's case was published. What the professional readings described so far have in common is that they all had primarily a cognitive purpose: almost all of the cited authors appropriated Lovat's case because they were convinced that, for one reason or another, Lovat's case would speak to the scientific field to which they sought to contribute with their publications. Within the described interpretive communities, Lovat's individual case essentially functioned as one piece of a puzzle that helped to answer unsolved scientific questions and to contribute to the making of different bodies of scientific knowledge.

CHAPTER 7

Popular Readings: Moral Education through Literary Entertainment

Parallel to its circulation in scientific debates, the narrative of Lovat's self-crucifixion transcended the realms of science and was disseminated through various popular publications. These publications, ranging from newspapers and periodicals to review journals and books, did not address specific professional observers, like the ones examined before. Instead, they sought to reach a much broader reading public. This chapter describes how Lovat's case travelled from the medical context into the field of journalism and literary debates and, by travelling within literary genres, to a great extent lost its epistemic functions. As mentioned in the introduction to this book, focusing on the popular readings in a separate chapter, I am not arguing that there is a clear-cut distinction between epistemic and literary genres. It is clear that the professional readings of Lovat's case influenced the lay reception in several ways and vice versa. However, considering the different goals which editors and authors pursued with Lovat's case in popular publications, this focus allows us to recognize exactly the permeable boundaries of genres and their dynamics between different readerships.

Whether Lovat's case was understood as a serious contribution to a specific body of scientific knowledge or rather as a piece of literature depended on the one hand on how it was framed. The publications where the narrative appeared themselves followed the conventions of certain genres which had an impact on readers' expectations. *How* readers encountered and read Lovat's case was therefore conditioned by the specific medium in which the case was included. On the other hand, it also depended on the readers' individual interest in the case. As in the case of the professional readings, the popular readings can be distinguished in different interpretive communities, as editors and authors were interested in different aspects of Lovat's case, with religion, madness and suicide remaining the main themes. These were topics that editors and literary writers had dealt with extensively since the late eighteenth century. Narratives concerning these themes spoke to nineteenth-century readers because they potentially concerned everyone. Reading about deviance from socially accepted norms was both threatening and reassuring for readers. What distinguishes popular readings of Lovat's case from professional discussions described above is, therefore, not so much the topics that were associated with

© KONINKLIJKE BRILL NV, LEIDEN, 2019 | DOI:10.1163/9789004353602_009

it, but the different goal editors and writers pursued. Instead of the formation of a specific body of knowledge, narratives such as Lovat's self-crucifixion were meant to morally educate the readership through literary entertainment and were used to shape certain views, values and attitudes concerning deviance and norm in specific cultural and national contexts. Last but not least, the popular readings of Lovat's case reveal how the narrative served the aims of nineteenth-century popular journalism.

1   Lovat's Case in German Literary Journals

Due to Schlegel's effective networking, reviews and summaries of his German translation from 1807 soon appeared in various literary journals that aimed at the amusement and moral instruction of a literate readership. Although these journals were published in the early nineteenth century, they convey the spirit of older journals produced at the time of the German Enlightenment. For instance, Schlegel's translation was advertised with a review in the *Jenaische Allgemeine Literaturzeitung* in April 1808. Demonstrating the attention to Lovat's case in literary circles, the review was written by Christian August Vulpius, the brother of Goethe's wife Christiane, who was a librarian in Weimar.[1] In his review, Vulpius accentuates Lovat's self-mutilation and depicts the 'hero' of the narrative as a man who 'exceeds all legends'. With a certain irony he remarks that even saints like Saint Franciscus – 'with the exception of Origen' – would have to admit that Lovat's way of combating carnal desire was the most effective: 'Who combats his enemy in this way and who is able to extirpate the roots of the evil in such a hearty way is worth asking: What kind of man was he [Lovat]?'[2]

Similarly, in 1809 an abridged version of Schlegel's translation appeared in the magazine *Minerva*.[3] It was entitled 'Lovat. A Great Contribution to the

---

1   C.A. Vulpius, 'Geschichte der durch Mathieu Lovat zu Venedig im Jahr 1805 an sich selbst vollzogenen Kreuzigung, bekannt gemacht von Cesar Ruggieri ... Aus dem Französischen übersetzt und mit Anmerkungen versehen von Julius Heinrich Gottlieb Schlegel ...', *Jenaische Allgemeine Literaturzeitung*, vol. 93, 1808, 134.

2   Ibid.: 'So grossen Respect er auch vor den Heiligen, in Rücksicht der Art und Weise, gewisse Begierden zu bekämpfen, haben mochte: So werden doch dieselben, selbst der heil. Franciscus, trotz seinen Schnee- und Dornen-Experimenten, (den heil. Origenes ausgenommen) gestehen müssen, M. Lovat sey dem Übel, mit grosser Herzhaftigkeit, geradezu auf den Grund gekommen [...]. Wer seinem Feinde so zu begegnen, und die Wurzel des Übels so herzhaft auszurotten weiß, der verdient, daß man wenigstens – fragt: Welch ein Mensch war er – ?'

3   J.W. von Archenholz, 'Lovat. Ein großer Beytrag zur Verirrung des menschlichen Geistes', *Minerva. Ein Journal historischen und politischen Inhalts*, no. 2, 1809, 97–102.

Aberrations of the Human Mind', and emphasised the singularity and the in-credible sophistication of Lovat's actions. The author claims that 'the legends of saints and self-martyrs, up to Simeon Stylites who lived on a pillar for thirty years, contain nothing comparable to this well-thought off action',[4] and he calls Lovat's self-crucifixion 'an extraordinary, fabulous, virtuous incident'.[5] He assures that the narrative was not a fairytale.[6] In a slightly modified version, two more German journals picked up Schlegel's translation in 1811, the impor-tant *Morgenblatt für gebildete Staende*,[7] and, in the identical version, the *Archiv für Geographie, Historie, Staats- und Kriegskunst* published in Vienna.[8] Here, Lovat's case is presented as a rather entertaining 'miraculous' and 'pitiable' ex-ample of exaggerated 'religious melancholy'. Explicitly, it is 'the horrific and the extraordinary character of the act' (*das Schreckliche und Außerordentliche der That*) that was expected to attract and to instruct readers.[9]

Altogether, these examples suggest that editors of German Enlightened journals included Lovat's case first and foremost because of its sensationalist potential. In the eyes of the editors, the narrative of Lovat's self-emasculation and self-crucifixion had everything needed to stimulate the readers' sensation-alist curiosity, which was induced by reading about horrible, painful and cruel incidents.[10] For this purpose, editors used various literary devices and narra-tive techniques to enhance the dramatic and popular potential of Lovat's case. For instance, they told the story in the present tense, focused on the develop-ment of Lovat's character, emphasised its singularity, and compared it with

---

4   Ibid., 97: 'Die Legenden der Heiligen und Selbstmärtyrer bis zu Simon Stilita hinauf, der dreyßig Jahre auf einer Säule lebte, haben nichts Aehnliches aufzuweisen, als diese über-dachte Handlung [...]'.

5   Ibid., 98: '[...] ein sehr ausserordentliches, fabelhaftes, sittliches Ereignis, daß gewiß ganz einzig in seiner Art, unter den größten Verirrungen des menschlichen Geistes einen aus-gezeichneten Platz behauptet'.

6   Ibid., 101: '[...] da man sonst geneigt seyn könnte, das Ganze für ein Mährchen zu halten'.

7   Anonymous, 'Lovats Selbstkreuzigung', *Morgenblatt für gebildete Staende*, 23 September 1811, 910.

8   Anonymous, 'Lovats Selbstkreuzigung', *Archiv für Geographie, Historie, Staats-und Krieg-skunst*, 6 and 8 November 1811, 563.

9   Anonymous, *Lovats Selbstkreuzigung*, 910: 'Das Schreckliche und Außerordentliche der That, welche wir erzählen wollen, und die Seltenheit der Schrift worin die Details ent-halten sind, bestimmen uns, das Ganze mit aller Umständlichkeit anzuführen. Mathäus Lovat, ein Schuster in Venedig, ist ein eben so wunderbares, wie beweinenswerthes Beispiel religiöser auf den höchsten Grad gestiegener Melancholie'.

10   On this sensationalist 'joy of grief' (Lust am Grauen), which is a category from the eighteenth-century German discourse on the aesthetics of *Das Erhabene*, see A. Košenina, 'Von Bedlam nach Steinhof. Irrenhausbesuche in der Frühen Neuzeit und Moderne', *Zeitschrift Für Germanistik. Neue Folge*, vol. 17, 2007, 322–339, 322.

Biblical and legendary tales. The references to the legends of saints served to emphasise that Lovat's deeds were even more bizarre than those of famous Christian martyrs. At the same time, these references reveal a certain irony in the description of Lovat's case. Indirectly, the editors suggest that such an extreme way of practising religion was anachronistic, not to be taken seriously and contrary to an Enlightened understanding of religion.

Nevertheless, it was important for editors to assure their readers of the authenticity, i.e. the historical truth, of Lovat's case. One anonymous author of a review published in the *Allgemeine Literatur-Zeitung* claimed that,

> The story told in this little pamphlet may seem too fantastic to be have been invented. This implausibility, however, will soon disappear before the eyes of the attentive reader. For not only are all circumstances reported in the greatest detail, time and place precisely documented, and not only is everything told by a well-known informant, but the communication of all the individual circumstances and how they interrelate give the narrative a stamp of credibility, which, even if it was not so detailed, would eliminate every doubt about its historical truth.[11]

This comment shows that, notwithstanding the frequent emphasis on 'historical truth', editors believed that it was more important that the case narrative of Lovat's self-crucifixion was plausible, that it seemed authentic in the eyes of the readers. In his examination of the popular genre of eighteenth-century criminal case narratives, Alexander Košenina has stated that they typically oscillated between fact and fiction, that is, between historical documentation and literary adaptation. Authors considered plausibility more important than reality, and the 'psychological causality' of a narrative was more important than the sources it relied on.[12] This is also true for the appropriations of Lovat's case by editors of literary journals.

---

11   Anonymous, 'Geschichte der durch Mathieu Lovat zu Venedig im Jahr 1805 an sich selbst vollzogenen Kreuzigung, bekannt gemacht von Cesar Ruggieri ... Aus dem Französischen übersetzt und mit Anmerkungen versehen von Julius Heinrich Gottlieb Schlegel ...', *Allgemeine Literatur-Zeitung*, vol. 3, no. 355, 1808, 805–807, 805f.: 'Diese in dieser kleinen Schrift erzählte Geschichte ist zu unwahrscheinlich, als dass sie erdichtet seyn könnte. Jene Unwahrscheinlichkeit verschwindet indessen bald vor den Augen des aufmerksamen Lesers. Denn nicht allein sind alle Umstände mit der größten Genauigkeit angegeben, Zeit und Ort auf das genaueste bestimmt, und nicht allein ist alles von einem nahmhaften Gewährsmann erzählt; sondern auch die einzelnen Umstände und ihr Zusammenhang geben der Erzählung eine innere Beglaubigung, die, auch wenn die Erzählung nicht so detailliert wäre, alle Zweifel an ihrer historischen Wahrheit aufheben müsste'.

12   Košenina, *Literarische Anthropologie*, 57 and 61.

By enhancing its sensationalist potential in this way, editors ultimately used Lovat's case in the framework of the specific journals to engage with an increasing anthropological interest in human nature, which had emerged during the eighteenth century both at a professional and the popular level. In various ways, the literary adaptations of Lovat's case served to explore one fundamental question, namely: what sort of people are able to commit such cruel crimes against themselves, and why would they do it? Such an interest in the psychological nature of humans was central to the anthropological discourse that characterises German literary production in the eighteenth and early nineteenth century, which scholars of German literature commonly refer to as 'literary anthropology'.[13] In various genres, writers concentrated on the psychological exploration of individuals through literary writing, and case narratives such as Lovat's played a fundamental role in this context.

2   Lovat's Case as a Historical *cause célèbre*

The broader context for the circulation of Lovat's case in the German literary market is that case narratives from the realm of science became increasingly popular with a broader literate readership. The most prominent example of this tendency from the late eighteenth century is Karl Philipp Moritz's Enlightened empirical psychology (1783–1793), which is often cited as the beginning of psychological medicine and, by some literary scholars, even as the 'birthplace of the psychological' case history.[14] From 1783 onwards, Moritz edited a journal entitled *Gnothi Sauton, oder Magazin für Erfahrungsseelenkunde für Gelehrte und Ungelehrte* ('Know Thyself, or a Magazine for empirical Psychology for Scholars and Laymen'), in which he announced a programme of examining and describing mental disturbances.[15] Moritz's *Magazin* was the first German journal in which physicians, jurists, teachers, state officials, theologians and

---

13   On 'literary anthropology' see ibid. and N. Pethes, *Zöglinge der Natur. Der literarische Menschenversuch des 18. Jahrhunderts*, Göttingen, Wallstein, 2007.

14   Gailus, *A Case of Individuality*, 69; Michael Shepherd, *Psychiatric Journals*. Considering early modern medical case histories in which physicians consistently put much attention on the psychological conditions of patients, this label is too simplifying. On psychological themes in early modern case histories see for instance M. Kutzer, 'Liebeskranke Magd, tobsüchtiger Mönch, schwermütiger Handelsherr: "Psychiatrie" in den Observationes und Curationes des niederländischen "Hippokrates" Pieter van Foreest (1522–1592)', *Medizinhistorisches Journal*, vol. 30, no. 3, 1995, 245–273.

15   See the collective volume edited by Dickson, Goldman and Wingertszahn, *'Fakta, und kein moralisches Geschwätz'*.

philosophers as well as lay people were invited to publish individual reports about deviant and criminal individuals and their psychological motives, as well as about afflictions they experienced themselves.[16] These narratives dealt with a great variety of themes and were presented in various text genres, both epistemic and literary.[17] Taking into account the 'criss-crossing of a number of professional discourses' in Moritz's magazine, Gailus rightly concludes that '[t]he genre of the psychological case history did not emerge from the simple extension of medical discourse to mental problems but from the complex crossings of medical thought, (auto)biographical traditions, and juridical narratives'.[18]

The *Magazin für Erfahrungsseelenkunde* played a pioneering role in promoting the case history as a popular form of writing in the German-speaking context. As Yvonne Wübben has shown, Moritz's work as an editor essentially consisted in textual revisions. In order to 'derive knowledge from the particular'[19] and to stimulate 'reasoning in cases', he reworked other genres, in particular medical reports, and presented them in the form of a case narrative with the purpose of making particular knowledge fit a rule, that is to generalise from individual observations.[20] Moritz was not the only one to see the potential of authentic case reports from different fields of knowledge. In the following decades, several German writers used juridical and medical cases as a basis for their 'criminal narratives' (*Kriminalgeschichten*), which presented cases of crime, madness and suicide. Addressing a broader lay readership, these narratives were meant to explore the human soul and to thereby teach moral lessons. The genre of *Kriminalgeschichten* was very successful in the German book trade.[21] An early example of this trend is a collection with the telling title *Kriminalgeschichten* published by the Berlin lawyer Karl Müchler in 1792.[22] An example of a more famous literary adaptation of an authentic juridical case – as also emphasised in the title – is Friedrich Schiller's successful short

---

16   See the editors' preface in ibid., 7f.
17   See Wübben, *Writing Cases and Casuistic Reasoning*, 472.
18   Gailus, *A Case of Individuality*, 73.
19   Wübben, *Writing Cases and Casuistic Reasoning*, 485.
20   Ibid., 483.
21   A. Košenina, 'Schiller und die Tradition der (kriminal)psychologischen Fallgeschichte bei Goethe, Meißner, Moritz und Spieß', in A. Stašková (ed.), *Friedrich Schiller und Europa: Ästhetik, Politik, Geschichte*, Heidelberg, Winter, 2007, 119–139. See also the criminal narratives by A.G. Meißner, *Ausgewählte Kriminalgeschichten. Mit einem Nachwort von Alexander Košenina*, St. Ingbert, Röhrig, 2003, and the editorial comment by Košenina, 91–112.
22   K. Müchler, *Kriminalgeschichten. Aus gerichtlichen Akten gezogen (1792). Mit einem Nachwort herausgegeben von Alexander Košenina*, Hannover, Wehrhahn, 2011.

story *Verbrecher aus verlohrener Ehre. Eine wahre Geschichte* (1792).[23] With such publications, German writers clearly drew on the early modern tradition of publishing sensational legal cases.[24] However, rather than describing primarily the criminal actions and the punishments, as the early modern crime reports had done, they put a stronger focus on the individual characters, that is, the biographies and psychological motives of criminals.[25]

This emerging publishing context helps to explain why, in 1844, Lovat's case appeared in a collection of crime stories entitled *Der neue Pitaval*.[26] The title relates to an important European tradition of publishing collections of juridical case narratives. Between 1735 and 1745, the French jurist Francois Gayot de Pitaval had published his famous *Causes célèbres et intéressantes* in 20 volumes.[27] As the title suggests, the cases presented in this work claimed to be authentic as they derived directly from legal practice. At the same time, they tried to appeal to a broader public in that they focused primarily on the biographies and the psychological motives of the protagonists.[28] Gayot's work influenced the development of the literary production in Germany.[29] Friedrich Schiller wrote the preface to the German translation of Gayot's *Pitaval* in 1795, reflecting the great interest of German writers in criminal cases and in the republication of earlier case collections.[30] Ever since, German writers have continued to publish collections of modern criminal cases under the title *Pitaval*.[31]

Published in the middle of the nineteenth century, *Der neue Pitaval* in which Lovat's case appeared kept close to the model of Gayot's *Causes célèbres*

---

23   The narrative is included in the book, F. Schiller, *Der Geisterseher, Erzählungen und historische Charakteristiken*, Stuttgart, Reclam, 1958. The work had been published already in 1786 under the title *Der Verbrecher aus Infamie, eine wahre Geschichte*.

24   Wiltenburg, *True Crime*.

25   A. Košenina, 'Recht-gefällig. Frühneuzeitliche Verbrechensdarstellung zwischen Dokumentation und Unterhaltung', *Zeitschrift für Germanistik Neue Folge*, vol. 15, no. 1, 2005, 28–47, 29.

26   J.E. Hitzig and W. Häring (eds.), *Der neue Pitaval. Eine Sammlung der interessantesten Criminalgeschichten aller Länder aus älterer und neuerer Zeit*, vol. 6, Leipzig, Brockhaus, 1844. Lovat's case is on 283–295.

27   F.G. de Pitaval, *Causes célèbres et intéressantes, avec les jugements qui les ont decidées*, La Haye, J. Neaulme, 1735–1745. For the German translation see Pethes, *Zöglinge der Natur*, 271.

28   Ibid.

29   Košenina, *Fallgeschichten*, 283.

30   F.G. de Pitaval, *Merkwürdige Rechtsfälle als ein Beitrag zur Geschichte der Menschheit nach dem französischen Werk des Pitaval durch mehrere Verfasser ausgearbeitet und mit einer Vorrede begleitet, herausgegeben von Schiller*, Jena, Cuno, 1792–1795.

31   See for instance K. Herrmann, A. Levèvre, and R. Wolff (eds.), *Neuköllner Pitaval. Wahre Kriminalgeschichten aus Berlin*, Hamburg, Rotbuch, 1994.

but put a new emphasis on psychology. *Der neue Pitaval* was a large editorial project of 60 volumes, published over 20 years, that promised in its title to offer a collection 'of the most interesting criminal cases from all countries and from ancient and modern times'.[32] The editors Julius Eduard Hitzig and Georg Wilhelm Heinrich Häring were both lawyers by education. The first served at the Berlin Superior Court of Justice, edited professional journals and was a member of literary societies, while the latter was a novelist.[33] Nevertheless, they presented themselves as 'historians', and as such their aim was 'to collect and provide original material for criminologists, psychologists and historians', so that these would not need to go back to the sources themselves.[34] Explicitly, they hoped to shed light on the 'dark regions of horror' in order to satisfy legal, historical and psychological interests.[35]

Hitzig's and Häring's understanding of *Kriminalgeschichten* appears rather broad. Along with crime reports that related to formal legal procedures, they explicitly include cases of a general anthropological interest that had no legal consequences[36] in order to reflect on 'unusual developments in the criminals' faculty of judgement' as well as on 'specific genres of crimes within one nation'.[37] In their view, their selection of cases mirrors false contemporary developments as well as individual aberrations,[38] and is therefore of great psychological interest.[39] Similar to Moritz's call for participation in the *Magazin für Erfahrungsseelenkunde*, the editors invite their readers to send interesting cases (*Fälle*) to them, but they also remind them that cases that are considered *causes célèbres* in one specific place might not necessarily be regarded as such by a broader public.[40]

---

32   Hitzig and Häring, *Der neue Pitaval*, title page.

33   Under the name Willibald Alexis, Häring was known as a German novelist.

34   Hitzig and Häring, *Der neue Pitaval*, VIf.: 'Wir sind Historiker, dieser Gesichtspunkt muß, wie wir bereits aussprachen, der vorwaltende bleiben. Es ist unsere Aufgabe, in unserer Sammlung ein möglichst vollständiges und geläutertes Malterial aller merkwürdigen und charakteristischen Verbrechen, welche Criminalprocesse hervorrifen, auch wenn der Proceß nicht die Hauptsache blieb, zu liefern, ein Material, das für die Dauer, so hoffen wir, künftigen Criminalisten, Psychologen und Geschichtsschreibern von Werth sei, und ihnen die Mühe, auf die Quellen zurückzugehen erspart'.

35   Ibid., v: 'So viele Schachte wir schon angegraben, ist doch der Reichthum des noch nicht zu Tage Geförderten in diesen dunklen Schreckensregionen immer noch sehr groß [...]'.

36   Ibid., VI.

37   Ibid.: 'Das zu ergründende Geheimnis darf dort in der ungewöhnlichen Entwickelung der Geisteskräfte eines Verebechers gesucht werden, und andererseits haben gewisse specielle Gattungen von Verbechen in einer Nation [...] einen Anspruch auf Darstellung'.

38   Ibid., VII.

39   Ibid., XII.

40   Ibid., VIII: 'Fälle, die für einen Ort und eine Provinz cause célèbres sind, sind es darum noch nicht für das größere Publikum'.

Wrongly presuming that Lovat's case had not so far been discussed in Germany, the editors base their narrative on Ruggieri's original second Italian edition. In order to testify to the historical authenticity of the case, they also publish a reproduction of the original illustration representing Lovat on the cross on the front page of the book.[41] The editors comment that already in Italy, it seemed necessary to add a picture, 'to provide evidence for the senses in order to make the unbelievable more plausible'.[42] Stating that in all ages, religious fanaticism had produced extraordinary crimes and criminals, the editors include Lovat's case under the category of 'religious fanaticism',[43] as an appendix to a section containing 'warning examples of how fanaticism and enthusiasm arise exactly in the period of the most sober Enlightenment'.[44] They describe Lovat as an enthusiast whose 'limited mental capacities focused not on the joy and consolation of Christian belief, but more and more on the confused ideas of martyrdom'.[45] Correspondingly, they call Lovat's self-mutilation an 'attack of enthusiasm'.[46] For Häring and Hitzig, Lovat was not a suicide because he was longing for pain and not for death. Like Ruggieri and several other authors, they consider Lovat's case unique not only because of his deeds, but because of the thoughtful way in which he 'carried out his assassination against his own flesh and blood', without the help of others.[47] Interestingly, the editors use the vernacular name 'Matheo von Casale', referring to Lovat's home village. Possibly because they were interested primarily in Lovat's biographical background, they sought to stress his provenance in modest circumstances and rural culture. In contrast to Hoffbauer's account, they emphasise that Lovat's attempted self-crucifixion was *not* guided by insane vanity (*Eitelkeit*), but that it was all about his *serious* desire to experience the same pain as Christ

---

41   Ibid., XIII.

42   Ibid.: 'Auch in Italien hielt man damals, um Glauben für das Unerhörte zu finden, für noethig, es durch ein Bild der vollendeten Operation den Sinnen zur Anschauung zu bringen'.

43   Ibid., 283–295.

44   Ibid., XIII: '[...] zum warnenden Beispiele, wie Fanatismus und Schwärmerei, und in ihrer aberwitzigen Gestalt, sich gerade in der Periode der nüchternsten Aufklärung geltend machen können, ja wie ein Pol vielleicht den anderen anzieht'.

45   See ibid., 284: '[...] sein beschränkter Geist fixierte sich immer mehr, nicht in der Freudigkeit und dem Troste des Christenglaubens, sondern in den trüben Vorstellungen den [sic!] Martyriums'.

46   Ibid., 285: '[...] Anfalle von Schwärmerei [...]'.

47   Ibid, 294: 'Matheo von Casale war kein Selbstmörder, denn er suchte Qualen, nicht den Tod. Auch solcher Schwärmer hat die letztere Zeit einige hervorgebracht, keinen aber, der mit gleichem Vorbedacht, so nüchtern ohne Beihilfe und Aufmunterung ähnlich fanatisierter Glaubensgenossen, und mit solcher Ausdauer das Attentat gegen sein eigen Fleisch und Blut ins Werk setzte'.

had and to imitate his crucifixion.[48] They thus consider Lovat's longing for a perfect *imitatio Christi* to be the primary motivation for his action.

Despite the emphasis on the uniqueness of Lovat's case, in *Der neue Pitaval* the narrative of Lovat's self-crucifixion fulfils a didactic function not in itself, but through its inclusion within a series of cases. Together with a second case narrative, entitled *Die beiden Christusfamilien in Jöllenbeck*,[49] it serves as an appendix to a third narrative about a criminal enthusiast, entitled *Rosenfeld. Der neue Messias in Berlin*.[50] All three narratives deal with exaggerated religious zeal and the potential of enthusiasts to establish religious sects around them. Explaining why they have put together these three cases, the authors admit that the two appendix cases do not really fit in their collection because they relate to crimes without an ensuing juridical examination. However, they justify their decision by stating that

> every phenomenon is put in the right light only by looking at analogous cases. At times when there are violent fights between a literal belief and a false belief, it is good to be reminded of the false beliefs of a former period, providing a mirror in which one can detect the aberrations of the present time.[51]

In *Der neue Pitaval*, Lovat's case thus provides one cautionary example of religious 'aberration' among many others that the editors use in order to promote rational religion and prevent criminal acts. Consistent with their self-understanding as historians, Häring and Hitzig use the case as an historical example that teaches a moral lesson for the present. Accordingly, they make a critical comment about how Lovat's case was received in Venice at the time. They remark that 'luckily, the first people who looked after Matheo were physicians and not lawyers or clerics'[52] and that

---

48   Ibid., 298.
49   Ibid., 272–282: 'Die beiden Christusfamilien zu Jöllenbeck (Als Anhang zum Vorigen.), 1768–1780'.
50   Ibid., 232–271: 'Rosenfeld. Der neue Messias in Berlin, 1726–1782'.
51   Ibid., 272f.: 'Durch analoge Fälle tritt jede Erscheinung erst in ihr rechtes Licht, und in einer Zeit, wo die heftigsten Kämpfe zwischen dem Buchstabenglauben und dem Unglauben gefochten werden, ist es nicht unangemessen, uns die religiösen Verwirrungen einer überlebten Epoche vor Augen zu rufen, ein Spiegel, in dem wir vielleicht nur mit verändertem Costüm die Verwirrungen der Gegenwart wiedersehen'.
52   Ibid., 292.

[...] Matheo von Casale did not find any devotees in Venice; nor has his death initiated the formation of a sect. At the time of the French dominion over Italy, the atmosphere in Italy was just not like that. Because of its uniqueness, this crime against oneself is even the more remarkable.[53]

The editors further assume that thirty years later, rather than declaring Lovat as a fool, people probably would have initiated a process of canonisation because Lovat's action and his healing are 'not without miracles, actually, they are maybe more miraculous than the actions of some martyrs who were actually canonised'. Apparently, the editors conclude, there was no desire for new saints in Italy in 1805.[54]

Hitzig and Häring thus undertake a historical reading of Lovat's case in its original context that implies a certain notion of secularisation and medicalisation. They observe that a broader change had taken place in the social responses to comparable cases, from a positive religious interpretation that would consider a person like Lovat a saint, to a medical perspective which would identify him as insane. Furthermore, their assumption that thirty years later Lovat would have been regarded as a saint suggests that Häring and Hitzig were well aware that, compared to the early Napoleonic period, contemporary societies in Restoration Europe saw a renaissance and revaluation of religion in various societal realms – a development that some historians have described as a 'second confessional age'.[55] This critical perspective on historical and religious change is a further dimension of the popular readings of Lovat's case. Instead of presenting the case only as a medical, legal or theological problem removed from its original context, the editors of *Der neue Pitaval* highlight the historical dimension of the narrative and focus on the social responses to Lovat's case. As the example of *Der neue Pitaval* shows quite well, Lovat's case was thus appropriated successfully in various popular publications because it corresponded to the rising demand of a broader German readership for authentic case narratives. Editors of journals and of crime stories recognised its sensationalist potential and the possibility of using Lovat's case for moral education.

---

53   Ibid., 295.
54   Ibid., 293: 'Dreißig Jahre später hätte man wahrscheinlich einen Canonisationsproceß begonnen; denn ohne Wunder war seine That und seine Rettung nicht, wunderbarer vielleicht als die mancher wirklich heilig gesprochenen Märtyrer. Aber das Italien vom Jahre 1805 hatte kein Verlangen und Bedürfnis nach neuen Heiligen'.
55   See O. Blaschke, 'Abschied von der Säkularisierungslegende. Daten zur Karrierekurve der Religion (1800–1970) im zweiten konfessionellen Zeitalter: eine Parabel', *Zeitenblicke*, vol. 5, no. 1, 2006, http://www.zeitenblicke.de/2006/1/Blaschke, (accessed 7 June 2017).

3   Lovat's Case in British Periodicals: Sensationalist Curiosity

With its very large and commercial publishing business, Britain differed from
the other European countries at the time. 'Victorian print media' has been
identified as so powerful in shaping the characteristics of the British society
in this period that scholars have even maintained that '[t]he essence of nineteenth-century Britain might indeed be defined as a move towards a society's
"Being-in-Print"'.[56] This important role of print production – in particular of
newspapers, periodicals, magazines and books – in shaping and distributing popular and scientific knowledge was a prerequisite for the circulation of
Lovat's case in Britain. In line with the increasing interest of the medical elite
in mental diseases, there was a great popular interest in social non-conformity,
in both physical and behavioural deviance. A separate genre for such 'eccentric
biographies' emerged in the first half of the nineteenth century, and for several
reasons, Lovat's case fitted well into this genre and was propagated through it.

    Rick Rylance has observed two opposing trends in medical case narratives
in Victorian medical journals.[57] On the one hand, he describes a tendency towards depersonalisation and anonymisation of patients in case reports that
are orientated towards clear diagnoses and display a language that is increasingly specialised and technical.[58] While he sees these characteristics in relation with various nineteenth-century developments in medical practice and
science associated with the general goal of professionalisation,[59] he emphasises that, on the other hand, the notion of medicine as a 'theatre' and 'spectacle'
did not vanish from medical journals. Focusing on monstrous births, lunacy,
bizarre suicides and such phenomena, many case reports are characterised
by 'the sustained and substantial presence of the bizarre, the grotesque, the
freakish, and the comical' and serve both the transmission of medical knowledge and popular entertainment.[60] For Rylance, nineteenth-century medical
cases therefore have a 'porous form'[61] in which '[...] the dividing lines between
the entertaining and the instructive, the fantastic and the enlightening, are, as

---

56   King and Plunkett, *Victorian Print Media*, 1. On publishing in nineteenth-century Britain
      see also J.O. Jordan and R.L. Patten (eds.), *Literature in the Marketplace. Nineteenth-Century
      British Publishing and Reading Practices*, Cambridge, UK, Cambridge University Press,
      1995.
57   R. Rylance, 'The Theatre and the Granary: Observations on Nineteenth-Century Medical
      Narratives', *Literature and Medicine*, vol. 25, no. 2, 2006, 255–276.
58   Rylance, *The Theatre and the Granary*, 261. On this aspect see also Nolte, *Vom Verschwin-
      den der Laienperspektive*.
59   Ibid., 257f.
60   Ibid., 263.
61   Ibid., 269.

ever, difficult to draw with confidence'.[62] The ways that Lovat's case circulated in popular British print media are a clear example of this 'porousness'.

As described in Chapter 3, the narrative of Lovat's self-crucifixion had reached Britain via various newspapers for the first time in 1811, three years before the full English translation of Ruggieri's French original edition appeared in the journal *Pamphleteer* in 1814. The version published in 1811 in *The Tradesman* and in *The European Review and London Magazine* as well as in some other British journals is a good example showing that British editors employed similar literary techniques to German editors to make the narrative more appealing for a broader readership and to enhance its sensationalist potential. The anonymous author briefly summarises Lovat's case by exaggerating here and there, especially at the end, where he even goes so far as to add some inventions of his own. For example, he distinguishes three acts of Lovat's insanity: first, his self-mutilation, second, his self-crucifixion, and he invents a third one which he describes as follows:

> In his third exploit, he [Lovat] imagined himself to have fallen under the Divine displeasure for not having trusted to miraculous means of being fed: he determined to starve himself, but imagining one night he heard a voice commanding him to go forth and feed like Nebuchadnezzar with the beasts of the field, he disposed of every thing he had, retired to a desolate spot, and for fifteen months fed upon wild fruits, constantly crawling upon his hands and feet. These voluntary and repeated abstinences at length exhausted his body, and he died in 1810 [sic!].[63]

The passage contains a clear reference to the book of Daniel, which conveys one of the Biblical accounts of madness: King Nebuchadnezzar dreams of a big fruitful tree that, by heavenly order, is cut to the roots. Asked to interpret the dream, David predicts that Nebuchadnezzar will lose his kingdom, that he will be excluded from society and that he will be forced to live amongst animals, grazing like them. According to the Biblical account, the dream comes true. Nebuchadnezzar loses his power, is expelled from human society, and eats grass like an animal. When even his body has assumed animalistic forms, he looks up to heaven and praises God. Finally, he regains both his reason and his sovereign power, because he understands that God brings low the pride of men.[64]

---

62 Ibid., 264. On the relation between medical case narratives and the Victorian novel more generally see M. Kennedy, *Revising the Clinic. Vision and Representation in Victorian Medical Narrative and the Novel*, Columbus: Ohio State University Press, 2010.

63 Anonymous, 'Foreign Intelligence', *The European Magazine and London Review*, vol. 60, 1811, 387.

64 The Bible, Dan. 4:9–28.

This Biblical narrative conveys the old idea of madness as a divine punishment. Ignorance of God's omnipotence is equated with an animalistic state of being: unlike men, animals do not possess the power of reason, they do not look up to heaven and thus are unable to recognise God's will. The comparison of Lovat with Nebuchadnezzar's transformation into a beast thus contains a moral judgement, namely that Lovat was punished by madness because of his pride. It served to expel Lovat from the community of thinking humans, and to define his place within the realm of animals, i.e., on the side of unreason. Originally, the account that Lovat refused to eat was a medical observation made by Ruggieri in the Clinical School as was reported by Portalupi in San Servolo. Some of the alienists in France were particularly interested in this observation, because for them it was a clear symptom of religious madness.[65] In contrast, this narrative in the British periodical press explains Lovat's food abstinence by taking into account Lovat's perspective and by asserting that he had an alleged religious motive. Lovat's voluntary fasting, the anonymous editor claims, was inspired by an inner voice convincing him of the divine mission to imitate Nebuchadnezzar. While other authors presumed that the Church Father Origen and Saint Matthew might have served Lovat as examples for his self-castration and self-crucifixion, this author invents Nebuchadnezzar as another possible theological ideal that might have inspired Lovat to starve himself.

Through this Biblical framework of interpretation, the anonymous author managed to add a legendary tone to Lovat's case. Such a rhetorical allusion to Biblical verses was surely a strategy of writers to display erudition, but it also indicates that Biblical notions of madness, notwithstanding the prevalence of secularised and medicalised views, were still conveyed in popular culture in 1811. Among other things, they served the aim of making a narrative more sensational. In an important article on the 'Origins of Modern Sensationalism', Joy Wiltenburg has convincingly shown how sixteenth-century authors of crime reports employed a broad range of rhetorical techniques in order to appeal to the emotions of their readers. This was only partly done with view to commercial effects. Through crime reports in the form of broadsheets, sensationalism itself could also serve as a 'cultural agent' for various purposes that were specific to the respective political, social and cultural contexts.[66] One of the features that Wiltenburg identifies as typical of early modern sensationalist crime reports is their underlying religious message: 'The juridical conception of crime and punishment strongly paralleled the Christian scheme of sin'.[67]

---

65   See Chapter 5 of this book.
66   Wiltenburg, *True Crime*, 1379 and 1383.
67   Ibid., 1385.

Throughout the early modern period, references to Biblical narratives and religious interpretations of crimes were used to teach moral lessons and to thereby edify readers. The religious framework of interpretation fostered and enhanced the emotive nature of crime reports. With view to the historical development of sensationalism as a genre, Wiltenburg therefore suggests that the crime reports' '[...] explicit appeal to emotion underlines the kinship of these early works with the later popular press'.[68]

By the early nineteenth century, the field of literature had become more independent and less functional than it had been during the early modern period. Christian religion provided no longer the evident framework of interpretation, but it could be used in various 'secularised' ways to serve literary and aesthetic aims.[69] In the appropriation of Lovat's case in British newspapers, Nebuchadnezzar's transformation into an animal works as a powerful picture that is able to arouse both feelings of disgust and pity among readers. As such, it was used to mark Lovat not only as differing from the rest of mankind, but also as being punished by God because of his sins. In this sense, the comparison with Nebuchadnezzar also suggested to the readers that madness could be controlled and tamed by identifying the culprit. For readers seeking moral messages rather than a scientific explanation, such a moralising Biblical picture was definitely more appealing than a purely medical description of the case. The association with Biblical figures made Lovat an even more intriguing character, and it rendered the narrative more educative, sensational and therefore popular.

The need of editors for sensational case narratives fostered the circulation of Lovat's case in British periodicals for the coming decades. For instance, it was published in 1822 in *The Mirror of Literature, Amusement and Instruction*, a weekly periodical founded in the same year.[70] *The Mirror* offered a broad range of content. In terms of readership, the editors explicitly tried to reach lower classes, as their objective was '[t]o afford the greatest quantity of "Amusement and Instruction" at the lowest possible expense, and to enable readers in the humblest circumstances to become acquainted with the current and

---

68   Ibid., 1379.
69   On the 'secularization' of literature in this period see A. Schöne, *Säkularisation als sprach-
      bildende Kraft. Studien zur Dichtung deutscher Pfarrersöhne*, Göttingen, Vandenhoeck
      & Ruprecht, 1958; S. Pott, *Medizin, Medizinethik und schöne Literatur. Studien zu Säku-
      larisierungsvorgängen vom 17. bis zum frühen 19. Jahrhundert*, Berlin, Walter de Gruyter,
      2002.
70   Anonymous, 'Self-Crucifixion of Matthew Lovat', *The Mirror of Literature, Amusement,
      and Instruction*, vol. 1, no. 6, 1823, 81–84.

expensive literature of the day [...]'.[71] Again in a slightly changed version, an engraving of Lovat's crucifixion attempt was published together with the narrative on the front page of a December issue of *The Mirror*. The opening lines read: 'The circumstance which the above engraving represents, is one of the most extraordinary and deplorable instances of self-delusion on record'. Appealing to the readers' sensationalist curiosity, Lovat's case served as a hook for this particular issue of the recently founded magazine (see illustration 9).

No matter how many years had past since the incident of Lovat's self-crucifixion in 1805 in Venice, British editors seemed to have considered Lovat's case as a perfect front-page story for recently founded periodicals. Almost 30 years after the publication in *The Mirror*, both the identical narrative and a new copy of the illustration appeared on the cover page of the *Terrific Record; and Chronicle of Remarkable and Interesting Events, &c.* in 1849, another weekly journal was sold for one penny (see illustration 10).[72]

In addition to those publications that explicitly aimed at 'amusement and instruction' of a broader readership through the description of curious characters, British publications that focused more strictly on crimes and calamities also discussed Lovat's case. *The Terrific Register; or Record of Crimes, Judgements, Providences, and Calamities*,[73] published in 1825, included a series of extraordinary criminal cases in the form of short case narratives. It provided a very reduced version of the original narrative under the title 'Extraordinary Case of a Man Who Crucified Himself', and presented Lovat's crucifixion as one of the most 'wonderful torments which fanaticism and insanity have led man to inflict upon themselves', and as 'a most curious and singular phenomenon in the history of the human mind'.[74] Comparable to the German *Pitaval*, publications like *The Terrific Register* resembled earlier legal case collections in that they used similar sensationalist features to enhance emotional resonance. Unlike earlier crime reports, however, those of the nineteenth century focused not so much on the victim but on the wrongdoer.[75] This increasing attention to the individual, its history and mental condition is also an important feature of the genre of 'eccentric biographies' which included Lovat's case in their repertory.

---

71   Anonymous, 'Preface', *The Mirror of Literature, Amusement, and Instruction*, vol. 1, no. 1, 1823.

72   Anonymous, 'Self-Crucifixion of Matthew Lovat', *The Terrific Record; and Chronicle of Remarkable and Interesting Events &c.*, vol. 1, no. 14, 1849, 209–212.

73   Anonymous, 'Extraordinary Case of a Man Who Crucified Himself', *The Terrific Register; or Record of Crimes, Judgements, Providences, and Calamities*, vol. 2, 1825, 384–350.

74   Ibid., 348f.

75   Wiltenburg, *True Crime*, 1398f.

The Mirror
OF
LITERATURE, AMUSEMENT, AND INSTRUCTION.

No. VI.]   SATURDAY, DECEMBER 7, 1822.   [PRICE 2d.

SELF-CRUCIFIXION
OF
Matthew Lovat.

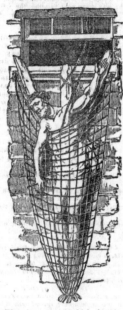

The circumstance which the above engraving represents, is one of the most extraordinary and deplorable instances of self-delusion on record. Matthew Lovat was born at Casale, a hamlet belonging to the parish of Soldo, in the territory of Belluno, of poor parents, employed in the coarsest and most laborious works of husbandry, and fixed to a place remote from almost all society. His imagination was so forcibly smitten with the view of the easy and comfortable lives of the rector and his curate, who were the only persons in the whole parish exempted from the labours of

Vol. I.

the field, and who engrossed all the power and consequence which the little world wherein Matthew lived presented to his eyes, that he made an effort to prepare himself for the priesthood, and placed himself under the tuition of the curate, who taught him to read and to write a little. But the poverty of his family was an effectual bar to his desire; he was obliged to renounce study for ever, and to betake himself to the trade of a shoemaker.

Having become a shoemaker from necessity, he never succeeded either as a neat or expeditious workman. The sedentary life, and the silence to which apprentices are condemned in the shops of the masters abroad, formed in him the habit of meditation, and rendered him gloomy and taciturn. As his age increased, he became subject, in the spring, to giddiness in his head, and eruptions of a leprous appearance showed themselves on his face and hands.

Until the month of July, 1802, Matthew Lovat did nothing extraordinary. His life was regular and uniform, his habits were simple, and nothing distinguished him, but an extreme degree of devotion. He spoke on no other subject than the affairs of the church. Its festivals and fasts, with sermons, saints, &c. constituted the topics of his conversation. It was at this date, that, in imitation of the early devotees, he determined to disarm the tempter, by mutilating himself. He effected his purpose without having anticipated the species of celebrity which the operation was to procure for him; and which compelled the poor creature to keep himself shut up in his house, from which he did not venture to stir for some time, not even to go to mass. At length, on the 13th of November, in the same year, he went to Venice, where a younger brother, named Angelo, conducted Matthew to the house of a widow, the relict of Andrew Osgualda, with whom he lodged, until the 21st of September in the following year, working assiduously at his trade, and without exhibiting any signs of madness. But on the above-mentioned day, he made an attempt to crucify himself, in the middle of the street called

G

ILLUSTRATION 9   Anonymous, 'Self-Crucifixion of Matthew Lovat', *The Mirror of Literature, Amusement, and Instruction*, 1822.

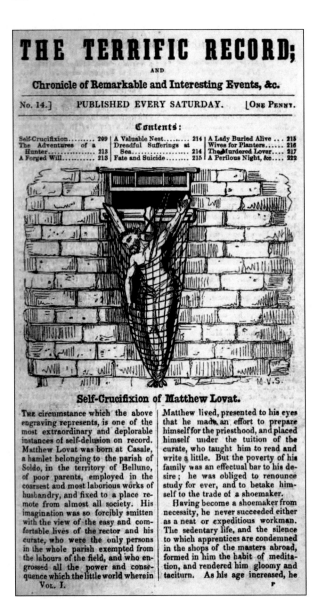

THE TERRIFIC RECORD;

AND

Chronicle of Remarkable and Interesting Events, &c.

No. 14.]   PUBLISHED EVERY SATURDAY.   [One Penny.

Contents:

Self-Crucifixion of Matthew Lovat.

The circumstance which the above engraving represents, is one of the most extraordinary and deplorable instances of self-delusion on record. Matthew Lovat was born at Casale, a hamlet belonging to the parish of Soldo, in the territory of Belluno, of poor parents, employed in the coarsest and most laborious works of husbandry, and fixed to a place remote from almost all society. His imagination was so forcibly smitten with the view of the easy and comfortable lives of the rector and his curate, who were the only persons in the whole parish exempted from the labours of the field, and who engrossed all the power and consequence which the little world wherein

Matthew lived, presented to his eyes that he made an effort to prepare himself for the priesthood, and placed himself under the tuition of the curate, who taught him to read and write a little. But the poverty of his family was an effectual bar to his desire; he was obliged to renounce study for ever, and to betake himself to the trade of a shoemaker.

Having become a shoemaker from necessity, he never succeeded either as a neat or expeditious workman. The sedentary life, and the silence to which apprentices are condemned in the shops of the masters abroad, formed in him the habit of meditation, and rendered him gloomy and taciturn. As his age increased, he

Vol. I.   P

ILLUSTRATION 10   Anonymous, 'Self-Crucifixion of Matthew
Lovat', *The Terrific Record*, 1849.

4   Lovat's Case in the British 'Eccentric Biographies'

In recent research, the label 'eccentric biography' serves to summarise various texts from the late eighteenth and nineteenth centuries that deal with the lives and deeds of so-called 'remarkable' characters, or extraordinary events. Scholars have examined different kinds of periodicals and books that shaped this genre in various ways.[76] Publications dealing explicitly with 'eccentric lives' became very popular in the British book trade during the first half of the nineteenth century.[77] The eccentric biographies represent a British specificity in that they combined the Europe-wide attention to physical and social deviance with a specific nineteenth-century national debate on what contemporary authors called 'British eccentricity'. According to James Gregory, the term 'eccentricity' had '[...] entered the language (if not common discourse) as a description of personal attributes or qualities [...]' already by the end of the seventeenth century.[78] At the beginning of the nineteenth century, the term appeared in various titles of periodicals and books that dealt with so-called remarkable or curious characters, lives or biographies. The publication of one single work was often followed by several reprints and new editions throughout the nineteenth century. Editors copied single narratives or entire contents from existent publications and recycled them in reprints, as plagiarism was common practice.[79] The eccentric biographies appeared in both expensive and cheaper versions and tried to reach different audiences: costly editions with high quality engravings were particularly precious for the learned elite and their collections, but the greater part of eccentric biographies addressed the bourgeois family who appreciated the moral lessons and entertainment contained in them.[80]

Gregory sees the origins of the genre as lying in the general public interest in 'physical and behavioural abnormality' since the invention of the printing press. The great interest in extraordinary natural phenomena was famously expressed in Francis Bacon's call for a collection of wonders of human nature, as

---

76   J. Gregory, 'Eccentric Biography and the Victorians', *Biography*, vol. 30, no. 3, 2007, 342–376, 352.

77   J. Gregory, 'Eccentric Lives: Character, Characters, and Curiosities in Britain, c. 1760–1900', in W. Ernst (ed.), *Histories of the Normal and of the Abnormal. Social and Cultural Histories of Norms and Normativity*, London and New York, Routledge, 2006, 72–100, 73.

78   Ibid., 74.

79   Gregory talks about around sixty works, see ibid.

80   Gregory, *Eccentric Biography and the Victorians*, 352.

it was likewise the motivation for the early modern *Wunderkammern*.[81] The individual titles of late eighteenth- and early nineteenth-century publications demonstrate their strong affiliation with this early modern interest in collecting wondrous and unique phenomena, in particular those that bear the adjectives 'wonderful' and 'extraordinary' in their title, and those that are explicitly called 'museum'.[82] The sensational magazine *The New Wonderful Magazine and Marvellous Chronicle,* first published in 1793, had been trend-setting. Shortly before the publication of this monthly periodical, a handbill was distributed to announce it:

> An entire new magazine: On Friday, February 1, 1793, will be Published, (price only Sixpence) Elegantly Printed on a Superfine Paper, and Embellished with a most Beautiful Frontispiece, finely Engraved by a Capital Artist, The Wonderful Magazine, and Marvellous Chronicle of extraordinary productions and events In Nature and Art: Consisting Entirely of Matters which come under the Denominations of Miraculous! Queer! Odd! Strange! Supernatural! Whimsical! Absurd! Out of the way! and Unaccountable! Including Many surprising Escapes from Death and Dangers, strange Discoveries of long-concealed Murders, and a vast Variety of other Matters equally curious and surprizing.[83]

As this handbill reveals, such publications used similar rhetorical strategies as early modern sensationalist crime accounts, as editors made use of exclamatory adjectives in the titles in order to emphasise 'the emotive quality of content', and to 'enhance visceral effect'.[84] The handbill also emphasised the alleged authentic sources of such compilations: 'The hole collected from the Writings of the most approved Historians, Travellers, Philosophers, and Physicians, of all Ages and Countries'.[85]

---

81   Gregory, *Eccentric Lives,* 73f. On the early modern interest in wonders see for instance Daston Park, *Wonders and the Order of Nature 1150–1750* and Da Costa, *The Singular and the Making of Knowledge.*

82   Gregory, *Eccentric Lives,* 73.

83   Anonymous, *An Entire New Magazine: On Friday, February 1, 1793, Will Be Published, (Price Only Sixpence) Elegantly Printed on a Superfine Paper...* London: Printed for the Proprietors, sold by C. Johnson, No. 14, and the Other Booksellers in Paternoster-Row; and may be had of all Booksellers and Newscarriers in England, Wales, Scotland, and Ireland, 1793.

84   Wiltenburg, *True Crime,* 1382.

85   Anonymous, *An Entire New Magazine.*

William Granger's and James Caulfield's *The New Wonderful Museum, and Extraordinary Magazine*[86] (1802), and Kirby's *The Wonderful and Scientific Museum; or, Magazine of Remarkable Characters*[87] (1803) as well as many other British publications from the early nineteenth century had a similar agenda as proposed by the cited handbill. A telling example of the general programme of such publications is Henry Wilson's *The Eccentric Mirror: Reflecting a Faithful and Interesting Delineation of Male and Female Characters, Ancient and Modern*.[88] In the preface to the first volume published in 1806, it says:

> It has been justly observed by the prince of British poets, that 'The proper study of mankind is MAN'. It is with a view to promote and facilitate this important study, that the Editor of these volumes presents to the public a series of lives of such individuals of either sex, as have been distinguished by any extraordinary circumstances from the mass of society. They embrace authentic biographical accounts of persons remarkable for longevity, unusual size, strength, singular habits and manners, adventures, virtues and vices; in short, of all such as have gained celebrity or notoriety, by deviating in a remarkable degree from the ordinary course of human existence.[89]

This programme is representative not only because of the reference to Alexander Pope's *Essay on Man* (1733), an allusion that was to become a commonplace in comparable publications.[90] It also contains the usual affirmation of authenticity as well as the common claim that the collection embraced characters of

---

86 W. Granger (ed.), *The New Wonderful Museum, and Extraordinary Magazine: Being a Complete Repository of All the Wonders, Curiosities, and Rarities of Nature and Art, from the Beginning of the World to the Present Year 1802*, vol. 1, London, R.S. Kirby, 1802.

87 R.S. Kirby (ed.), *The Wonderful and Scientific Museum; or, Magazine of Remarkable Characters; Including all the Curiosities of Nature and Art, from the Remotest Period to the Present Time, Drawn from Every Authentic Source*, vol. 1, London, T. Keating, 1803, IIIf.

88 H. Wilson (ed.), *The Eccentric Mirror: Reflecting a Faithful and Interesting Delineation of Male and Female Characters, Ancient and Modern, Who Have Been Particularly Distinguished by Extraordinary Qualifications, Talents, and Propensities, Natural or Aquired, Comprehending Singular Instances of Longevity, Conformation, Bulk, Stature, Powers of Mind and of Body, Wonderful Exploits, Adventures, Habits, Propensities, Enterprising Pursuits, &c.&c.&c*, vol. 1, London, James Cundee, 1806.

89 Ibid., III.

90 Gregory, *Eccentric Lives*, 88. For the citation see A. Pope, 'An Essay on Men', in H.F. Cary (ed.), *The Poetical Works of Alexander Pope*, London, William Smith, 1839, 216–248: 'Know then thyself, presume not God to scan;/ The proper study of mankind is Man'.

'every age' and 'every country', both dead and alive.[91] Likewise, the emphasis that the magazine includes 'many valuable and expensive foreign publications'[92] is a common feature of publications alike.

This passage reveals the main criterion for a character to be included in such a collection, namely a significant deviance from social norms, be it physical or behavioural, and celebrity thereby achieved. The fact that Lovat's case appeared in many eccentric biographies indicates that in the eyes of many editors, he was such an eccentric character because he fulfilled these requirements perfectly. Editors usually cited the complete English translation published in 1814 by *The Pamphleteer*, but in most cases, they provided a reduced version and let the narrative end with Lovat's death in San Servolo. As a result, they left out the medical explanations and diagnostic terms with which Ruggieri had concluded his original text. This loss of expert terminology with the aim of being intelligible to all characterises many of the popular readings of Lovat's case and is an important signal for the gradual transformation from an epistemic to a more literary genre.[93]

The first editor to adopt Lovat's case after it had appeared in *The Pamphleteer* was John Cecil. In 1819, Cecil published his *Sixty Curious Authentic Narratives and Anecdotes Respecting Extraordinary Characters: Illustrative of the Tendency of Credulity, and Fanaticism*[94] in which he put the focus on characters whose deeds were motivated by religious ideas. Cecil had a clear didactic purpose in mind. He was eager to emphasise that his stories were not only meant to entertain, but also to instruct, since, as he states in the foreword,

> [...] in the science of life, as well as in every other, it is necessary to become acquainted with the exception to the general rule. To estimate properly what is, we must possess some knowledge of what *may* be, and

---

91 Wilson, *The Eccentric Mirror*, IIIf.: '[...] this faithful Mirror represents without distortion only such characters as have really existed, and such events as have actually happened. It reflects the image of the most surprizing human phenomena, of the greatest prodigies, in every age and in every country, that have commanded the particular notice of their contemporaries; and exhibits a delineation not only of characters that have quitted this mortal stage, but of many whose living eminence entitles them to a place in this Collection'.

92 Ibid., IV.

93 On intelligibility as a characteristic of science popularisation see Schwarz, *Bilden, Überzeugen, Unterhalten*, 222.

94 J. Cecil, *Sixty Curious Authentic Narratives and Anecdotes Respecting Extraordinary Characters: Illustrative of the Tendency of Credulity, and Fanaticism; Exemplifying the Imperfection of Circumstantial Evidence; and Recording Singular Instances of Voluntary Human Suffering, and Interesting Occurrences*, London, William Hone, 1819.

the information is only to be acquired by an attention to the memorable and peculiar, which *have been*.[95]

Thus, like the German authors who had promoted the knowledge of man under the label of an empirical science of the soul (*Erfahrungsseelenkunde*), British authors claimed that, in order to explore the nature of man, one must look at every possible deviation of the human nature in both past and present.

In Cecil's book, Lovat's case is presented under the column 'Voluntary Human Suffering'.[96] As Cecil explains in the foreword, this category '[...] display[s] a few examples of a species of misery arising out of the perversity of human nature. It would be difficult to invent greater torments than mankind inflicts upon itself, when impelled by baleful and superstitious ideas of the benevolent Creator of all things'.[97] In Cecil's view, religion in general, and especially religious institutions, had to be blamed as one, if not *the* main source for human misery eventually leading to madness and self-destruction. Because of his emphasis on the *voluntary* admission to religious institutions, religious belief appears as a matter of choice.[98] In Cecil's collection, extreme religious zeal is therefore not so much regarded as a pathological aberration, but rather as self-inflicted. It is this moral warning that narratives such as Lovat's crucifixion attempt were supposed to convey in Cecil's book.

Other eccentric biographies which presented Lovat's case contained no such explicit instructions for a moral reading, but just printed one story after the other without any further comment. This is the case with *Kirby's Wonderful and Eccentric Museum; or, Magazine of Remarkable Characters*,[99] published in 1820, in which Lovat's case is reproduced in the complete authorised version of the *Pamphleteer*. Nevertheless, the editor provided instruction through the selection and order of case narratives, reporting about '[t]hat which is truly

---

95 Ibid., 111.

96 Ibid., 279.

97 Ibid., Vf.

98 Ibid.: The editor remarks that '[*t*]*he* word *voluntary,* however, as here applied, is not strictly to be confined to the individuals who suffer, but is to be interpreted as significant of misery, originating from institutions to which Sects and Nations *voluntarily* and conscientiously submit'.

99 R.S. Kirby, *Kirby's Wonderful and Eccentric Museum; or, Magazine of Remarkable Characters. Including all the Curiosities of Nature and Art from the Remotest Period to the Present Time*, vol. 5, London, R.S. Kirby, 1820, 274–287. Kirby's collection embraced six volumes with the first edition starting in 1803. Apparently, Kirby borrowed the idea of such a collection from one of the earliest examples of this genre, the collection by William Granger that Kirby himself had printed: Granger, *The New Wonderful Museum, and Extraordinary Magazine*. This shows the sometimes double function of printers who were in possession of plenty material and not seldom acted as editors themselves.

curious, positively, or relatively wonderful', and 'collect[ed] from the inex-
haustible regions of animate or inanimate nature; from the records of history,
or the improvements of art'.[100] The sheer quantity of Kirby's narratives showed
that such individuals or events were not unique at all but existed in great
numbers and therefore reflected part of human nature. In this sense, they normalised the eccentric characters they described. As Gregory rightly suggests,
'[a] central idea emerging from eccentric material is that *eccentricity is part of
the normal*'.[101] Moreover, the numerous engravings in Kirby's collection provided visual entertainment for readers. Like in an actual museum, each character was displayed with an appropriate illustration showing the unusual body
or the extraordinary behaviour described in the respective narratives. Like all
the other editors who provided an illustration of Lovat's case, Kirby had to ar-
range for a completely new engraving while remaining as true as possible to
Ruggieri's original illustration (see illustration 11).

The American book market was totally dominated by unlicensed copies of
British material well into the nineteenth century.[102] Due to American reprints
of British publications, single narratives or whole case collections reappeared
on the American book market.[103] This is why we find the narrative of Lovat's
self-crucifixion in American publications as well. That American editors readily combined British material with American sources[104] is confirmed by *The
Sketch Book of Character; or, Curious and Authentic Narratives and Anecdotes
Respecting Extraordinary Individuals*, a publication which was launched in
1835 in Philadelphia and appears to be a direct copy of Cecil's *Sixty Curious and
Authentic Narratives and Anecdotes Respecting Extraordinary Characters*.[105]

---

100   Citations from the foreword of the first edition, see Kirby, *The Wonderful and Scientific
      Museum*, III.

101   Gregory, *Eccentric Lives*, 83.

102   On copyright see J.J. Barnes and Patience P. Barnes, 'Copyright', in S. Mitchell (ed.), *Victo-
      rian Britain: An Encyclopedia*, New York, Garland, 1988, 192–193; J.J. Barnes, *Authors, Pub-
      lishers and Politicians: The Quest for an Anglo-American Copyright Agreement 1815–1854*,
      Columbus, OH, Ohio State University Press, 2016 and J. Feather, *Publishing, Piracy and
      Politics: An Historical Study of Copyright in Britain*, London, Mansell, 1994.

103   Gregory, *Eccentric Biography and the Victorians*, 349f. See for instance D. Fraser (ed.),
      *The American Magazine of Wonders, and Marvellous Chronicle, Intended as a Record of
      Accounts of the Most Extraordinary Productions, Events, and Occurrences, in Providence,
      Nature, and Art, That Have Been Witnessed at Any Time in Europe and America*, New York,
      Southwick and Pelsue, 1809.

104   Gregory, *Eccentric Lives*, 78.

105   Anonymous, *The Sketch Book of Character; or, Curious and Authentic Narratives and
      Anecdotes Respecting Extraordinary Individuals; Exemplifying the Imperfections of Cir-
      cumstantial Evidence: Illustrative of the Tendency of Credulty and Fanaticism: and Record-
      ing Singular Instances of Voluntary Human Suffering and Interesting Occurrences*, vol. 2,
      Philadelphia, Carey & A. Hart, 1835.

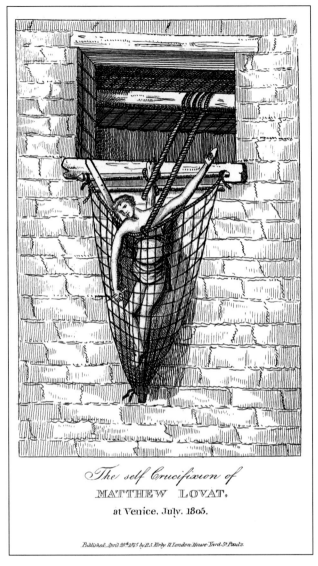

The self Crucifixion of
MATTHEW LOVAT,
at Venice, July, 1805.

Published, April 28th 1815 by P.S Kirby 11 London House Yard St Pauls.

ILLUSTRATION 11   Kirby, *Kirby's Wonderful and Eccentric Museum*,
1820.

As shown before, this was one of the first British publications which had presented Lovat's case among other 'eccentric characters'. If one compares the two editions, small changes in the arrangement of contents are detectable, but all the narratives are identical.[106]

In the second half of the nineteenth century, the practice of recycling older eccentric biographies continued. Thanks to numerous new editions, Lovat's case was transmitted in ever new variations of the same genre. For instance, John Watts included it in his *The Museum of Remarkable and Interesting Events*, which embraced *Historical and Other Accounts of Adventures, Incidents of Travels and Voyages, Scenes of Peril, and Escapes, Military Achievements, Eccentric Personages, Noble Examples of Fortitude and Patriotism, with Various Other Entertaining Narratives, Anecdotes, etc. etc.*. Explicitly 'designed as a book of leisure reading for all classes',[107] this collection was inspired by the contemporary idea that history teaches important lessons and is able to morally improve individuals.[108] Watts was therefore eager to declare that, 'The selection of them [narratives, M.B.] was made not from the extravagant and distorted caricatures of fiction, but from the authentic and well attested records of sober reality [...]'.[109] On the frontispiece of his collection, he claimed that 'Truth is sometimes more strange than fiction'.[110] Referring to the original context of his sources was, however, not important to him.

The inclusion of Lovat in the British canon of remarkable characters is signalled most clearly by Henry Wilson's *The Book of Wonderful Characters: Memoirs and Anecdotes of Remarkable and Eccentric Persons in All Ages and*

---

106   Like in Cecil's book, Lovat's case is included in the category 'Voluntary Human Suffering', and the introduction reads likewise: 'Matthew Lovat presents an extraordinary and deplorable instance of religious melancholy [...]', see ibid., 137–141.

107   J. Watts, *The Museum of Remarkable and Interesting Events, Containig Historical and Other Accounts of Adventures, Incidents of Travels and Voyages, Scenes of Peril, and Escapes, Military Achievements, Eccentric Personages, Noble Examples of Fortitude and Patriotism, with Various Other Entertaining Narratives, Anecdotes, etc.etc... Designed as a Book of Leisure Reading for All Classes*, vol. 1, Cleveland, OH, Sanford & Hayward, 1844, 25–30.

108   See ibid., III: 'Leaving the natural world, we find in the records of history the elements of a still higher interest, and the objects of more permanent and commanding passions, than even the proud sublimities of nature can produce. Amid the excitement of heroic fortitude, unconquerable energy, and bold and perilous adventure, accompanied with all the enchantment of diversified and overwhelming emotion, and the endless variety of good and ill which distinguish the more tragic scenes of life, we rise above ourselves and become conscious of capabilities of feeling and action which slept unexercised before, but which when once awakened are for ever wakeful. Such is the interest which many of the following narratives are adapted to excite. They embrace some of the most sublime and affecting developments of history'.

109   Ibid.

110   Ibid, frontispiece.

Countries published in 1869.[111] This was a very successful new edition of a huge collection of remarkable characters with portraits that were originally provided by James Caulfield (1764–1826), an editor who had made a name for himself with various similar publications.[112] After his death, Henry Wilson, who himself had published several editions of 'wonderful characters' in the 1820s,[113] continued to recycle Caulfield's material. *Wonderful Characters* appeared until 1873 with at least eleven different publishers;[114] the edition of 1869 being printed by John Camden Hotten, 'chiefly from the text by Henry Wilson and James Caulfield'. This particular edition arranged the narratives in alphabetical order and contained costly partly coloured engravings, one portrait for each narrative. The entry 'Matthew Lovat. Who crucified himself' accordingly appears under the letter L.[115] Like in most of the other British popular publications, the last diagnostic part of the original narrative is omitted, so that the story ends with Lovat's death in San Servolo. However, it was important to Wilson to stress the almost literal reproduction of his sources, as a comment following the introduction reveals: 'It is proper to state that the several biographies in this work have not been modernized in any way, but are given in very nearly the exact words of the original narrative. There is a piquancy about the old narrations which seems to harmonize with the subject of "Wonderful characters" far better than the cold modern treatment of such a theme'.[116] Of course, in Lovat's case, the 'original' narrative to which Wilson referred was not Ruggieri's *Storia della crocifissione* but that of the English translation published in the *Pamphleteer*.

By the second half of the nineteenth century, Lovat's case had become part of the genre's classics. The ongoing interest in Lovat's case can be related to

---

111   H. Wilson, *The Book of Wonderful Characters: Memoirs and Anecdotes of Remarkable and Eccentric Persons in All Ages and Countries. Chiefly from the Text by Henry Wilson and James Caulfield*, London, John Camden Hotten, Piccadilly, 1869, 55–63.

112   W. Granger et al., *The New, Original and Complete Wonderful Museum and Magazine Extraordinary: Being a Complete Repository of All the Wonders, Curiosities, and Rarities of Nature and Art, from the Beginning of the World to the Present Year ... Including, among the Greatest Variety of Other Valuable Matter in this Line of Literature (from an Illustrated Edition of the Rev. Mr. James Granger's Celebrated Biographical History) Memoirs and Portraits of the Most Singular and Remarkable Persons ...*, London, M. Allen, 1802–1808. See also J. Caulfield, *Portraits, Memoirs and Characters of Remarkable Persons, from the Reign of King Edward the Third to the Revolution*, London, Caulfield & Herbert, 1794–1795.

113   H. Wilson, *Wonderful Characters: Comprising Memoirs and Anecdotes of the Most Remarkable Persons of every Age and Nation*, London, J. Robins, 1821–1827; H. Wilson, *Fifty Wonderful Portraits*, London, J. Robins, 1821–26.

114   Gregory, *Eccentric Biography and the Victorians*, 347.

115   Wilson, *The Book of Wonderful Characters*, 55.

116   Ibid., xx.

specific shifts in the genre of eccentric biographies itself. Firstly, as Gregory has observed, in the first decades of the nineteenth century, there was an equal interest in both physical and behavioural deviance. By contrast, 'modern works of eccentric biography no longer possess[ed] the range of curiosities', in that they focused more on non-conformist social behaviour than on physical aberrations.[117] As Lovat's case was not a story about physical deformity but about an extraordinary action allegedly caused by mental disorder, the narrative remained equally interesting in this slightly altered debate. Secondly, later eccentric biographies suggest that there was a rising concern about a decline of eccentric characters in British society. In the preface to the 1869 *Book of Wonderful Characters*, the editor claims that, because of the egalitarianism of the modern age, eccentric biographies are now even more necessary than before:

> The biographies of men who have essentially differed from the rest of the human race, either by their having been born with some peculiar congenital defect, or possessing an eccentricity of character, which inevitably impels them to overleap and trespass from the boundaries of the beaten highway of conventional life, have been in all times eagerly sought after by the curious inquirer into human nature. [...] There is a great change, too, in the manners and customs of the people of England, that renders a book like this still more interesting at the present time. We have nearly lost all, and are daily losing what little remains of, our individuality; all people and all places seem now to be alike [...] Indeed, the tendency of the present day, in England, is directly opposed to the spirit of individual exclusiveness, which, as the great encourager of eccentricity of character, once prevailed over all the country.[118]

As this comment suggests, general societal changes provoked a sense of nostalgia regarding individuality and eccentricity. As Gregory remarks, '[i]t was felt that eccentricity waned locally and nationally, and that early-nineteenth century characters lacked successors. Connoisseurs of the eccentric explained this apparent diminution variously. The extension of railways and popular education, or developments in policing, or the establishment of asylums for the mentally ill, provided reasons for the disappearance of village and urban "characters"'.[119] Despite this concern for a decline of eccentric characters,

---

117   Gregory, *Eccentric Lives*, 90.
118   Wilson, *The Book of Wonderful Characters*, I–III.
119   Gregory, *Eccentric Biography and the Victorians*, 359.

however, '[...] eccentrics survived in a range of texts and reprints'[120] and successful British writers such as Charles Dickens were inspired by the collections
of eccentric characters published by Caulfield, Kirby and others.[121] The public
interest in physical deformation continued to be satisfied in the so-called freak
shows, i.e., public exhibitions of individuals that deviated from physical or social
norms. In fact, many of the 'unusual bodies' that were presented in British print
media belonged to still living individuals who were exposed in such shows.[122]

By the second half of the nineteenth century, the genre had contributed to
a very positive connotation of eccentricity. In the last collection that brought
'new' contents, John Timbs' *English Eccentrics and Eccentricities*, published in
1866,[123] the editor emphasises '[...] how often do we find eccentricity in the
minds of persons of good understanding', and '[...] that with oddity of character may co-exist much goodness of heart'.[124] With such a positive view on
eccentricity, Timbs and other editors joined a liberal idea that the philosopher
and economist John Stuart Mill had expressed a few years before in his essay
On Liberty from 1859.[125] Discussing the importance of individuality and eccentricity for a society's well-being and progress, Mill argues that,

> [...] exceptional individuals, instead of being deterred, should be
> encouraged in acting differently from the mass. In other times there was
> no advantage in their doing so, unless they acted not only differently, but
> better. In this age the mere example of non-conformity, the mere refusal
> to bend the knee to custom, is itself a service. Precisely because the tyr-
> anny of opinion is such as to make eccentricity a reproach, it is desirable,
> in order to break through that tyranny, that people should be eccentric.
> Eccentricity has always abounded when and where strength of character
> has abounded; and the amount of eccentricity in a society has generally
> been proportional to the amount of genius, mental vigour, and moral

120   Ibid., 360.
121   Ibid., 357. On Dickens see J.S. Saville, 'Eccentricity as Englishness in David Copperfield',
      Studies in English Literature 1500–1900, vol. 42, no. 4, 2002, 781–797, 783ff.
122   Gregory, *Eccentric Lives*, 84. On freak shows see M. Tromp (ed.), *Victorian Freaks. The So-
      cial Context of Freakery in Britain*, Columbus, OH, The Ohio State University Press, 2008
      and B. Stammberger, *Monster und Freaks. Eine Wissensgeschichte außergewöhnlicher Kör-
      per im 19. Jahrhundert*, Bielefeld, transcript, 2011.
123   J. Timbs (ed.), *English Eccentrics and Eccentricities*, vol. 1, London, Richard Bentley, 1866.
      Gregory comes to the same conclusion in his *Eccentric Biography and the Victorians*, 345.
124   Timbs, *English Eccentrics and Eccentricities*, IIf.
125   J.S. Mill, *On Liberty*, Boston, Ticknor and Fields, 1863.

courage that it contained. That so few now dare to be eccentric, marks the chief danger of the time.[126]

In Britain, thus, eccentricity came to be associated with 'strength of character' and 'genius', and came to be viewed as something desirable, useful, even an expression of individuality and liberty. This positive view on social 'otherness' was closely related to the fear of a mass society in the industrial age that would bring about social egalitarianism and a 'tyranny of opinion'. And yet, the celebration of the idea of individuality as a specificity of the British was not new, but a common feature of the genre. In 1806, for example, the editors of *The Eccentric Mirror* already claimed that '[i]t is universally admitted that no country in the world produces so many humourists and eccentric characters as the British islands. This acknowledgement is an indirect eulogy on the political constitution and the laws under which the English enjoy the happiness of living, and by which each individual is suffered to gratify every whim, fancy, and caprice, provided it be not prejudicial to his fellow-creatures'.[127] British eccentricity was thus explained by the political independence and liberty and a constitution that supposedly allowed each individual to live out his or her 'eccentricities', as long as they did not infringe upon another person's freedom. As Julia F. Saville has emphasised, the idea of eccentric characters was closely related to the idea of a national character: 'Since character stood as a manifestation of individual freedom within a nation that prided itself on the liberty of its citizens, to be *a character* in the sense of feeling free to assert one's individuality was simultaneously to participate in defining the *national character* as free'.[128] Eccentricity thus formed part of the construction of a national identity.[129] In this sense, the eccentric biography genre also signals a novel notion of individuality. Matthias Pohlig has shown that, in close connection with the

---

126   Ibid., 129f.
127   See Anonymous, 'Henry Lee Warner, Esq', in H. Wilson (ed.), *The Eccentric Mirror: Reflecting a Faithful and Interesting Delienation of Male and Female Characters, Ancient and Modern, Who Have Been Particularly Distinguished by Extraordinary Qualifications, Talents, and Propensities, Natural or Aquired, Comprehending Singular Instances of Longevity, Conformation, Bulk, Stature, Powers of Mind and of Body, Wonderful Exploits, Adventures, Habits, Propensities, Enterprising Pursuits, &c.&c.&c*, vol. 1, London, James Cundee, 1806, 22.
128   Saville, *Eccentricity as Englishness in David Copperfield*, 782.
129   Gregory shows that the construction of national identity in Britain also had local peculiarities, see J. Gregory, '"Local Characters": Eccentricity and the North-East in the Nineteenth Century', *Northern History*, vol. 42, no. 1, 2005, 163–186. See also P. Langford, *Englishness Identified. Manners and Character 1650–1850*, Oxford, Oxford University Press, 2000, especially the chapter on 'Eccentricity', 267–311.

political upheavals caused by the Napoleonic Wars and due to the pluralisation of social contexts and the loss of moral and social barriers, a novel idea of the individual emerged in European societies that differed remarkably from the understanding of individuality during the *ancien regime*. If in pre-modern Europe the individual was bound to powerful authorities and collective loyalties, now, it was considered unique, free and able to master his own fate according to his or her own will.[130]

It might seem confusing that a Venetian shoemaker should make a career as a British eccentric, but, as many editors emphasised in the titles, they were proud to include characters 'from every age and nation' in their collections. Apparently, this was a way pointing to the universal laws of human nature that brought about eccentric characters independent of time and space.[131] The origin and context of Lovat's story was not important, because 'Eccentric biographies were anecdotal rather than analytical, and made no attempt to examine cultural factors that might contribute to eccentricity [...]'.[132] It was more important that editors provided sensational and fast-selling material rather than offering a convincing analysis of the original narratives. By providing a sensational story together with a disturbing illustration of the crucified Lovat, Ruggieri himself had facilitated a popular reception of Lovat's case in Britain. In a country in which biographical portraiture and visual portraits of deviant characters were very popular and had a long tradition, this strategy bore fruit.

The circulation of Lovat's case in the eccentric biographies also illuminates the link between the British popular debate on eccentricity and the medical discourse on insanity. The debates indeed overlapped when the eccentric character in question was considered insane. In these cases, 'eccentric' was actually used as a 'synonym for madness'.[133] However, in contrast to medical authors, writers of eccentric biographies were not interested in mental diseases per se, or in the definition of an individual as insane. Instead, they appreciated the extraordinary ideas and deeds of a person. As we have seen before, 'good understanding' and 'goodness of the heart'[134] was not at all seen as contradicting eccentricity – but it would very likely have been considered incompatible with pathological insanity. Eccentric characters were even believed to surpass the wisdom of the learned and reasonable. As John Timbs put it, '[...] your

---

130   Pohlig, *Individuum und Sattelzeit*, 267–269.
131   Gregory, *Eccentric Lives*, 89.
132   Ibid.
133   Gregory, 'Local Characters', 172: 'In other cases, the label of "eccentric" represented an alternative to "lunatic". Eccentricity inhabited the borderland between sanity and insanity; indeed it could be a synonym for madness'.
134   Timbs, *English Eccentrics and Eccentricities*, IIIf.

strange fellow, though, according to the lexicographer, he be outlandish, odd, queer, and eccentric, may possess claims to our notice which the man who is ever studying the fitness of things would not so readily present'.[135] Hence, within the framework of the eccentric biographies, Lovat was admired for his sophisticated deeds and his singular beliefs rather than accused of insanity. What kind of madness or disease he had actually suffered from was not important for the editors. This is why in many of the examples cited in this chapter, the last part of the narrative containing Ruggieri's diagnostic suggestions was omitted, and the focus was laid on his astonishing performance.

5   Lovat's Case as a Popular Anecdote

As shown in the previous pages, we find a variety of popular readings of Lovat's case in Germany and Britain which coexisted and sometimes corresponded with professional readings. In France, by contrast, the professional appropriations of Lovat's case clearly prevailed. Only towards the end of the nineteenth century did the case narrative also take on more popular forms and reach a wider lay readership in France. One example is particularly revealing because it shows another explicit transformation of genre, namely that from a medical case history to a literary anecdote. In 1871, Lovat's case appeared in a French publication called *Dictionnaire encyclopédique d'anecdotes modernes, anciennes, françaises et étrangères*.[136] The editor's declared aim was to overcome lacunas and errors in existent collections of anecdotes, and to build the 'classic repertory of the genre'.[137] For this purpose, the dictionary included anecdotes regarding 'French history and the history of the past centuries, the biography of important men in its different genres'; moreover, it included those anecdotes 'that have somehow become classics [...]'.[138]

---

135   Ibid.
136   E. Guérard, 'Crucifiement volontaire', in E. Guérard (ed.), *Dictionnaire encyclopédique d'anecdotes modernes, anciennes, françaises et étrangères*, vol. 1, Paris, Firmin-Diderot, 1872, 287.
137   E. Guérard, 'Introduction', in E. Guérard (ed.), *Dictionnaire encyclopédique d'anecdotes modernes, anciennes, françaises et étrangères*, vol. 1, Paris, Firmin-Diderot, 1872, I–X, X: '[...] le répertoire classique du genre'. The original plan was a 'universal dictionary' including all anecdotes of all times and places, see ibid., v.
138   Ibid.: '[...] nous avons préféré celles qui intéressent particulièrement l'histoire de France et l'historie des dernier siècles, la biographie des hommes célèbres dans les divers genres. Nous n'avons pas cru devoir exclure les anecdotes devenues en quelque sorte classiques, et qui sont comme la base de tout dictionnaire analogue [...]'.

The editor legitimises his vast editorial project by referring to the common 'taste for anecdotes' as well as to the special fondness of the French for similar genres that boomed in eighteenth- and nineteenth-century France: 'to please the crowd and to get consent and be understood, morality is put into narratives, experience in sayings, tragedy in sentences, history in selected excerpts, and politics in couplets'.[139] He claims that,

> the anecdote is made to please everybody [...] One likes to see the flipside of the cards and medals, to encounter important persons in dressing gowns, and to look behind the curtains of the story. [...] even if historically false, it often has this moral truth which made Aristotle write that poetry is often more true than history [...].[140]

The entries in the dictionary embrace all kinds of small forms of prose: anecdotes, short stories, aphorisms, legends, sayings, and jokes, which were taken from various publications: other dictionaries, historical works, travel accounts, newspapers as well as scientific publications.[141] As to anecdotes without author, the editor explains that these are those which '[...] have become a sort of common and banal property [...] By travelling and travelling, they have lost their home, and I have found them in a state of vagabondage, far from their birth place, without any mark that would allow me to make a guess about their origin'.[142] Stressing the anthropomorphic metaphor further, the editor points to the problem that, somewhere along their way, some narratives had lost their authenticity: because of the existence of numerous unauthorised

---

139 Ibid., III: 'Pour plaire à la foule et s'en faire accepter et comprendre, la morale se met en récits, l'expérience en dictons, la tragédie en sentences, l'histoire en morceaux choisis, et la politique en couplets'.

140 Ibid., If.: 'L'anecdote est faite pour plaire à tous [...]. On aime à voir le dessous des cartes et le revers des médailles, à rencontrer les grands hommes en robe de chambre, et à pénétrer dans les coulisses de l'histoire. [...] même historiquement fausse, elle peut revendiquer souvent cette vérité morale qui a fait écrire à Aristote que la poésie est plus vraie que l'histoire [...]'.

141 Ibid., VII.

142 Ibid., VIIf.: 'Les anecdotes dont la source n'est point indiquée sont celles qui n'ont aucune importance, qu'on retrouve partout, qui sont devenues une sorte de propriété commune et banale, sans qu'on sache d'où elles viennent, du moins sans qu'on puisse retrouver leur rédaction primitive; ou bien enfin celles dont la rédaction est propre à ce recueil, soit parce qu'il a fallu les abréger ou les condenser, soit pour toute autre raison. Quelquefois, surtout par certaines anecdotes modernes qui n'ont point le caractère historique, il n'a pas été possible de remonter à la source. De pérégrinations en pérégrinations elles s'étaient dépaysées, et je les trouvais à l'état de vagabondage, loin du lieu natal, sans aucune marque qui permit d'en deviner l'origine'.

copies,[143] but also because of their 'adaptation to another time and another role', as 'some of them have travelled even for centuries and centuries and from country to country by changing their costume at every stage'.[144]

Included under the letter C and entitled Voluntary Crucifixion (*Crucifiement volontaire*),[145] the narrative of Lovat's self-crucifixion is presented under the described category of homeless and vagabonding anecdotes without author that 'travel' about. At the end of the narrative, instead of an author's name, it says 'national opinion',[146] indicating the popularity of the narrative with the French by that time. In the framework of this encyclopaedic dictionary, Lovat's case was therefore completely dissociated from any scientific and medical context and transformed into a popular anecdote that told the history of an isolated event: a remarkable self-crucifixion attempt. For this reason, many of the formal features that originally had made Ruggieri's *Histoire du crucifiement* recognisable as a medical case history in the form of the *observatio* had completely disappeared. Most telling for this transformation, there was no reference to the author, and it no longer mattered if the narrative was fictional or corresponded to real incidents. If at the beginning of the century, Ruggieri's case history was a rare pamphlet that contained specialist knowledge and circulated in the professional circle of physicians and the new specialists of mental diseases, towards the end of the century, parallel to its canonisation as a famous example of religious madness in French psychiatry, the narrative of Lovat's self-crucifixion had become 'common and banal property', that is popular knowledge.

---

143 Ibid., VIIIf.: 'Ces plagiats se pratiquent si continuellement, si universellement et sur une si large échelle, que, pendant la composition de ce Dictionnaire, il m'arrivait chaque jour de reconnaître et de saluer au passage les trois-quarts [...]'.

144 Ibid., VII: '[...] des adaptions à un autre temps et à un autre personnage. Il en est qui ont voyagé ainsi de siècles en siècles et de pays en pays, en changeant de costume à chaque étape'.

145 Guérard, *Crucifiement volontaire*, 287.

146 Ibid.

Epilogue

This book has examined how Lovat's case was read and understood by particular groups, in particular ways, at particular times. It was inspired by the
call made long ago by the literary scholar André Jolles to write the history of
the multiple journeys and metamorphoses of one particular case.[1] This endeavour was encouraged by a dynamic and growing interdisciplinary research
field concerning the case as a style of thinking and a particular form of writing
that has developed with astonishing productivity over the last few decades. In
particular, my study of the history of Lovat's case has profited from existing
scholarship on the medical case history as an epistemic genre as well as from
the insights offered by literary scholars regarding the role of medical cases in
fiction.

I have suggested in this book that rather than comparing national contexts
of reception, it is more illuminating to focus on the main themes connected
with Lovat's case, and to distinguish different interpretive communities. However, the many appropriations of Lovat's case also provide a lens on the national contexts in which they circulated. The Italian, German, British and French
readership required different meanings of Lovat's case and, accordingly, produced different readings, which can roughly be summarized as follows. The
German reception was many-voiced: German readers looked at Lovat's case
from the perspectives of religion, philosophy, criminology, medicine and psychiatry, which indicates the entanglement of these discourses in early nineteenth-century Germany. A striking aspect of the German readings is that most
of them conveyed the idea that Lovat was a typical enthusiast (*Schwärmer*),
which bespeaks the importance of this notion in the confessional history of
the German states. The French readership, by contrast, turned out to be much
more homogenous, as it was predominantly professional and medical: here,
Lovat's case was received almost exclusively by the circle of the Parisian *aliénistes* who were concerned with establishing the study and treatment of mental diseases as a new medical specialty. For French psychiatrists, Lovat's case
confirmed the diagnosis of religious madness, i.e., it implied a consensus on
a specific clinical picture within their professional interpretive community.
Italian readings mostly looked at Lovat's case from a medical perspective and
classified him as a suicide victim. In quantitative terms, Italian readings were
comparatively rare – the case soon travelled away from its origin. It is significant that many Italian commentators on Lovat's case became acquainted with

---

1 Jolles, *Einfache Formen*, 182.

© KONINKLIJKE BRILL NV, LEIDEN, 2019 | DOI:10.1163/9789004353602_010

it only through the reading of French publications, which indicates the su-
premacy of nineteenth-century French psychiatry and the exemplary function
French psychiatrists had for Italian physicians. Finally, the English readings
turned out to be the most particular and self-contained compared with the
German, French and the Italian appropriations of Lovat's case: the interpretive
communities within which Lovat's case circulated in Britain predominantly
included a lay readership interested in biographies of 'eccentric characters'.
The precondition for the British readings was thus the popularity of a specific
literary genre which helped to foster a sense of patriotism and to construct
national identity. Reproductions of the original illustration showing Lovat on
the cross played a prominent role in this context because the tradition of the
genre required portraits. In the British case, reflections on national identity
determined the specific readings of Lovat's case to a much larger extent than
it was the case in the other countries. Through the specific framing of Lovat's
case as an 'eccentric', he could be appropriated as a British national character,
despite the fact that he was originally an 'Italian' case.

The perspective on Lovat's case as one that travels within and between different audiences reveals, however, that nineteenth-century scientific and lay
discourses can neither be confined to political and territorial, nor to linguistic
boundaries: through scientific networks, exchange and translation of scientific
publications as well as through an increasing circulation of popular newspapers and magazines, authors influenced their ideas reciprocally and readers
shared common reading experiences. In this way, they all contributed to debates that by nature were transnational.

In terms of methodology, my decision to make one particular medical case
the object of investigation presents some obvious problems. Everyone familiar
with the current academic debate on cases is aware that a single case never
fully corresponds to a rule, and that, in turn, the generalities drawn from particular cases never capture the single case with all its peculiarities. This is true
for the different contemporary readings of Lovat's case, and it is also true for
this book. While it explains how and why Lovat's *particular* case was productive and travelled in specific contexts, it does not provide us with a rule as to
how medical cases in nineteenth-century Europe *generally* travelled. Taking
into account the intrinsic singularity of cases, the psychoanalyst Winnicott
wrote in 1968 that, 'One case proves nothing, but it may illustrate much'.[2] If we
take this for granted, we may still ask what it is, then, that the history of Lovat's
case illustrates?

---

2   D.W. Winnicott, 'Physical and Emotional Disturbances in an Adolescent Girl', in C. Winnicott,
    R. Shephard, and M. Davis (eds.), *Psychoanalytic Explorations*, Cambridge, MA, Harvard
    University Press, 1968, 369–374, 369.

One answer is that the journeys of Lovat's case described in this book high-light the role of the audience, that is, of readers, for the question of how cases work: a case is only what people see in it, think about it and make of it.[3] Lovat's self-crucifixion would have been an extraordinary local event with hardly any impact, if Ruggieri had not decided to write down and publish his case history in 1806. And even this text would have remained without further influence, if there had not been readers who were attracted by it and responded to it, and thereby multiplied and conveyed the narrative to further readers. Hence, it is the readers who gave significance to Lovat's case and who made that its signifi-cance continuously changed, from time to time and from place to place. Here, the readers' social and professional contexts – their interpretive communities – mattered as did the form of publication in which they inserted the case when rewriting and republishing it. In short, the journey of Lovat's case illustrates that the case history, despite its independent narrative form, is necessarily a dependent genre. Both its significance and function depend on its material and conceptual framing.[4] What this framing looks like and how it affects the particular case narrative, however, varies, and is always a conscious choice of authors and editors who read and then rewrite the narrative in different ways.

Moreover, the entangled history of Lovat's case illustrates the simple fact that – as it is true for all published narratives – the meaning and message of medical cases cannot be controlled. The first author of Lovat's case, Cesare Ruggieri, selected a specific epistemic genre to present his text, the form of the *storia*, corresponding to the early modern Latin *observatio*. For him, it was a tool to acquire and to transmit empirical medical knowledge. In his narrative, he therefore suggested how to understand the case from a medical perspective. However, as the journey of Lovat's case shows, the genre of the medical case history is not a stable format, but can be adjusted and appropriated for differ-ent purposes. The first author's original reading and intention may or may not be pursued in this process of transformation. Once it is published, he loses control how and by whom his narrative is read, and how it is understood – new readers, authors, editors take his place. In this way, new and multiple layers of meaning are added to the case.

The journey of Lovat's case therefore also illustrates what case narratives do for the writers (both scientific and lay), who work with them. For scholars from

---

3 Brian Hurwitz has recently pointed to the importance of audience for the workings of clini-cal case reports in modern medicine, see Hurwitz, *Narrative Constructs in Modern Clinical Case Reporting*, 72f.

4 Christiane Frey calls this the 'simultaneity of functional dependence and formal indepen-dence' ('Gleichzeitigkeit von funktionaler Abhängigkeit und formaler Unabhängigkeit'), Frey, *Fallgeschichte*, 283.

various professional fields, Lovat's case helped them to sustain their scientific arguments. The narrative thus worked as a piece of evidence that illustrates and thereby confirms (or sometimes contradicts) a more general claim. For this purpose, they had to make it relevant for their interpretive community by highlighting, adding or downplaying different narrative elements. As Mary S. Morgan has recently described the workings of narrative science, this is '[...] a process of throwing out and taking in both possible explanations and shards of evidence during successive re-descriptions in order to make a fruitful fit between the scientist's projections and their experience [...]'.[5] From a history of science perspective, the focus on the role of scientific authors and editors in the various rewritings of Lovat's case, and on the interpretive communities they built, confirms the importance of social context in the making of narrative knowledge: 'What counts as explanation, and understanding, within a science depends less on a universal ideal, than on what satisfies the scientific norms and values and shared knowledge set of a community. The scientist as narrator – constructing a narrative of a particular sort, aimed at reaching an audience of other scientists within a particular context – sits at the centre of such scientific activity'.[6] In the case of travelling medical cases such as Lovat's, 'authorship' appears to be a collective endeavour rather than reducible to a single original author.

For the various authors and editors of popular publications, in contrast, Lovat's case helped them to achieve other things, which had less to do with the exigencies of the medical market than with the market and dynamics of nineteenth-century popular journalism and literature, and with the demands of a broader reading public. This book has shown that the fertile soil which made Lovat's case travel so well was the growing preference of nineteenth-century editors and readers for short narrative forms, which is discussed in recent scholarship of media history as the boom of 'the short and the brief'.[7] These short narrative forms, which in Lovat's case range from newspaper articles and the eccentric biographies to crime stories and anecdotes, frequently draw on case knowledge by means of narrative techniques such as excerpting, recycling, abbreviation and condensation. They are presented to the readership through the vehicles of larger formats, such as encyclopaedias, anthologies or collections of one particular genre, which collect, subsume and organise the short

---

5   M.S. Morgan, 'Introduction. Narrative Science and Narrative Knowing. Introduction to Special Issue on Narrative Science', *Studies in History and Philosophy of Science*, vol. 62, 2017, 1–5, 2.

6   Ibid., 4.

7   M. Gamper and R. Mayer (eds.), *Kurz&Knapp. Zur Mediengeschichte kleiner Formen vom 17. Jahrhundert bis zur Gegenwart*, Bielefeld, transcript, 2017.

narratives they embrace, and direct the readers' attention as to how to read them.[8] Depending on its epistemic or literary character, the particular framing determines the rewritings of a case narrative, and if it is perceived as pertaining to specialist or rather popular knowledge. In this regard, therefore, the journeys of Lovat's case illuminate the complex interdependencies between a short narrative form and larger formats, and the effects that the insertion of a case in larger formats can have. Paying attention to the relationship and exchange between epistemic and literary genres in this way also shows how the production and the reception of case knowledge are interrelated – popular and scientific knowledge about the case appear as two sides of the same coin.

With regard to the onging scholarly discussion on cases, this book suggests that writing the history of individual case narratives can fruitfully complement a distant reading of the medical case as an epistemic genre over the centuries.[9] It enriches our understanding of the case as a form of knowing, thinking and writing in that it sheds light on the productivity of individual cases, and on how authors and editors thought in and worked with cases at specific points in time and in specific social contexts. Looking through the lens of particular cases and tracing their stories in a nutshell gives colour to theoretical discussions about the nature of cases. Which particular cases scholars consider worth examining, however, probably depends not only on the cases' historical career, but also on contemporary interests and research agendas. As mentioned in the introduction to this book, it was not only in the nineteenth century that Lovat's case travelled between readers. The narrative of his self-crucifixion continues to circulate, adapting itself to and interacting with the media formats and genres of today. The Internet plays a crucial role here. It disseminates both scientific and popular readings of Lovat's case to a global audience, thereby enabling more and more readers to become authors of Lovat's case by publishing about it in shorter or longer forms. As in the nineteenth century, the case appears in different framings, some more epistemic, others more literary in character. Twentieth-first-century readers may encounter Lovat's case not only in bookshops, but also when reading blogs about Venetian history,[10]

---

8   See M. Gamper and R. Mayer, 'Erzählen, Wissen und kleine Formen. Eine Einleitung', in M. Gamper and R. Mayer (eds.), *Kurz&Knapp. Zur Mediengeschichte kleiner Formen vom 17. Jahrhundert bis zur Gegenwart*, Bielefeld, transcript, 2017, 7–22.

9   Pomata, *The Medical Case Narrative*.

10   Anonymous, 'L' autocrocifissione di Mattio Lovat', *Cercodiamanti*, [web blog], 21 April 2014, http://dipoco.altervista.org/l-autocrocifissione-mattio-lovat/, (accessed 10 September 2017).

Italian literature,[11] or psychiatry.[12] Thanks to digitalisation projects of libraries, they might also find copies of Ruggieri's original case history. Thus, Lovat's case keeps on morphing into different narrative forms, appealing to different readerships with different reading habits. In this way, the case remains alive as a commodity and discursive event even in the twentyfirst century.

---

11   Alessandra, 'Marco e Mattio', *Libri nella mente,* [web blog], 21 May 2016, https://librinellamente.wordpress.com/2016/05/21/marco-e-mattio/, (accessed 10 September 2017); D. Ginevra, 'Mattio Lovat, l'autocrocifisso', *Pensiero spensierato,* [web blog], 8 October 2011, http://www.pensierospensierato.net/2011/10/mattio-lovat-lautocrocifisso/, (accessed 10 September 2017).

12   G. Castigliego, 'L'indicibile tenerezza della sofferenza', *Il sole 24 ore,* [web blog], 19 March 2016, http://giulianocastigliego.nova100.ilsole24ore.com/2016/03/19/lindicibile-tenerezza -della-sofferenza/?refresh_ce=1, (accessed 10 September 2017).

Bibliography

1   Manuscript Sources

Archivio dell' Ateneo Veneto (=*ATV*)

ATV, Società Veneta di Medicina, b. 1, fasc. 1 (=anni 1789–1810, Statuti e regolamenti).

ATV, Società Veneta di Medicina, b. 1, fasc. 2 (=anni 1790–1811, Relazioni sull'attività della società e verbali delle sedute; Rese di conti, cariche onorarie).

ATV, Società Veneta di Medicina, b. 1, fasc. 4 (=anni 1792 a 1810, Atti riguardanti la sede della società e a sua chiesa).

ATV, Società di Medicina, b. 2, fasc. V a (=anni 1790–1810, Lavori accademici).

ATV, Ateneo Veneto, b. 8.1 (=anni 1808–1862, Elenchi dei soci, prospetti e relazioni).

ATV, Ateneo Veneto, b. 28 (=anni 1812–1817, Attività letteraria e scientifica, memorie e studi).

ATV, Ateneo Veneto, Adunanze/processi verbali, b. 13 (=anni 1812–1826, Corpo accademico, adunanze, relazioni annuali) (a register for these files is available).

Archivio di Stato di Venezia (=*ASV*)

ASV, Prefettura dell'Adriatico (1806–1814), b. 85 (=anno 1807).

ASV, Direzione Generale di Polizia, Indice del Protocollo, reg. 15 (=anno 1805; dal 19 gennaio al 31. agosto) (=The registri are the inevitable medium through which the protocols can be used. The registri are classified per year, each listing the names of the cases treated by the police in alphabetical order).

ASV, Direzione Generale di Polizia, atti, bb. 54–58 (=anno 1805).

ASV, Direzione Generale Polizia, protocolli degli esibiti, b. 18 (=anno 1805; 7.V-5.VIII, protocollo 2761–5207).

ASV, Direzione Generale Polizia, Protocolli degli esibiti, b. 19 (=anno 1805; 5.VIII-31.XII, protocollo 5208–8659).

ASV, Prima Dominazione Austriaca, Governo generale, Protocollo degli esibiti del governo, No. 74 (=anno 1805, dal 1. al 31. lulio).

ASV, Deputazione alle cause pie, b. 33 (=anno 1803).

ASV, Archivio Notarile Testamenti, b. 234.

ASV, Miscellanea Legislativa, b. 1722–1797.

Archivio Comunale di Venezia (=*ACV*)

ACV, Serie Anagrafe, Prima ominazione Austriaca, anagrafi generale (1805).

Archivio di San Servolo (=*ASS*)

ASS, Registri Generali, 1 (=Elenco A dei maniaci entrati dal 25 ottobre 1725 a tutto il 24 settembre 1812).

ASS, Libro dei morti dal 1 marzo 1798 a tutto il 2 febbraio 1825.

ASS, Documenti settecenteschi 1759–1799, b. 584.

ASS, Maniaci, Atti, b. 2, fasc. 1–9 (=anni 1803–1810).

ASS, Rapporti Sanitari, b. 1, fasc. 1 (=anni 1805–1810).

Biblioteca e Archivio del Museo Correr di Venezia (=BMC)

BMC, Cod. Cicogna, 2999, fasc.12 (s.d.) (=Regolamento dell'ateneo veneto, manuscripts by Gaetano Ruggieri).

BMC, Direzione Generale di Polizia, documenti, 1–146, anni 1799–1823.

Padova, Archivio Generale di Ateneo, Archivio dell'Ottocento

Padova, Archivio Generale di Ateneo, Archivio dell'Ottocento, Atti del rettorato, 1817, b. 17 (manuscript autograph of Cesare Ruggieri).

Paris, Bibliothèque Interuniversitaire de Santé (=BIU)

BIU, Société médicale d'Émulation, Procès-verbeaux des séances de la société, Carton 1: 1811–1831 et 1837, Ms 2194.

BIU, Société médicale d'Émulation, Registres divers provenant de la société médicale d'émulation. Tome Ier. Procès verbaux du 7 février 1810 au 19 octobre 1831, Ms 2191.

BIU, Société médicale d'Émulation, Registres diverses provenant de la société médicale d'émulation. Registre de présence aux séances (1797–1868), MS 2193.

Paris, Bibliothèque de l'Académie nationale de Médecine

Biographic dossier of Charles Marc, MS 552 (1424).

Fouzia, Fennouri-Ghalloudi, *Charles-Chrétien Henri Marc 1771–1840. Un pionnier de la psychiatrie médico-légale en France* (Memoire pour le D.I.S. de psychiatrie, Université de Caen, 1993), MS 76237.

2   Printed Sources

Adelmann, Georg, *Über die Krankheiten der Künstler und Handwerker nach den Tabellen für kranke Gesellen der Künstler und Handwerker in Würzburg von den Jahren 1786 bis 1802 nebst einigen allgemeinen Bemerkungen*, Würzburg, Bey den Gebrüdern Stahel, 1803.

Adelon, Nicolas-Philibert et al. (eds.), *Dictionnaire de médecine par MM. Adelon, Béclard, Biett et al.*, Paris, Béchet Jeune, 1821–1828.

Adelon, Nicolas-Philibert et al. (eds.), *Dictionnaire de médecine ou répertoire général des sciences médicales considérées sous le rapport théorique et pratique, par MM. Adelon, Béclard, Bérard, Biett et al.*, Paris, Béchet Jeune et Labé, 1832–1846.

Aglietti, Francesco (ed.), *Giornale per servire alla storia ragionata della medicina di questo secolo*, Venice, nella Stamperia Pasquali, 1783–1793.

Aglietti, Francesco, *Saggio sopra la costanza delle leggi fondamentali dell'arte medica. Discorso accademico di Francesco Aglietti P.P. di clinica*, Venice, Dalla Stamperia Palese, 1804.

Alibert, Jean-Louis, *Monographie des dermatoses ou précis théorique et pratique des maladies de la peau*, Paris, Daynac, 1832.

Alibert, Jean-Louis, *Précis théorique et pratique sur les maladies de la peau*, vol. 2, Paris, Chez Caille et Ravier, 1818.

Amoretti, Carlo, 'Ai leggitori. L'editore', in Carlo Amoretti (ed.), *Nuova scelta di opuscoli interessanti sulle scienze e sulle arti tratti dagli atti delle accademie, e dalle altre collezioni filosofiche e letterarie, dalle opere piu recenti inglesi, tedesche, francesi, latine, e italiane, e da' manoscritti originali, e inediti*, vol. 1, no. 6, Milan, Presso Giacomo Agnelli successore Marelli Librajo-Stampatore in S. Margherita, 1804–1807.

Amoretti, Carlo, *Opuscoli scelti sulle scienze e sulle arti, tratti dagli atti delle accademie e dalle altre collezioni filosofiche e letterarie dalle opere più recenti inglesi, tedesche, francesi, latine, e italiane, e da manoscritti originali, e inediti*, Milan, presso Giuseppe Marelli, 1778–1803.

Anonymous, 'Amoretti, Karl', in von Wurzbach, Constantin (ed.), *Biographisches Lexikon des Kaiserthums Österreich*, vol. 1, Vienna, L.C. Zamarsti, 1856, 31–32.

Anonymous, *An Entire New Magazine: On Friday, February 1, 1793, Will Be Published, (Price Only Sixpence) Elegantly Printed on a Superfine Paper...* London: Printed for the Proprietors, sold by C. Johnson, No. 14, and the Other Booksellers in Paternoster-Row; and may be had of all Booksellers and Newscarriers in England, Wales, Scotland, and Ireland, 1793, 1793a.

Anonymous (ed.), *Beyträge zur Geschichte der Verirrungen des menschlichen Geistes und der Thorheiten gelehrter Männer*, Leipzig, Bruder&Hoffmann, 1809a.

Anonymous, 'Blennorée produite par une cause singulière', *Journal général de médecine, de chirurgie et de pharmacie, françaises et étrangères; ou recueil périodique de la société de médecine de Paris*, vol. 60, 1817, 94–98.

Anonymous, 'Cajetan Strambio, Abhandlungen über das Pellagra', in Nicolai, Friedrich (ed.), *Neue allgemeine deutsche Bibliothek*, Kiel, Carl-Ernst Bohn, 1797, 157–158.

Anonymous, 'Die Leipziger Büchermesse', *Morgenblatt für gebildete Stände*, 16 June 1821, 189–192.

Anonymous, 'Enthusiasterey', in Zedler, Johann Heinrich (ed.), *Grosses vollständiges Universallexikon aller Wissenschaften und Künste*, vol. 8, Leipzig and Halle, Johann Heinrich Zedler, 1734a, 1285–1290.

Anonymous, 'Extraordinary Case of a Man Who Crucified Himself', *The Terrific Register; or Record of Crimes, Judgements, Providences, and Calamities*, vol. 2, 1825, 384–350.

Anonymous, 'Fanatici', in Zedler, Johann Heinrich (ed.), *Grosses vollständiges Universallexikon aller Wissenschaften und Künste*, vol. 9, Leipzig and Halle, Johann Heinrich Zedler, 1734b, 212.

Anonymous, 'Foreign Intelligence', *The European Magazine and London Review*, vol. 60, 1811a, 387.

Anonymous, '*Geschichte der durch Mathieu Lovat zu Venedig im Jahr 1805 an sich selbst vollzogenen Kreuzigung*, bekannt gemacht von Cesar Ruggieri ... Aus dem Französischen übersetzt und mit Anmerkungen versehen von Julius Heinrich Gottlieb Schlegel ...', *Allgemeine Literatur-Zeitung*, vol. 3, no. 355, 1808, 805–807.

Anonymous, 'Henry Lee Warner, Esq', in Wilson, Henry (ed.), *The Eccentric Mirror: Reflecting a Faithful and Interesting Delienation of Male and Female Characters, Ancient and Modern, Who Have Been Particularly Distinguished by Extraordinary Qualifications, Talents, and Propensities, Natural or Aquired, Comprehending Singular Instances of Longevity, Conformation, Bulk, Stature, Powers of Mind and of Body, Wonderful Exploits, Adventures, Habits, Propensities, Enterprising Pursuits, &c.&c.&c*, vol. 1, London, James Cundee, 1806, 22.

Anonymous, 'Histoire d'une blennorrhée accompagnée d'ulcères, produite par le LÉCHEMENT d'un chien (traduit de l'italien)', in Alard, Marie and Charles Chrétien Henri Marc (eds.), *Bulletin des sciences médicales. Publié au nom de la société médicale d'émulation de Paris, séant à l'école de médecine, et rédigé par M. Alard, secrétaire général, et par M. Marc, adjoint à la rédaction*, vol. 8, Paris, Chez Crochard, 1811b, 174–179.

Anonymous, 'Introduction', in *The European Magazine and London Review: Containing the Literature, History, Politics, Arts, Manners & Amusements of the Age*, vol. 2, 1782.

Anonymous (ed.), *L'esprit des journaux français et étrangers, par une société de gens de lettres*, Brussels, De Weissenbruch, 1809b.

Anonymous, 'Lovats Selbstkreuzigung', *Morgenblatt für gebildete Staende*, 23 September 1811c, 910.

Anonymous, 'Lovats Selbstkreuzigung', *Archiv für Geographie, Historie, Staats-und Kriegskunst*, 6 and 8 November 1811d, 563.

Anonymous (ed.), *Mercure de France. Journal littéraire et politique*, vol. 38, Paris, Arthus-Bertrand, 1809c.

Anonymous, 'Michaeli Gherardini, Geschichte des Pellagra, aus dem Ital.', in Nicolai, Friedrich (ed.), *Neue allgemeine deutsche Bibliothek*, Kiel, Carl-Ernst Bohn, 1793b, 90–91.

Anonymous, 'Preface', *The Pamphleteer. Respectfully Dedicated to Both Houses of Parliament. To Be Continued Occasionally, at an Average of Four or Five Numbers Annually*, vol. 1, no. 1, 1813, III–XI.

Anonymous, 'Preface', *The Mirror of Literature, Amusement, and Instruction*, vol. 1, no. 1, 1823a.

Anonymous, 'Schwärmer, diejenigen Fanatici genennt', in Zedler, Johann Heinrich (ed.), *Grosses vollständiges Universallexikon aller Wissenschaften und Künste*, vol. 35, Leipzig and Halle, Johann Heinrich Zedler, 1743, 1795.

Anonymous, 'Self-Crucifixion of Matthew Lovat', *The Mirror of Literature, Amusement, and Instruction*, vol. 1, no. 6, 1823b, 81–84.

Anonymous, 'Self-Crucifixion of Matthew Lovat', *The Terrific Record; and Chronicle of Remarkable and Interesting Events &c.*, vol. 1, no. 14, 1849, 209–212.

Anonymous, *The Sketch Book of Character; or, Curious and Authentic Narratives and Anecdotes Respecting Extraordinary Individuals; Exemplifying the Imperfections of Circumstantial Evidence: Illustrative of the Tendency of Credulty and Fanaticism: and Recording Singular Instances of Voluntary Human Suffering and Interesting Occurrences*, vol. 2, Philadelphia, Carey & A. Hart, 1835.

Anonymous, *Sopra il suicidio. Saggio filosofico, pubblicato con annotazioni da G.V.*, Venice, Nella tipografia Picotti, 1824.

Anonymous, 'Variétés médicales, dictionnaire des sciences médicales par une société de médecins et de chirurgiens, avis des editeurs', *Bibliothèque médicale ou recueil périodique d'extraits des meilleurs ouvrages de médecine et de chirurgie. Par une société de médecins*, vol. 35, 1812, 129–131.

Anonymous, 'Verschnittener um des Himmelreichs willen', in Zedler, Johann Heinrich (ed.), *Grosses vollständiges Universallexikon aller Wissenschaften und Künste*, vol. 47, Leipzig and Halle, Johann Heinrich Zedler, 1746, 1722.

Anonymous, 'Von den Folgen eines unrichtig geleiteten Religions-Unterrichtes. Eine belehrende Erzählung für Aeltern und Erzieher', *Der Correspondent der Volksschullehrer. Eine pädagogische Zeitschrift*, vol. 1, 1831, 3–21.

Anonymous, 'Wund-Artzt', in Zedler, Johann Heinrich (ed.), *Grosses vollständiges Universallexikon aller Wissenschaften und Künste*, vol. 59, Leipzig and Halle, Johann Heinrich Zedler, 1749, 1490–1511.

Archambault, Théophile, 'Lypémanie suicide. Tentative de suicide par section de la verge. – Observation communiquée par M. le docteur Archambault, médecin de la maison royale de Charenton', in Jules Baillarger, Laurent Alexis Philibert Cerise, and François Achille Longet (eds.), *Annales médico-psychologiques. Journal destiné à récueillir tous les documents relatifs à l'aliénation mentale, aux névroses, et à la médecine légale des aliénés, par MM. les docteurs Baillarger, Cerise et Moreau*, Paris, Victor Masson, 1852.

Ateneo Veneto, *L'ateneo veneto nel suo primo centenario 1812–1912*, Venice, Ateneo Veneto, 1912.

Auzouy, Théodore, 'Art. IV. – On Lesions of the Cutaneous Sensibility among the Insane', in Forbes Winslow (ed.), *The Journal of Psychological Medicine and Mental Pathology*, vol. 13, London, John Churchill, 1860, 68–82.

Auzouy, Théodore, 'Des troubles fonctionnels de la peau et de l'action de l'électricité chez les aliénés', in Jules Baillarger, Laurent Alexis Philibert Cerise, and

Jacques-Joseph Moreau (eds.), *Annales médico-psychologiques. Journal destiné à récueillir tous les documents relatifs à l'aliénation mentale, aux névroses, et à la médecine légale des aliénés, par MM. les docteurs Baillarger, Cerise et Moreau,* Paris, Victor Masson, 1859, 527–563.

Baillarger, Jules, Laurent Alexis Philibert Cerise, and François Achille Longet (eds.), *Annales médico-psychologiques. Journal de l'anatomie, de la physiologie, et de la pathologie du système nerveux, destiné particulièrement à recueillier tous les documents relatifs à la science des rapports du physique et du moral, à la pathologie mentale, à la médecine légale des aliénés, et à la clinique des névroses,* Paris, Victor Masson, 1843.

Baillarger, Jules, Laurent Alexis Philibert Cerise, and Jacques-Joseph Moreau (eds.), *Annales médico-psychologiques. Journal destiné à récueillir tous les documents relatifs à l'aliénation mentale, aux névroses, et à la médecine légale des aliénés, par MM. les docteurs Baillarger, Cerise et Moreau,* Paris, Victor Masson, 1859, 527–563.

Ballet, Gilbert (ed.), *Traité de pathologie mentale,* Paris, Octave Doin, 1903.

Barnes, Thomas, *Memoirs of the Literary and Philosophical Society of Manchester,* vol. 2, Manchester, T. Cadell, 1785.

Bembo, Pier Luigi, *Delle istituzioni di beneficenza nella città e provincia di Venezia. Studii storico economico-statistici,* Venice, Nella Tipografia di P. Naratovich, 1859.

Bernardi, Francesco, *Prospetto storico-critico dell'origine, facoltà, diversi stati, progressi, e vicende dell collegio medico-chirurgico, e dell'arte chirurgica in Venezia. Arricchito d'aneddoti interessanti l'italiana letteratura, utilissimo alla disciplina dell'arte medica ed alla comun salute,* Venice, Dalle stampe del cittadino Domenico Costantini, 1797.

Brach, Bernhard, *Lehrbuch der gerichtlichen Medizin,* Cologne, Franz Carl Eisen, 1850.

Brièrre de Boismont, Alexandre, *Du suicide et de la folie suicide: considérés dans leurs rapports avec la statistique, la médecine et la philosophie,* Paris and New York, Baillière, 1856.

Brièrre de Boismont, Alexandre, *La pellagre et de la folie pellagreuse, observations recueillies au grand hôpital de Milan. Mémoire lu à l'académie des sciences dans sa séance du 30 novembre 1830,* Paris, Baillière, 1834.

Browne, William Alexander Francis, 'Endemic Degeneration. By W.A.F. Browne, Commissioner in Luncay for Scotland', in John Charles Bucknill (ed.), *The Journal of Mental Science. Published by Authority of the Association of Medical Officers of Asylums and Hospitals for the Insane,* vol 7, London, John Churchill, 1861, 61–76.

Caldani, Floriano, *Discorso funebre recitato nella chiesa di Santa Maria de' servi di Padova il giorno XV di febbrajo dell'anno MDCCCXXVIII nelle solenni esequie del Professore Cesare Ruggieri professore di clinica chirurgia nell'I.R. università colla descrizione della sezione anatomica del suo cadavere,* Padua, Coi Tipi della Minerva, 1828.

Callisen, Angelo, *Medicinisches Schriftsteller-Lexikon der jetzt lebenden Aerzte, Wundärzte, Geburtshelfer, Apotheker, und Naturforscher aller gebildeten Völker*, vol. 17, Copenhagen, Reitzl, 1833.

Caluci, Eugenio, *L'omicidio-suicidio. Cenni critici*, Venice, Fontana, 1884.

Caulfield, James, *Portraits, Memoirs and Characters of Remarkable Persons, from the Reign of King Edward the Third to the Revolution*, London, Caulfield & Herbert, 1794–1795.

Cazaban, Pierre-Prosper, *Recherches et observations sur la pellagre, dans l'arrondissement de Saint-Sever (Landes)*, Paris, Rignoux, 1848.

Cecil, John, *Sixty Curious Authentic Narratives and Anecdotes Respecting Extraordinary Characters: Illustrative of the Tendency of Credulity, and Fanaticism; Exemplifying the Imperfection of Circumstantial Evidence; and Recording Singular Instances of Voluntary Human Suffering, and Interesting Occurrences*, London, William Hone, 1819.

Chiarugi, Vincenzo, *Della pazzia in genere, e in specie: trattato medico-analitico: con una centuria di osservazioni*, Florence, Presso Luigi Carlieri, 1793–1794.

Collenbusch, Daniel, *Der Rathgeber für alle Stände, in Angelegenheiten, welche die Gesundheit, den Vermögenserwerbstand und den Lebensgenuß betreffen*, Schneeberg, In der neuen Verlagshandlung, 1802.

Comandini, Alfredo, *L'Italia nei cento anni del secolo XIX (1801–1900) giorno per giorno illustrata*, vol. 1, Milan, Antonio Vallardi, 1900–1901.

Comparetti, Andrea, *Riscontro clinico nel nuovo spedale. Regolamenti medico-pratici*, Padua, Nella Stamperia Penada, 1799.

Comparetti, Andrea, *Saggio della scuola clinica nello spedale di Padova*, Padua, Nella Stamperia Penada, 1793.

Corniani, Giambattista, *I secoli della letteratura italiana dopo il suo risorgimento*, vol. VII, Turin, Unione Tipografico-Editrice Torinese, 1855.

Courbon-Pérusel, Antoine, *Essai sur la manière d'observer les maladies. Dissertation présentée et soutenue à l'école de médecine de Paris*, Paris, Migneret, 1803.

Dandolo, Girolamo, *La caduta della repubblica di Venezia ed i suoi ultimi cinquant'anni*, Venice, Coi tipi di Pietro Naratovich, 1855.

De la Roche, Daniel and Philippe Petit Radel (eds.), *Encyclopédie méthodique, chirurgie, publié par une société de médecins*, vols. 1 and 2, Paris, Panckoucke, 1790–1792.

De la Roche, Daniel and Philippe Petit Radel (eds.), *Encyclopédie méthodique, chirurgie, publié par une société de médecins*, vol. 3, Paris, H. Agasse, 1798–1799.

De Pitaval, François Gayot, *Causes célèbres et intéressantes, avec les jugements qui les ont decidées*, La Haye, J. Neaulme, 1735–1745.

De Pitaval, François Gayot, *Merkwürdige Rechtsfälle a ls ein Beitrag zur Geschichte der Menschheit nach dem französischen Werk des Pitaval durch mehrere Verfasser ausgearbeitet und mit einer Vorrede begleitet, herausgegeben von Schiller*, Jena, Cuno, 1792–1795.

Del Chiappa, Giuseppe Antonio, *Della stretissima unione della medicina e della chirurgia. Lezione accademica tenuta nella grand'aula dell'imp. r. università di Pavia il dì 14 dicembre in occasione di laure dottorale*, Pavia, Nella Tipografia di Pietro Bizzoni successore di Bolzani, 1820.

Desportes, Emile, *Du refus de manger chez les aliénés*, Thesis, Faculté de Médicine de Paris, 1864.

Dickens, Charles, William Harrison Ainsworth, and Albert Smith (eds.), *Bentley's Miscellany*, vol. 1, London, Richard Bentley, 1837.

Dickens, Charles, William Harrison Ainsworth, and Albert Smith (eds.), *Bentley's Miscellany*, vol. 4, New York, Jemima M. Mason, 1839.

Diez, Carl August, *Der Selbstmord, seine Ursachen und Arten vom Standpunkte der Psychologie und der Erfahrung*, Tübingen, In der Laubb'schen Buchhandlung, 1838.

Esquirol, Jean-Étienne, 'Démonomanie', in Antoine Jacques Louis Jourdan et al. (eds.), *Dictionnaire des sciences médicales. Par une société de médecins et de chirurgiens*, vol. 8, Paris, Panckoucke, 1814, 294–316.

Esquirol, Jean-Étienne, *Des maladies mentales considérées sous les rapports médical, hygienique et médico-légal* [...] *Accompagnées de 27 planches gravées*, Paris, Chez J.-B. Baillère, 1838.

Esquirol, Jean-Étienne, *Des maladies mentales (1838)*, vol. 1, ed. Thérèse Lempérière, Toulouse, Privat, 1998.

Esquirol, Jean-Étienne, 'Mélancolie', in Antoine Jacques Louis Jourdan et al. (eds.), *Dictionnaire des sciences médicales. Par une société de médecins et de chirurgie*ns, vol. 32, Paris, Panckoucke, 1819a, 147–183.

Esquirol, Jean-Étienne, 'Monomanie', in Antoine Jacques Louis Jourdan et al. (eds.), *Dictionnaire des sciences médicales. Par une société de médecins et de chirurgie*ns, vol. 34, Paris, Panckoucke, 1819b, 34–115.

Esquirol, Jean-Étienne, 'Suicide', in Antoine Jacques Louis Jourdan et al. (eds.), *Dictionnaire des sciences médicales. Par une société de médecins et de chirurgie*ns, vol. 13, Paris, Panckoucke, 1821, 213–283.

Falret, Jean-Pierre, *De l'hypochondrie et du suicide. Considérations sur les causes, le siège et le traitement de ces maladies, sur les moyens d'en arreter les progrès et d'en prévenir le développement*, Paris, Croullebois, 1822.

Falret, Jean-Pierre, *De l'utilité de la religion dans le traitement des maladies mentales et dans les asiles d'aliénés. Extrait des annales médico-psychologiques, article intitulé: Visite à l'établissement d'aliénés d'illenau et conditions générales sur les asiles d'aliénés*, Paris, Bourgogne et Martinet, 1845.

Fettleworth, Holden, *Neue Erfindung für S., Schuhe u. Stiefeln mittelst einer Maschine stehend zu verfertigen*, Leipzig, s.n., 1805.

Fodéré, François-Emmanuel, *Essai théorique et pratique de pneumatologie humaine, ou recherches sur la nature, les causes et le traitement des flatuosités et des diverses vésanies, telles que l'extase, le somnambulisme, la magi-manie, et autres qui ont pour phénomène principal l'insensibilité, et qui ne peuvent s'expliquer par les simples connaissances de l'organisme*, Strasbourg, Février, 1829.

Fossati, A., *Del suicidio nei suoi rapporti colla medicina legale, colla filosofia, colla storia. Dissertazione inaugurale cui per conseguire la laureau dottorale in medicina nell'i.r. università di Pavia nel mese di settembre MDCCCXXXI*, Milan, Presso Luigi Nervetti, 1831.

Foville, Antonio, *Note sur la mégalomanie ou lypémanie partielle, avec prédominance du délire des grandeurs*, Paris, Imprimerie de l'Étoile, 1888.

Fraser, Donald (ed.), *The American Magazine of Wonders, and Marvellous Chronicle, Intended as a Record of Accounts of the Most Extraordinary Productions, Events, and Occurrences, in Providence, Nature, and Art, That Have Been Witnessed at Any Time in Europe and America*, New York, Southwick and Pelsue, 1809.

Galeazzi, Giuseppe and Giuseppe Marelli (eds.), *Scelta di opuscoli interessanti tradotti da varie lingue*, Milan, Marelli, 1775–1777.

Gallée, Petrus-Franciscus, *De capitis humeri luxatione et colli ejusdem fractura simultanea. Dissertatio anatomico-chirurgica*, Paris, Typis Michaelis Lambert, 1786.

Gehlen, Adolf Ferdinand (ed.), *Journal für die Chemie, Physik und Mineralogie*, vol. 4, Berlin, Realschulbuchhandlung, 1807, 51.

Granger, James, *A Biographical History of England, from Egbert the Great to the Revolution: Consisting of Characters Disposed in Different Classes, and Adapted to a Methodical Catalogue of Engraved British Heads. Intended as an Essay Towards Reducing our Biography to System, and a Help to the Knowledge of Portraits. Interspersed with a Variety of Anecdotes, and Memoirs of a Great Number of Persons*, London, T. Davies, 1769.

Granger, William et al., *The New, Original and Complete Wonderful Museum and Magazine Extraordinary: Being a Complete Repository of all the Wonders, Curiosities, and Rarities of Nature and Art, from the Beginning of the World to the Present Year ... Including, among the Greatest Variety of other Valuable Matter in this Line of Literature (from an Illustrated Edition of the Rev. Mr. James Granger's Celebrated Biographical History) Memoirs and Portraits of the Most Singular and Remarkable Persons ...*, London, M. Allen, 1802–1808.

Granger, William (ed.), *The New Wonderful Museum, and Extraordinary Magazine: Being a Complete Repository of All the Wonders, Curiosities, and Rarities of Nature and Art, From the Beginning of the World to the Present Year 1802*, vol. 1, London, R.S. Kirby, 1802.

Graperon, Jean-Baptiste-Étienne (ed.), *Bulletin des sciences médicales. Publié au nom de la société médicale d'émulation de Paris*, vol. 1, Paris, Chez Crochard, 1807.

Graperon, Jean-Baptiste-Étienne (ed.), *Bulletin des sciences médicales. Publié au nom de la société médicale d'émulation de Paris, séant à l'école de médecine*, vol. 2, Paris, Chez Crochard, 1808.

Griesinger, Wilhelm, *Die Pathologie und Therapie der psychischen Krankheiten*, Stuttgart, A. Krabbe, 1861.

Guérard, Edmond, 'Crucifiement volontaire', in Edmond Guérard (ed.), *Dictionnaire encyclopédique d'anecdotes modernes, anciennes, françaises et étrangères*, vol. 1, Paris, Firmin-Diderot, 1872a, 287.

Guérard, Edmond 'Introduction', in Edmond Guérard (ed.), *Dictionnaire encyclopédique d'anecdotes modernes, anciennes, françaises et étrangères*, vol. 1, Paris, Firmin-Diderot, 1872b, I–X.

Haurenski, Erich, *Der Teufel ein Bibelerklärer? Oder Beitrag zur Entscheidung über das Zwingende einer vernunftgemässen Christenthums-und Bibelansicht sowie das Staats-und sittengefährliche des Gegenteils*, Altenburg, Johann Karl Gottfried Wagner, 1834.

Henke, Adolf, *Lehrbuch der gerichtlichen Medizin. Zum Behufe akademischer Vorlesungen und zum Gebrauch für gerichtliche Ärzte und Rechtsgelehrte*, Berlin, Ferdinand Dümmler, 1832.

Herbst, Feridnand Ignaz (ed.), *Merkwürdige Beispiele religiöser Schwärmerei. Gesammelt und als Supplement des kathol. Exempelbuches,* vol. 3, Regensburg, Georg Joseph Manz, 1845.

Hitzig, Julius Eduard and Wilhelm Häring (eds.), *Der neue Pitaval. Eine Sammlung der interessantesten Criminalgeschichten aller Länder aus älterer und neuerer Zeit*, vol. 6, Leipzig, Brockhaus, 1844.

Hoffbauer, Johann Christoph, *Die Psychologie in ihren Hauptanwendungen auf die Rechtspflege nach den allgemeinen Gesichtspunkten der Gesetzgebung; oder, Die sogenannte gerichtliche Arzneywissenschaft nach ihrem psychologischen Theile*, Halle, Schimmelpfennig, 1808.

Hoffbauer, Johann Christoph, *Psychologische Untersuchungen über den Wahnsinn und die übrigen Arten der Verzückung und die Behandlung derselben*, Halle, Bey Hemmerde und Schwetschke, 1807.

Hoffbauer, Johann Christoph, *Über den Selbstmord, seine Arten und Ursachen*, Lemgo, Verlag der Meyerschen Hofbuchhandlung, 1842.

Hoffbauer, Johann Christoph, *Untersuchungen über die Krankheiten der Seele und die verwandten Zustände*, Halle, Bey Joh. Gottfr. Trampens Erben, 1802–1807.

Hoffbauer, Johann Christoph, 'Welches sind die Ursachen der in neuerer Zeit so sehr überhand nehmenden Selbstmorde und welche Mittel sind zu deren Verhütung anzuwenden?', in Albrecht Erlenmeyr et al. (eds.), *Archiv der Deutschen Gesellschaft für Psychiatrie und gerichtliche Psychologie*, vol. 2, Neuwied, J.H. Heuser, 1859, 15, 1–138.

Hohnbaum, Karl, 'Der Selbstmord', in *Blätter für literarische Unterhaltung, Erster Band*, Leipzig, F.A. Brockhaus, 1845, 453–466.

Horn, Ernst (ed.), *Vollständiges Universal-Register des Archivs für medizinische Erfahrung im Gebiete der praktischen Medizin und Staatsarzneikunde*, vol. 58, Berlin, G. Reimer, 1819.

Horne, Richard, 'Analysis of Crime. Being an Attempt to Distinguish Its Chief Causes, in Answer to the Statistical Deductions of M. Guerry, and the Rev. Whitworth Bussell; the Former Finding that Popular Education Did Not Prevent Crime – the Latter That It Was the Cause of Crime', in Forbes Winslow (ed.), *The Journal of Psychological Medicine and Mental Pathology*, vol. 3, London, John Churchill, 1850, 94–123.

Ideler, Karl Wilhelm, *Biographien Geisteskranker in ihrer psychologischen Entwickelung dargestellt*, Berlin, Schroeder, 1841.

Ideler, Karl Wilhelm, *Die Geisteskrankheiten in Beziehung zur Rechtspflege von C.C. Marc, Leibarzte des Königs der Franzosen etc.etc. Deutsch bearbeitet und mit Anmerkungen begleitet. Ein Handbuch für Gerichts-Aerzte und Juristen*, Berlin, Voss'sche Buchhandlung, 1843–1844.

Ideler, Karl Wilhelm, *Versuch einer Theorie des religiösen Wahnsinns. Ein Beitrag zur Kritik der religiösen Wirren der Gegenwart. Erster Theil: Die Erscheinungen des religiösen Wahnsinns*, Halle, Schwetschke und Sohn, 1848.

Ideler, Karl Wilhelm, *Versuch einer Theorie des religiösen Wahnsinns. Ein Beitrag zur Kritik der religiösen Wirren der Gegenwart. 2. Theil: Die Entwickelung des religiösen Wahnsinns*, Halle, Schwetschke und Sohn, 1850.

Isensee, Emil, *Neuere und neueste Geschichte der Heilwissenschaften und ihrer Literatur*, Berlin, Albert Nauck & Comp., 1834.

Jackson's Oxford Journal, vol. 16, 1811.

Jourdan, Antoine Jacques Louis et al. (eds.), *Dictionnaire des sciences médicales. Par une société de médecins et de chirurgiens*, vol. 37, Paris, Panckoucke, 1819.

Jourdan, Antoine Jacques Louis, *Dissertation sur la pellagre, présentée et soutenue à la faculté de médecine de Paris, le 18 décembre 1819, pour obtenir le grade de Docteur en médecine*, Paris, Didot Jeune, 1819.

Journal universel des sciences médicales, quatorzième année, vol. 63, 1829.

Jubinal, Achill, *Notice biographique sur le Docteur Charles-Chrétien-Henri Marc*, Paris, Laurent Thoinon et Cie, 1865.

Kirby, Ralph Smith, *Kirby's Wonderful and Eccentric Museum; or, Magazine of Remarkable Characters. Including all the Curiosities of Nature and Art from the Remotest Period to the Present Time*, vol. 5, London, R.S. Kirby, 1820.

Kirby, Ralph Smith (ed.), *The Wonderful and Scientific Museum; or, Magazine of Remarkable Characters; Including All the Curiosities of Nature and Art, from the Remotest Period to the Present Time, Drawn from Every Authentic Source*, vol. 1, London, T. Keating, 1803.

Klassik, Stiftung Weimar (ed.), *Briefe an Goethe. Gesamtausgabe in Regestform,* http://ora-web.swkk.de/swk-db/goeregest/index.html, (accessed 7 July 2017).

Kleinert, Carl Ferdinand (ed.), *Allgemeines Repertorium der gesammten deutschen medizinisch-chirurgischen Journalistik,* vol. 4, no. 9, 1830.

Knape, Christoph and August Friedrich Hecker, *Kritische Jahrbücher der Staatsarznei-kunde für das 19. Jahrhundert,* Berlin, Bei Friedrich Maurer, 1809.

Kopp, Johann Heinrich (ed.), *Jahrbuch der Staatsarzneykunde,* vol. 1, Frankfurt, Bei Johann Christian Hermann, 1808.

Kraepelin, Emil, *Compendium der Psychiatrie zum Gebrauche für Studierende und Ärzte,* Leipzig, Ambr. Abel, 1883.

Krügelstein, Franz Christian Karl, 'Agende zum Gebrauch für Gerichtsärzte bei Untersuchung und Begutachtung der Krankheit der Selbstmörder. Nach eignen und fremden Beobachtungen und Erfahrungen bearbeitet', *Annalen der Staats-Arzneikunde,* vol. 5, no. 1, 1840, 673–775.

La Société medicale d'Émulation (ed.), *Mémoires de la société medicale d'émulation, séante à l'école de médecine de Paris. Pour l'an Ve de la république,* Paris, Chez Maradan, 1798a.

La Société medicale d'Émulation (ed.), *Mémoires de la société medicale d'émulation, séante à l'école de médecine de Paris. Pour l'an Ve de la république,* Paris, Chez Maradan, 1798b.

La Société medicale d'Émulation (ed.), *Mémoires de la société medicale d'émulation, séante à l'école de médecine de Paris. Pour l'année 1816,* Paris, Chez Crochard, Gabon, 1817.

La Société medicale d'Émulation, 'Règlement de la société médicale d'émulation de Paris', in Graperon, Jean-Baptiste-Étienne (ed.), *Bulletin des sciences médicales. Publié au nom de la société médicale d'émulation de Paris, séant à l'école de médecine,* vol. 1, Paris, Chez Crochard, 1807, 8–18.

Lenz, Jakob Michael Reinhold, *Der Hofmeister oder Vortheile der Privaterziehung. Eine Komödie,* Leipzig, Weygandsche Buchhandlung, 1774.

Levacher de La Feutrie, Thomas, *Recherches sur la pellagre, affection cutanée endémique dans la Lombardie,* Paris, Crapart, Caille et Ravier, 1805.

Levi, Mosè Giuseppe, *Biografia di Gaetano Alfonso Ruggieri, medico e letterato veneziano. Scritta da Mosè Giuseppe Levi, medico e letta nel veneto ateneo la tornata del giorno 19 dicembre 1836,* s.l., s.n., 1836.

Levi, Mosè Giuseppe (ed.), *Dizionario classico di medicina interna ed esterna. Prima tradizione italiana di M. Giuseppe Levi,* Venice, G. Antonelli, 1831–1846.

Levi, Mosè Giuseppe, *Ricordo intorno agli incliti medici chirughi e farmacisti che praticarono loro arte in Venezia dopo il 1740 raccolti aumentati e pubblicati da M.G. Levi...,* Venice, Tipografia di Giuseppe Antonelli, 1835.

Levi, Mosè Giuseppe, 'Ruggieri Cesare, ua vita', in Mosè Giuseppe Levi (ed.), *Dizionario classico di medicina interna ed esterna. Prima tradizione italiana di M. Giuseppe Levi*, Venice, G. Antonelli, 1838, 520–523.

Levi, Mosè Giuseppe, 'Suicidio', in Mosè Giuseppe Levi (ed.), *Dizionario classico di medicina interna ed esterna. Prima tradizione italiana di M. Giuseppe Levi*, Venice, G. Antonelli, 1839, 477–562.

Lorthiois, Marie Michel Edmond Joseph, *De l'automutilation. Mutilations et suicides étrangères*, Paris, Vigot Frères, 1908.

Marc, Charles Chrétien Henri, 'Castration. Considérée sur le rapport de la médecine légale e de la hygiène publique', in Antoine Jacques Louis Jourdan et al. (eds.), *Dictionnaire des sciences médicales. Par une société de médecins et de chirurgiens*, vol. 4, Paris, Panckoucke, 1812, 278.

Marc, Charles Chrétien Henri, 'Consultation délibérée à Paris sur l'état mentale du Pièrre Rivière', *Annales d'hygiène publique et de médecine légale*, vol. 15, no. 1, 1836, 202–205.

Marc, Charles Chrétien Henri, *De la folie considérée dans ses rapports avec les questions medico-judiciaires*, vol. 1 Paris, J.-B. Baillière, 1840.

Marc, Charles Chrétien Henri, 'Introduction', *Annales d'hygiène publique et de médecine légale*, vol. 1, no. 1, 1829, XXXVIII–XXXIX.

Marc, Charles Chrétien Henri, 'Mélancolie religieuse. Rapport fait à la société médicale d'emulation, par M. le docteur MARC, sur une brochure ayant pour titre: Histoire du crucifiement exécuté par sa propre personne, par Mathieu Lovat; communiquée au public, dans une Lettre de César RUGGIERI, docteur en médecine et professur de clinique chirurgicale à Venise, écrite à un médecin de ses amis', in Marie Alard and Charles Chrétien Henri Marc (eds.), *Bulletin des sciences médicales publié au nom de la société médicale d'émulation de Paris, séant à l'école de médecine, et rédigé par M. Alard, secrétaire général, et par M. Marc, adjoint à la rédaction*, vol. 8, Paris, Chez Crochard, 1811, 5–17.

Marchant, Gerard, *Recherches sur les aliénés*, Toulouse, Bonnal et Gobrac, 1845.

Marchant, Léon, *Étude de la pellagre des landes...rapport au conseil central de salubrité du département de la Gironde*, Bordeaux, impr. de P. Faye, 1840.

Matthey, Andrey, *Nouvelles recherches sur les maladies de l'esprit, précédées de considerations sur les difficultés de l'art de guérir*, Paris and Geneva, Paschoud, 1816.

Maury, Alfred, 'Les mystiques extatiques et les stigmatisés', in Jules Baillarger, Laurent Alexis Philibert Cerise, and Jacques-Joseph Moreau (eds.), *Annales médico-psychologiques. Journal destiné à récueillir tous les documents relatifs à l'aliénation mentale, aux névroses, et à la médecine légale des aliénés, par MM. les docteurs Baillarger, Cerise et Moreau*, Paris, Victor Masson, 1855, 181–232.

Maury, Alfred, *Les mystiques extatiques et les stigmatisés*, Paris, Martinet, 1845–1855.

Mill, John Stuart, *On Liberty*, Boston, Ticknor and Fields, 1863.

Millingen, John Gideon, *Curiosities of Medical Experience*, London, Richard Bentley, 1839a.

Millingen, John Gideon, 'Remarkable Suicides' by Dr. Millingen, the Author of "Curiosities of Medical Experience"', in Charles Dickens, William Harrison Ainsworth, and Albert Smith (eds.), *Bentley's Miscellany*, vol. 4, New York, Jemima M. Mason, 1839b, 516–528.

Moreau, Jean-Jacques, *Suicides et crimes étranges*, Paris, Société d'éditions scientifiques, 1899.

Morel, Bénédicte-Auguste, *Études cliniques. Traité théorique et pratique des maladies mentales considérées dans leur nature, leur traitement, et dans leur rapport avec la médecine légale des aliénés*, vol. 2, Paris, Victor Masson et Baillière, 1853.

Moschini, Giannantonio, *Della letteratura veneziana del secolo XVIII fino ai giorni nostri*, vol. 4, Venice, Dalla Stamperia Palese, 1808.

Nicoulou, Élie, *Essai sur la mégalomanie*, Bordeaux, Mourau, 1886.

Osiander, Friedrich Benjamin, *Über den Selbstmord, seine Ursachen, Arten, medicinisch-gerichtliche Untersuchung und die Mittel gegen denselben: Eine Schrift sowohl für Policei- und Justiz-Beamte, als für gerichtliche Aerzte und Wundärzte, für Psychologen und Volkslehrer*, Hannover, Hahn, 1813.

Pavanetto, Lara, *Crocifissione di Matteo Lovat*, Catania, Villagio Maori, 2017.

Perfect, William, *Annals of Insanity, Comprising a Selection of Curious and Interesting Cases in the Different Species of Lunacy, Melancholy, or Madness with the Modes of Practice in the Medical and Moral Treatment, as Adopted in the Cure of Each*, London, Chalmers, 1800.

Pezzi, Pietro, *Discorso pronunciato dal vice-presidente Pezzi alla società di medicina di Venezia nella prima sessione di settembre dell'anno 1807 diciottesimo della sua istituzione prima della sua riforma*, Venice, Per Giuseppe Picotti, Stampatore della suddettta Società, 1808.

Pilgrim, Charles Winfield, 'A Study of Suicide', in William Jay Youmans (ed.), *The Popular Science Monthly*, vol. 35, New York, D. Appleton and Company, 1889, 303–313.

Pinel, Philippe, *L'aliénation mentale ou la manie. Traité médico-philosophique*, Paris, Chez Richard, Caille et Ravier, 1800.

Pinel, Philippe, 'Mémoire sur la manie périodique ou intermittente par Ph. Pinel, professeur à l'école de médecin de Paris', in La Société medicale d'Émulation (ed.), *Mémoires de la société medicale d'émulation, séante à l'école de médecine de Paris. Pour l'an Ve de la république*, Paris, Chez Maradan, 1798.

Pinel, Philippe, *Traité medico-philosophique sur l'aliénation mentale*, Paris, Brosson, 1809.

Pope, Alexander, 'An Essay on Men', in Henry Francis Cary (ed.), *The Poetical Works of Alexander Pope*, London, William Smith, 1839, 216–248.

Portalupi, Giovanni Luigi, *Storia ragionata dell'enorme tumore del nobile signore Luigi Tedeschidi Verona estirpato nel giorno 26 giugno 1823 da Fr. Gio. Luigi Portalupi*, Venice, Tipografia Armena di S. Lazzaro, 1823.

Ramazzini, Bernardino, *De morbis artificum diatriba*, Mutinae, Typis Antonii Capponi, impressoris episcopalis, 1700.

Regnault, Elias, *Du degré de compétence des médecins dans les questions judiciaires relatives aux aliénations mentales*, Paris, B. Warée, 1828.

Reil, Johann Christian and Hoffbauer Johann Christoph, *Beyträge zur Beförderung einer Kurmethode auf psychischem Wege*, vol. 1, Halle, In der Curt'schen Buchhandlung, 1808.

Reil, Johann Christian and Hoffbauer Johann Christoph, *Beyträge zur Beförderung einer Kurmethode auf psychischem Wege*, vol. 2, Halle, In der Curt'schen Buchhandlung, 1812.

Rousseau, Jean-Jacques, *Emile, où, de l'éducation*, Paris, Garnier Frères, 1961.

Ruggieri, Cesare, *Aneurisma vastissimo dell'aorta, causa di morte in un operato di pietra. Osservazione del Signor Dottore Cesare Ruggieri professore di chirurgia in Venezia*, Padua, Nella Tipografia del Seminario, 1814a.

Ruggieri, Cesare, *De kruissiging van Matthieu Lovat, aan zich zelven volbragt te Venetie, in den jaare 1805, medegedeeld door Cesare Ruggieri; volgens de hoogduitsche overzetting, naar het fransch, met de aanmerkingen van J.H.G. Schlegel, en ook van den nederduitschen vertaaler*, Amsterdam, Esveldt-Holtrop, 1807a.

Ruggieri, Cesare, *Dei doveri di chi studia e di chi esercita la medicina. Discorso inaugurale letto nella grande aula dell'imp.reg.università di Padova nel giorno XXX novembre MDCCCXXIII dal Dott. Cesare Ruggieri p.o. prof. di clinica, terapia speciale e di operazioni chirurgiche*, Padua, Nella tipografia del seminario, 1824.

Ruggieri, Cesare, 'Dei polipo dell'ano', in Mosè Giuseppe Levi (ed.), *Dizionario classico di medicina interna ed esterna. Prima tradizione italiana di M. Giuseppe Levi*, Venice, G. Antonelli, 1837a, 228–231.

Ruggieri, Cesare, 'Del processo litotomico di Lecat seguito dal dottor Francesco Pajola', in Mosè Giuseppe Levi (ed.), *Dizionario classico di medicina interna ed esterna. Prima tradizione italiana di M. Giuseppe Levi*, Venice, G. Antonelli, 1835a, 318–320.

Ruggieri, Cesare, 'Delle variazioni riguardanti la esecuzione del taglio nell'apparecchio laterale fatto da più accreditati autori italiani', Mosè Giuseppe Levi (ed.), *Dizionario classico di medicina interna ed esterna. Prima tradizione italiana di M. Giuseppe Levi*, Venice, G. Antonelli, 1835b, 686–688.

Ruggieri, Cesare, *Dizionario enciclopedico di chirurgia. Tradotto dal francese in italiano ed accresciuto di aggiunte e note di Cesare Ruggieri medico fisico e chirurgo e regio pubblico professore di clinica chirurgica in Venezia*, Padua, Nella Stamperia del Seminario presso Tommaso Bettinelli, 1805–1810.

Ruggieri, Cesare, *Dizionario enciclopedico di chirurgia. Tradotto dal francese in italiano ed accresciuto di aggiunte e note di Cesare Ruggieri medico fisico e chirurgo e regio pubblico professore di clinica chirurgica in Venezia,* vol. 3, Padua, Nella Stamperia del Seminario presso Tommaso Bettinelli, 1806.

Ruggieri, Cesare, *Dizionario enciclopedico di chirurgia. Tradotto dal francese in italiano ed accresciuto di aggiunte e note, Spiegazione delle tavole del dizionario enciclopedico di chirurgia dei signori Petit-Radel, e Allan,* vol. 4, Padua, Nella Stamperia del Seminario presso Tommaso Bettinelli, 1810.

Ruggieri, Cesare, 'Dolore spasmodico riccorrente alla parte interna dell'anti-braccio sinistro, che apportò la piegatura della mano sull'anti-braccio medesimo con contrazione di tutte le dita; osservazione Medico-chirurgica', *Nuovi commentarj di medicina e di chirurgia pubblicati dai Signori Valeriano Luigi Brera Cesareo-Regio Consigliere, Cesare Ruggieri, e Floriano Caldani professori di medicina e chirurgia nell'imperiale regia università di Padova etc.,* vol. 1, no. 3, 1818, 97–104.

Ruggieri, Cesare, *Geschichte der durch Mathieu Lovat zu Venedig im Jahr 1805 an sich selbst vollzogenen Kreuzigung. Bekannt gemacht von Cesar Ruggieri [...] Aus dem Französischen übersetzt und mit Anmerkungen versehen von Julius Heinrich Gottlieb Schlegel [...],* Rudolstadt, Klüger, 1807b.

Ruggieri, Cesare, *Histoire du crucifiement éxécuté sur sa propre personne par Mathieu Lovat, communiqué au public dans une lettre de César Ruggieri docteur en medecine et professeur de chirurgie clynique à Venise. A un medecin son ami,* s.l., s.n., s.d.

Ruggieri, Cesare, *Mathieu Lovat's Selbstkreuzigung zu Venedig im J. 1805. A.d.F. von dem Hofrath und Ritter Julius Heinrich Gottlieb Schlegel. Unveränderte, wohlfeile Ausgabe,* Meiningen, In der Reyßnerschen Hofbuchhandlung, 1821.

Ruggieri, Cesare, 'Narrative of the Crucifixion of Matthew Lovat Executed by His Own Hands at Venice, in the Month of July, 1805. Originally Communicated to the Public by Cesare Ruggieri, M.D. Professor of Clynical Surgery at Venice, in a Letter to a Medical Friend. Now First Translated into English', *The Pamphleteer. Respectfully dedicated to both houses of Parliament,* vol. 3, no. 6, 361–375.

Ruggieri, Cesare, 'Pellagra. Malattia della pelle chiamata anche da alcuni dermatagra [...]', in Cesare Ruggieri (ed.), *Dizionario enciclopedico di chirurgia. Tradotto dal francese in italiano ed accresciuto di aggiunte e note,* vol. 4, Padua, Nella Stamperia del Seminario presso Tommaso Bettinelli, 1808, 105–122.

Ruggieri, Cesare, *Prolusione intorno ai progressi ed avvanzamenti della chirurgia recitata nel sacro collegio de' medici fisici di Venezia per l'apertura della scuola di clinica chirurgica dal Dr. Cesare Ruggieri medico fisico, e r. prof. della scuola suddetta, il giorno 25. agosto 1803,* Venice, Per Gio, Antonio Perlini, 1803.

Ruggieri, Cesare, *Selbstkreuzigung: der Fall Matteo Lovat,* Munich, Belleville, 1984.

Ruggieri, Cesare, 'Storia della crocifissione di Matteo Lovat da se stesso eseguita. Comunicata in lettera da Cesare Ruggieri. Medico fisico, e di clinica chirurgica a

Venezia. Ad un medico suo amico', in Carlo Amoretti (ed.), *Nuova scelta di opus-coli interessanti sulle scienze e sulle arti tratti dagli atti delle accademie, e dalle altre collezioni filosofiche e letterarie, dalle opere piu recenti inglesi, tedesche, francesi, latine, e italiane, e da' manoscritti originali, e inediti*, vol. 1, no. 6, Milan, Presso Giacomo Agnelli successore Marelli Librajo-Stampatore in S. Margherita, 1804–1807, 403–412.

Ruggieri, Cesare, *Storia della crocifissione di Mattio Lovat da se stesso eseguita. Comunicata in lettera da Cesare Ruggieri medico fisico, e di clinica chirurgica in Venezia elettore nel collegio dei dotti, socio corrispondente delle accademie i.r. giuseppina medico-chirurgica di Vienna, reale di Madrid, della facoltà e società medica d'emulazione di Parigi ec.ec. Ad un medico suo amico*, Venice, Nella Stamperia Fracasso, 1814b.

Ruggieri, Cesare, *Storia della crocifissione di Mattio Lovat da se stesso eseguita*, Crema, Amici del Museo, Arti grafiche, 1996.

Ruggieri, Cesare, *Storia di una blennorea prodotta da lambimento canino associata ad ulceri, ec. di Cesare Ruggieri, medico fisico, p.p. di clinca chirurgia in Venezia, elettore nel collegio dei dotti, socio corrispondente delle accademie i.r. giuseppina medico-chirugica di Vienna, reale di Madrid, della facoltà e società medica d'emulazione di Parigi ec.ec.*, Venice, Nella Stamperia Fracasso, 1814c.

Ruggieri, Cesare, *Storia ragionata di una donna avente gran parte del corpo coperta di pelle e pelo nero*, Venice, Tipografia Picotti, 1815a.

Ruggieri, Cesare, 'Storia ragionata di una donna avente gran parte del corpo coperta di pelle e pelo nero', in Mosè Giuseppe Levi (ed.), *Dizionario classico di medicina interna ed esterna. Prima tradizione italiana di M. Giuseppe Levi*, Venice, G. Antonelli, 1837b.

Ruggieri, Cesare, *Storia ragionata di una donna avente gran parte del corpo coperta di pelle e pelo nero di Cesare Ruggieri medico fisico p.o.p. di clinica, terapia speciale ed operazioni chirurgiche nell'i. r. università di Padova, già elettore nel collegio dei dotti, socio corrispondente delle accademie imp. r. giussepina medico-chirurgica di Vienna, reale di Madrid, della facoltà e società medica d'emulazione di Parigi, ec. ec. ec. Edizione seconda*, Padua, dalla Tipografia della Minerva, dalla Nuova società tipografica in ditta N. Zanon Bettoni e compagni, 1822.

Ruggieri, Cesare, 'Taglio laterale eseguito alla parte destra del perineo', in Mosè Giuseppe Levi (ed.), *Dizionario classico di medicina interna ed esterna. Prima tradizione italiana di M. Giuseppe Levi*, Venice, G. Antonelli, 1835c, 699–701.

Ruggieri, Gaetano (ed.), *Esercitazioni scientifiche e letterarie dell'ateneo di Venezia*, Venice, Presso G. Picotti, 1827–1829.

Ruggieri, Gaetano, 'Ricordi storici sull'ateneo di Venezia, compilati dal Dott. Gaetano A. Ruggieri, membro ordinario, e vice-presidente', in Gaetano Ruggieri (ed.), *Esercitazioni scientifiche e letterarie dell'ateneo di Venezia*, vol. 1, Venice, Presso G. Picotti, 1827, 2–16.

Ruggeri [sic!], Gaetano, *Riflessioni intorno ad una memoria del p. trivigiano Giambattista Marzari, intitolata della pellagra e della maniera die estirparla in Italia,* Padua, Nella tipografia del Seminario, 1815b.

Ruggieri, Gaetano (ed.), *Sessioni pubbliche dell'ateneo veneto,* Venice, Vitarelli, 1812–1817.

Savoldello, Giovanni Batista, *Relazione della gravissima mortal malattia sofferta dalla neofita Elena Savorgnan e della sua perfetta guarigione istantanea ottenuta da Dio per intercessione de' Santi Martiri di Concordia estesa da Giovanni Battista Savoldello maestro e prefetto del pio luogo de' catumeni di Venezia e corredata di documenti autentici estratti dal processo istituito nella reverendissima cura patriarcale capitolare,* Venice, Nella Stamperia di Andrea Santini, 1807.

Schiller, Friedrich, *Der Geisterseher, Erzählungen und historische Charakteristiken,* Stuttgart, Reclam, 1958.

Schlegel, Julius Heinrich Gottlieb (ed.), *Briefe einiger Ärzte in Italien über das Pellagra. Aus dem Italienischen übersetzt und mit beygefügter Literatur,* Jena, Joh. Christ. Gottfr. Göpferdt, 1807a.

Schlegel, Julius Heinrich Gottlieb, *Materialien für die Staatsarzneiwissenschaft und praktische Heilkunde,* Jena, Goepferdt, 1800–1803.

Schlegel, Julius Heinrich Gottlieb, *Reise durch das mittägliche Deutschland und einen Theil von Italien. Mit Kupfern,* Gießen and Wetzlar, Tasche und Müller, 1807b.

Sforza Benvenuti, Francesco, 'Ruggieri Cesare', in Francescoi Sforza Benvenuti (ed.), *Dizionario biografico cremasco,* Crema, Forni, 1888, 247–248.

Società Scientifiche e Letterarie formanti l'ateneo Veneto (ed.), *Relazioni accademiche delle società scientifiche e letterarie formanti l'ATENEO VENETO. Prima pubblica sessione 21 novembre 1812,* Venice, Nella Tipografia Picotti, 1812.

Société de Médecins (ed.), *Bibliothèque médicale ou recueil périodique d'extraits des meilleurs ouvrages de médecine et de chirurgie. Par une société de médecins,* vol. 1, 1803.

Société de Médecins (ed.), *Bibliothèque médicale ou recueil périodique d'extraits des meilleurs ouvrages de médecine et de chirurgie. Par une société de médecins,* vol. 33, 1811.

Société Royale (ed.), *Journal général de médecine, de chirurgie et de pharmacie, françaises et étrangères; ou recueil périodique de la société de médecine de Paris,* Paris, Croullebois, T. Barrois jeune, 1802–1830.

Société Royale (ed.), *Recueil périodique de la société de médecine de Paris,* Paris, Croullebois & Barrois, 1797–1802.

Spieß, Christian Heinrich, *Biographien der Selbstmörder,* Göttingen, Wallstein, 2005.

Spieß, Christian Heinrich, *Biographien der Wahnsinnigen,* Leipzig, Voß, 1796.

Sydenham, Thomas, *Medical Observations Concerning the History and the Cure of Acute Diseases. Translated from the Latin Edition of Dr. Greenhill with a Life of the Author by R.G. Latham,* London, Sydenham Society, 1848.

Tartra, A.-E. (ed.), *Bulletin des sciences médicales. Publié au nom de la société médicale d'émulation de Paris, séant à l'école de médecine, et rédigé par M. Alard, secrétaire général, et par M. Marc, adjoint à la rédaction*, vol. 6, Paris, Chez Crochard, 1810.

Taruffi, Cesare, *Hermaphrodismus und Zeugungsunfähigkeit. Eine systematische Darstellung der menschlichen Geschlechtsorgane von Prof. Cesare Taruffi, autorisierte deutsche Ausgabe von Dr. med. R. Täuscher mit Abbildungen*, Berlin, Verlag von H. Barsford Tissier, 1903.

The European Magazine and London Review, Containing Traits, Views, Biography, Anecdotes, Literature, History, Politics, Arts, Manners, and Amusements of the Age, vol. 60, 1811.

The Leeds Mercury, vol. 16, 1811.

The London Dispatch and People's Political and Social Reformer, vol. 17, 1839.

The Scots Magazine and Edinburgh Literary Miscellany Being a General Repertory of Literature, History, and Politics, vol. 76, 1814.

*The Tradesman; or, Commercial Magazine: Including Subjects Relating to Commerce, Foreign and Domestic, Together with Suggestions for New Commercial Connexions; Expositions of History and Processes of Manufactories...*vol. 8, 1811.

Théophile Roussel, Jean-Baptiste Victor, *De la pellagre, de son origine, de ses progrès, de son existence en France, de ses causes et de son traitement curatif et préservatif*, Paris, Bureau de l'Encyclopédie médicale, 1845.

Théophile Roussel, Jean-Baptiste Victor, *Histoire d'un cas de pellagre observé à l'hôpital Saint-Louis, dans le service de M. Gibert*, Paris, impr. de Moquet et Hauquelin, 1842.

Timbs, John (ed.), *English Eccentrics and Eccentricities*, vol. 1, London, Richard Bentley, 1866.

Vassalli, Sebastiano, *Marco e Mattio*, Turin, Einaudi, 1992.

Voigt, Bernhard Friedrich, *Neuer Nekrolog der Deutschen*, vol. 18, no. 1, Weimar, Bernh. Friedr. Voigt, 1842.

Voisin, Felix, *Des causes morales et physiques des maladies mentales: et de quelques autres affections nerveuses telles que l'hystérie, la nymphomanie et la satyriaisis*, Paris, Chez J.-B.- Baillière, 1826.

Von Archenholz, Joahnn Wilhelm, 'Lovat. Ein großer Beytrag zur Verirrung des menschlichen Geistes', *Minerva. Ein Journal historischen und politischen Inhalts*, no. 2, 1809, 97–102.

Vulpius, Christian August, '*Geschichte der durch Mathieu Lovat zu Venedig im Jahr 1805 an sich selbst vollzogenen Kreuzigung*, bekannt gemacht von Cesar Ruggieri ... Aus dem Französischen übersetzt und mit Anmerkungen versehen von Julius Heinrich Gottlieb Schlegel ...', *Jenaische Allgemeine Literaturzeitung*, vol. 93, 1808, 134.

Watts, John, *The Museum of Remarkable and Interesting Events, Containig Historical and Other Accounts of Adventures, Incidents of Travels and Voyages, Scenes of Peril*, *and Escapes, Military Achievements, Eccentric Personages, Noble Examples of Fortitude and Patriotism, with Various Other Entertaining Narratives, Anecdotes, etc.etc... Designed as a Book of Leisure Reading for All Classes*, vol. 1, Cleveland, OH, Sanford & Hayward, 1844.

Wessenberg, Ignaz Heinrich, *Ueber Schwärmerei. Historisch-philosophische Betrachtungen mit Rücksicht auf die jetzige Zeit,* Heilbronn, Claßische Buchhandlung, 1835.

Wilson, Henry, *Fifty Wonderful Portraits*, London, J. Robins, 1821–26.

Wilson, Henry, *The Book of Wonderful Characters: Memoirs and Anecdotes of Remarkable and Eccentric Persons in All Ages and Countries. Chiefly from the Text by Henry Wilson and James Caulfield*, London, John Camden Hotten, Piccadilly, 1869.

Wilson, Henry (ed.), *The Eccentric Mirror: Reflecting a Faithful and Interesting Delienation of Male and Female Characters, Ancient and Modern, Who Have Been Particularly Distinguished by Extraordinary Qualifications, Talents, and Propensities, Natural or Aquired, Comprehending Singular Instances of Longevity, Conformation, Bulk, Stature, Powers of Mind and of Body, Wonderful Exploits, Adventures, Habits, Propensities, Enterprising Pursuits, &c.&c.&c*, vol. 1, London, James Cundee, 1806.

Wilson, Henry, *Wonderful Characters: Comprising Memoirs and Anecdotes of the Most Remarkable Persons of Every Age and Nation*, London, J. Robins, 1821–1827.

Winslow, Forbes, *The Anatomy of Suicide*, London, Henry Renshaw, 1840.

Winslow, Forbes (ed.), *The Journal of Psychological Medicine and Mental Pathology*, vol. 1, London, John Churchill, 1848.

Youmans, William Jay (ed.), *The Popular Science Monthly*, vol. 1, New York, D. Appleton and Company, 1872.

Zannini, Paolo, *Biografia di Francesco Aglietti*, Padua, Coi tipi della Minerva, 1836.

Zimmermann, Johann Georg, *Von der Erfahrung in der Arzneykunst. Neue Auflage*, Zurich, Orell, 1777.

Zyro, Ferdinand Friedrich, *Wissenschaftlich-praktische Beurtheilung des Selbstmords nach allen seinen Beziehungen als Lebensspiegel für unsere Zeit*, Bern, Chur and Leipzig, J.F.J. Dalp, 1837.

3   Literature

Ackerknecht, Erwin H., 'Die Pariser Spitäler von 1800 als Ausgangspunkt einer neuen Medizin', *Ciba-Sympoisum 7*, 1959, 98–105.

Ackerknecht, Erwin H., *Medicine at the Paris Hospital, 1794–1848*, Baltimore, Johns Hopkins University Press, 1967.

Alberti, Samuel J.M.M., 'Objects and the Museum', *Isis*, vol. 96, no. 4, 2005, 559–571.

Alessandra, 'Marco e Mattio', *Libri nella mente,* [web blog], 21 May 2016, https://librinellamente.wordpress.com/2016/05/21/marco-e-mattio/, (accessed 10 September 2017).

Andrews, J., 'Cause or Symptom? Contentions Surrounding Religious Melancholy and Mental Medicine in Late-Georgian Britain', *Studies in the Literary Imagination*, vol. 44, no. 2, 2011, 63–91.

Andrews, Jonathan, 'Winslow, Forbes Benignus (1810–1874)', *Oxford Dictionary of National Biography*, 2004, http://www.oxforddnb.com/view/article/29752, (accessed 20 July 2017).

Ankeny, Rachel A., 'The Case Study in Medicine', in Miriam Solomon, Jeremy R. Simon, and Harold Kincaid (eds.), *The Routledge Companion to Philosophy of Medicine*, New York and London, Routledge, 2017, 310–318.

Ankeny, Rachel A., 'The Overlooked Role of Cases in Casual Attribution in Medicine', *Philosophy of Science*, vol. 81, no. 5, 2014, 999–1011.

Ankeny, Rachel A., 'Using Cases to Establish Novel Diagnoses: Creating Generic Facts by Making Particular Facts Travel Together', in Peter Howlett and Mary S. Morgan (eds.), *How Well Do Facts Travel? The Dissemination of Reliable Knowledge*, Cambridge, UK, Cambridge University Press, 2011, 252–273.

Anonymous, 'L' autocrocifissione di Mattio Lovat', *Cercodiamanti*, [web blog], 21 April 2014, http://dipoco.altervista.org/l-autocrocifissione-mattio-lovat/, (accessed 10 September 2017).

Apple, Rima D., Gregory J. Downe, and Stephen L. Vaughn (eds.), *Science in Print: Essays on the History of Science and the Culture of Print*, Madison, University of Wisconsin Press, 2012.

Archivio di Stato di Venezia (ed.), *Difesa della sanità a Venezia, secoli XIII–XIX, catalogo della mostra documentaria*, Venice, Ministero per i beni culturali e ambientali, 1979.

Aschauer, Lucia, Horst Grunder, and Tobias Gutmann (eds.), *Fallgeschichten. Text- und Wissensformen exemplarischer Narrative in der Kultur der Moderne*, Würzburg, Königshausen&Neumann, 2015.

Bachleitner, Norbert, '"Übersetzungsfabriken". Das deutsche Übersetzungswesen in der ersten Hälfte des 19. Jahrhunderts', *Internationales Archiv für Sozialgeschichte der deutschen Literatur (IASL)*, vol. 14, no. 1, 1989, 1–49.

Bähr, Andreas and Hans Medick (eds.), *Sterben von eigener Hand: Selbsttötung als kulturelle Praxis*, Cologne, Böhlau, 2005.

Bandirali, Simone (ed.), *Storia della crocifissione di Mattio Lovat da se stesso eseguita, postfazione di Sebastiano Vassalli*, Crema, Amici del Museo, Arti grafiche, 2000, 1996.

Bandorf, Melchior Josef, 'Reil, Johann Christian', in Historische Kommission bei der Bayerischen Akademie der Wissenschaften (ed.), *Allgemeine Deutsche Biographie*, vol. 27, Munich, Duncker & Humblot, 1888, 700–701.

Barbagli, Marzio, *Farewell to the World. A History of Suicide*, Cambridge, UK, Polity Press, 2015.

Barnes, James J., *Authors, Publishers and Politicians: The Quest for an Anglo-American Copyright Agreement 1815–1854*, Columbus, OH, Ohio State University Press, 2016.

Barnes, James J. and Patience P. Barnes, 'Copyright', in Sally Mitchell (ed.), *Victorian Britain: An Encyclopedia*, New York, Garland, 1988, 192–193.

Bautz, Friedrich Wilhelm, 'Böhme, Jacob, Mystiker und Naturphilosoph', in Friedrich Wilhelm Bautz (ed.), *Biographisch-Bibliographisches Kirchenlexikon*, vol. 1, Hamm, Traugott Bautz, 1990, 661–665.

Benassati, Giuseppina and Daniela Savoia (eds.), *L'Italia nei cento anni. Libri e stampe della biblioteca di alfredo comandini,* Bologna, grafis, 1998.

Berengo, Marino (ed.), *Giornali veneziani del settecento*, Milan, Feltrinelli, 1962.

Bernardi, Paolo L., 'Introduction: A Culture of Death: Suicide in Italy in the Long Nineteenth Century 1798–1915', in Paolo L. Bernardi and Anita Virga (eds.), *Voglio morire! Suicide in Italian Literature, Culture and Society 1789–1919,* Cambridge, UK, Cambridge Scholars Publishing, 2013a, 1–26.

Bernardi, Paolo L. and Anita Virga (eds.), *Voglio morire! Suicide in Italian Literature, Culture and Society 1789–1919,* Cambridge, UK, Cambridge Scholars Publishing, 2013b.

Bianco, Elisa, 'Suicidi di primo ottocento: Riflessioni sulla liceità della morte volontaria nell'Italia preunitaria', in Paolo L. Bernardi and Anita Virga (eds.), *Voglio morire! Suicide in Italian Literature, Culture and Society 1789–1919,* Cambridge, UK, Cambridge Scholars Publishing, 2013, 85–114.

Blanchard, Pascal et al. (eds.), *Exhibitions: L'invention du sauvage*, Paris, Actes Sud, 2011.

Blaschke, Olaf, 'Abschied von der Säkularisierungslegende. Daten zur Karrierekurve der Religion (1800–1970) im zweiten konfessionellen Zeitalter: eine Parabel', *zeitenblicke*, vol. 5, no. 1, 2006, http://www.zeitenblicke.de/2006/1/Blaschke, (accessed 7 June 2017).

Boden, Petra and Dorit Müller (eds.), *Populäres Wissen im medialen Wandel seit 1850*, Berlin, Kadmos Kulturverlag, 2009.

Böning, Holger, 'Weltaneignung durch ein neues Publikum. Zeitungen und Zeitschriften als Medientypen der Moderne', *Historische Zeitschrift. Beihefte*, Vol. 41, 2010, 105–134.

Bowie, Angus M., 'The Death of Priam: Allegory and History in the *Aenedid*', *Classical Quarterly*, vol. 40, no. 2, 1990, 470–481.

Brambilla, Elena, *Corpi invasi e viaggi dell'anima. Santità, possessione, esorcismo dalla teologia barocca alla medicina illuminista*, Rome, viella, 2010.

Brancaccio, Maria Teresa, Eric J. Engstrom, and David Lederer, 'The Politics of Suicide: Historical Perspectives on Suicidology before Durkheim. An Introduction', *Journal of Social History*, vol. 46, no. 3, 2013, 607–619.

Braun, Karl, *Die Krankheit Onania. Körperangst und die Anfänge moderner Sexualität im 18. Jahrhundert*, Frankfurt, campus, 1995.

Bräunlein, Peter J., *Passion/Pasyon. Rituale des Schmerzes im europäischen und philippinischen Christentum*, Munich, Wilhelm Fink, 2010.

Bredekamp, Horst, *Repräsentation und Bildmagie in der Renaissance als Formproblem*, Munich: Carl Friedrich von Siemens Stiftung, 1984.

Breuer, Dieter, 'Origenes im 18. Jahrhundert in Deutschland', *Seminar. A Journal of Germanic Studies*, vol. 21, 1985, 1–30.

Brian, Charles S. and Chane R. Mull, 'Pellagra Pre-Goldberger: Rupert Blue, Fleming Sandwith, and The "Vitamine Hypothesis"', *Transactions of the American Clinical an Climatological Association*, vol. 126, 2015, 20–45.

Brown, Horatio, *The Venetian Printing Press, 1469–1800*, New York, G.P. Putnam's Sons, 1891.

Burke, Peter, 'Cultures of Translations in Early Modern Europe', in Peter Burke and Ronnie Po-Chia Hsia (eds.), *Cultural Translation in Early Modern Europe*, Cambridge, UK, Cambridge University Press, 2007, 7–38.

Bynum, Caroline W., 'Fast, Feast, and Flesh: The Religious Significance of Food to Medieval Women', *Representations*, vol. 11, 1985, 1–25.

Bynum, Caroline W., *Holy Feast and Holy Fast. The Religious Significance of Food to Medieval Women*, Berkeley, University of California Press, 1987.

Bynum, William F. and Michael Neve, 'Hamlet on the Couch: Hamlet Is a Kind of Touchstone by Which to Measure Changing Opinion – Psychiatric and Otherwise – about Madness', *American Scientist*, vol. 74, no. 4, 1986, 390–396.

Bynum, William F. and Janice C. Wilson, 'Periodical Knowledge: Medical Journal and Their Editors in Nineteenth-Century Britain', in William F. Bynum, Stephen Lock, and Roy Porter (eds.), *Medical Journals and Medical Knowledge. Historical Essays*, London, Routledge, 1992, 29–48.

Bynum, William F., Stephen Lock, and Roy Porter (eds.), *Medical Journals and Medical Knowledge. Historical Essays*, London and New York, Routledge, 1992.

Carlino, Andrea, *Paper Bodies: A Catalogue of Anatomical Fugitive Sheets 1538–1687*, London, Wellcome Institute for the History of Medicine, 1999.

Carlino, Andrea and Michel Jeanneret (eds.), *Vulgariser la médecine. Du style médical en France et en Italie*, Geneva, Droz, 2009.

Carlino, Andrea and Alexandre Wenger (eds.), *Littérature et médecine. Approches et perspectives (XVIe–XIXe siècle)*, Geneva, Droz, 2007.

Carroll, Victoria, *Science and Eccentricity: Collecting, Writing and Performing Science for Early Nineteenth-Century Audiences*, London, Pickering & Chatto, 2008.

Carroy, Jaqueline, 'L'étude de cas psychologique et psychanalytique (XIXe siècle-début du XXe siècle)', in Jean-Claude Passeron and Jacques Revel (eds.), *Penser par cas*, Paris, EHESS, 2005, 201–228.

Carroy, Jaqueline, 'Observer, raconter ou ressuciter les rêves? "Maury guilotiné" en question', *Communication*, vol. 84, 2009, 137–149.

Castigliego, Giuliano, 'L'indicibile tenerezza della sofferenza', *Il sole 24 ore*, [web blog], 19 March 2016, http://giulianocastigliego.nova100.ilsole24ore.com/2016/03/19/lindicibile-tenerezza-della-sofferenza/?refresh_ce=1, (accessed 10 September 2017).

Castiglioni, Arturo, *Gli albori del giornalismo medico italiano*, Trieste, Tipografia del Lloyd triestino, 1923.

Cavallo, Guglielmo and Roger Chartier (eds.), *Histoire de la lecture dans le monde occidental*, Paris, Seuil, 1997.

Chartier, Roger, 'Laborers and Voyagers: From the Text to the Reader', *diacritics*, vol. 22, no. 2, 1992, 49–61.

Chartier, Roger, 'Texts, Printings, Readings', in Lynn Hunt (ed.), *The New Cultural History*, Berkeley, University of California Press, 1989, 154–175.

Chartier, Roger, *Forms and Meanings. Texts, Performances, and Audiences from Codex to Computer*, Philadelphia, University of Pennsylvania Press, 1995.

Connor, Jennifer J., 'Introduction. Book Culture and Medicine', *Canadian Bulletin of Medical History*, vol. 12, no. 2, 1995, 203–214.

Corbin, Alain, *Le monde retrouvée sur les traces d'un inconnu, 1798–1876*, Paris, Flammarion, 1998.

Crignon-De Oliveira, Claire, 'La mélancolie entre médecine et religion: d'une pathologie des comportements religieux à une pratique pathologique de la religion', *Gesnerus*, vol. 63, 2006, 46–60.

Cunningham, Andrew, 'Identifying Disease in the Past: Cutting the Gordian Knot', *Asclepio* vol. 54, 2002, 13–34.

Da Costa, Palmira Fontes, 'The Making of Extraordinary Facts: Authentication of Singularities of Nature at the Royal Society of London in the First Half of the Eighteenth Century', *Studies in History and Philosophy of Science*, vol. 33, 2002, 265–288.

Da Costa, Palmira Fontes, *The Singular and the Making of Knowledge at the Royal Society of London in the Eighteenth Century*, Newcastle upon Tyne, Cambridge Scholars Publishing, 2009.

Darnton, Robert, *The Business of Enlightenment. A Publishing History of the Encyclopédie, 1775–1800*, Cambridge, MA, Harvard University Press, 1979.

Daston, Lorraine (ed.), *Biographies of Scientific Objects*, Chicago, University of Chicago Press, 1999.

Daston, Lorraine, *Wunder, Beweise und Tatsachen. Zur Geschichte der Rationalität*, Frankfurt, Fischer, 2011.

Daston, Lorraine and Katherine Park, 'Unnatural Conceptions: The Study of Monsters in Sixteenth- and Seventeenth-Century France and England', *Past & Present*, no. 92, 1981, 20–54.

Daston, Lorraine and Katherine Park, *Wonders and the Order of Nature 1150–1750*, New York, Zone Books, 1998.

Daum, Andreas, *Wissenschaftspopularisierung im 19. Jahrhundert. Bürgerliche Kultur, naturwissenschaftliche Bildung und die deutsche Öffentlichkeit, 1848–1914*, Munich, R. Oldenbourg, 1998.

Davidson, Arnold, 'Miracles of Bodily Transformation, or, How St. Francis Received Stigmata', in Caroline A. Jones and Peter Galison (eds.), *Picturing Science and Producing Art*, New York and London, Routledge, 1998, 101–124.

Davis, John A., 'Health Care and Poor Relief in Southern Europe in the 18th and 19th Centuries', in Ole Peter Grell, Andrew Cunningham, and Bernd Roeck (eds.), *Health Care and Poor Relief in 18th and 19th Century Southern Europe*, Aldershot, Ashgate, 2005, 10–33.

Daxelmüller, Christoph, *Die Geschichte der Selbstkreuzigung von Franz von Assisi bis heute*, Düsseldorf, Patmos, 2001.

De Bernardi, Alberto, *Il mal della rosa. Denutrizione e pellagra nelle campagne italiane tra '800 e '900*, Milan, Franco Angeli, 1984.

De Bernardi, Alberto, 'Malattia mentale e trasformazioni sociali. La storia dei folli', in Alberto De Bernardi (ed.), *Follia, psichiatria e società. Istituzioni manicomiali, scienza psichiatrica e classi sociali nell'Italia moderna e contemporanea*, Milan, Franco Angeli, 1982, 11–32.

Della Peruta, Franco (ed.), *Storia d'Italia. Annali. Vol. 7: Malattia e Medicina*, Turin, Einaudi, 1984.

Dickson, Sheila, 'Die internationale Rezeption der Fallgeschichten im Magazin zur Erfahrungsseelenkunde', in Sheila Dickson, Stefan Goldman, and Christoph Wingertszahn (eds.), *'Fakta, und kein moralisches Geschwätz'. Zu den Fallgeschichten im 'Magazin für die Erfahrungsseelenkunde' (1783–1793)*, Göttingen, Wallstein, 2011, 256–276.

Didi-Huberman, Georges, *Invention de l'hystérie. Charcot et l'iconographie photographique de la Salpêtrière*, Paris, Macula, 1982.

Dinges, Martin, 'Zimmermann, Johann Georg', in Werner E. Gerabek et al. (eds.), *Enzyklopädie Medizingeschichte*, Berlin and New York, Walter de Gruyter, 2005, 1530.

Dinzelbacher, Peter, 'Diesseits der Metapher: Selbstkreuzigung und Stigmatisation als konkrete Kreuzesnachfolge', *Revue Mabillon*, vol. 7, 1996, 157–181.

Doyle, Julie, 'The Spectre of the Scalpel: The Historical Role of Surgery and Anatomy in Conceptions of Embodiment', *Body and Society*, vol. 14, no. 1, 2008, 9–30.

Durkheim, Emile, *Le suicide: Étude de sociologie*, Paris, Félix Alcan, 1897.

Düwell, Susanne, 'Populäre Falldarstellungen in Zeitschriften der Spätaufklärung: Der spektakuläre Fall des "Menschenfressers" Goldschmidt', in Susanne Düwell and Nicolas Pethes (eds.), *Fall – Fallgeschichte – Fallstudie. Theorie und Geschichte einer Wissensform*, Frankfurt, campus, 2014, 293–314.

Düwell, Susanne and Nicolas Pethes (eds.), *Fall – Fallgeschichte – Fallstudie. Theorie und Geschichte einer Wissensform*, Frankfurt, campus, 2014.

Düwell, Susanne and Nicolas Pethes, 'Noch nicht Wissen. Die Fallsammlung als Prototheorie in Zeitschriften der Spätaufklärung', in Michael Bies and Michael Gamper (eds.), *Literatur und Nicht-Wissen. Historische Konstellationen 1730–1930*, Zurich, Diaphanes, 2012, 131–148.

Eder, Franz X., 'Diskurs und Sexualpädagogik: Der deutschsprachige Onanie-Diskurs des späten 18. Jahrhunderts', *Paedagogica Historica*, vol. 39, no. 6, 2003, 719–735.

Eisenstein, Elizabeth L., *The Printing Press as an Agent of Change: Communications and Cultural Transformations in Early-Modern Europe*, Cambridge, UK, Cambridge University Press, 1994.

Feather, John, *A History of British Publishing*, London and New York, Routledge, 2006.

Feather, John, *Publishing, Piracy and Politics: An Historical Study of Copyright in Britain*, London, Mansell, 1994.

Feldmann, Detlef, *Die 'religiöse Melancholie' in der deutschsprachigen medizin-theologischen Literatur des ausgehenden 18. und frühen 19. Jahrhunderts*, Kiel, Diss. med., 1973.

Fischer-Homberger, Esther, *Medizin vor Gericht: Gerichtsmedizin von der Renaissance bis zur Aufklärung. Mit 70 illustrierenden Fallbeispielen, zusammengestellt von Cécile Ernst*, Bern, Hans Huber, 1983.

Fischer-Homberger, Esther, 'On the Medical History of the Doctrine of Imagination', *Psychological Medicine*, vol. 9, 1979, 619–628.

Fischer, Ernst, 'Buchmarkt', *Europäische Geschichte Online*, [website], 2010, http://ieg-ego.eu/de/threads/hintergruende/buchmarkt/ernst-fischer-buchmarkt, (accessed 12 July 2017).

Fish, Stanley, *Is There a Text in This Class? The Authority of Interpretive Communities*, Cambridge, MA, Harvard University Press, 1982.

Föcking, Marc, *Pathologia litteralis. Erzählte Wissenschaft und wissenschaftliches Erzählen im französischen 19. Jahrhundert*, Tübingen, Gunter Narr, 2002, 170–209.

Fondazione San Servolo I.R.S.E.S.C. (Istituto per le Ricerche e per gli Studi sull'EmarginazioneSocialeeCulturale),[website],http://www.fondazionesanservolo.it/html/fondazione.asp, (accessed 15 March 2016).

Forrester, John, 'If p – Then What? Thinking in Cases', *History of the Human Sciences*, vol. 9, no. 3, 1996, 1–25.

Forrester, John, *Thinking in Cases*, Cambridge and Malden, Polity Press, 2016.

Foucault, Michel, *Discipline and Punish: The Birth of the Prison*, London, Allen Lane, 1979.

Foucault, Michel, *La naissance de la clinique. Une archéologie du regard medical*, Paris, Presses universitaire de France, 1963.

Foucault, Michel, *Moi, Pierre Rivière, ayant égorgé ma mère, ma soeur et mon frère....
Un cas de parricide au XIXe siècle*, présenté par Michel Foucault, Paris, Gallimard,
1973.

Foucault, Michel, *Power, Truth, Strategy*, Sydney, Feral Publications, 2006.

Foucault, Michel, *The Birth of the Clinic: An Archaeology of Medical Perception*, London,
Routledge, 1997.

Frey, Christiane, 'Am Beispiel der Fallgeschichte. Zu Pinels "Traité medico-philosophique sur l'aliénation"', in Jens Ruchatz, Stefan Willer and Nicolas Pethes (eds.),
Das Beispiel. Epistemologie des Exemplarischen, Berlin, Kadmos Kulturverlag, 2007,
263–278.

Frey, Christiane, 'Fallgeschichte', in Roland Borgards et al. (eds.), *Literatur und Wissen.
Ein interdisziplinäres Handbuch*, Stuttgart and Weimar, Metzler, 2013, 282–287.

Furth, Charlotte, 'Introduction. Thinking with Cases', in Charlotte Furth, Judith T. Zeitlin, and Ping-chen Hsiung (eds.), *Thinking with Cases. Specialist Knowledge in Chinese Cultural History*, Honolulu, University of Hawaii Press, 2007, 1–27.

Gafner, Lina, Schreibarbeit. *Die alltägliche Wissenspraxis eines Bieler Arztes im 19.
Jahrhundert*, Tübingen: Mohr Siebeck, 2016.

Gailus, Andreas, 'A Case of Individuality. Karl Philipp Moritz and the Magazine for
Empirical Psycchology', *New German Critique*, no. 79, 2000, 67–105.

Galzigna, Mario, *La malattia morale. Alle origini della psichiatria moderna*, Venice,
Marsilio, 1988.

Galzigna, Mario (ed.), *Museo del manicomio di San Servolo. La follia reclusa*, Verona,
Arsenale Editrice, 2007.

Galzigna, Mario and Hrayr Terzian (eds.), *L'archivio della follia. Il manicomio di San Servolo e la nascita di una fondazione. Antologia di testi e documenti*, Venice, Marsilio,
1980.

Gamper, Michael and Ruth Mayer, 'Erzählen, Wissen und kleine Formen. Eine Einleitung', in Michael Gamper and Ruth Mayer (eds.), *Kurz&Knapp. Zur Mediengeschichte kleiner Formen vom 17. Jahrhundert bis zur Gegenwart*, Bielefeld, transcript,
2017, 7–22.

Gamper, Michael and Ruth Mayer (eds.), *Kurz&Knapp. Zur Mediengeschichte kleiner
Formen vom 17. Jahrhundert bis zur Gegenwart*, Bielefeld, transcript, 2017.

Gates, Barbara T., *Victorian Suicides. Mad Crimes and Sad Histories*, Princeton, Princeton University Press, 2013.

Gelfand, Toby, *Professionalizing Modern Medicine. Paris Surgeons and Medical Science
and Institutions in the 18th Century*, Westport, CT and London, Greenwood Press,
1980.

Gentilcore, David, '"Italic Scurvy", "Pellarina", "Pellagra": Medical Reactions to a New
Disease in Italy, 1770–1815', in Kevin Siena and Jonathan Reinarz (eds.), *A Medical
History of the Skin: Scratching the Surface*, London, Taylor&Francis, 2013, 57–69.

Gentilcore, David, 'Louis Sambon and the Clash of Pellagra Etiologies in Italy and the United States, 1905–1914', *Journal of the History of Medicine and Allied Sciences*, vol. 71, no. 1, 2016, 19–42.

Gentilcore, David, 'Peasants and Pellagra in Nineteenth-Century Italy', *History Today*, vol. 64, 2014, 32–38.

Geyer-Kordesch, Johanna, 'Medizinische Fallbeschreibungen und ihre Bedeutung in der Wissensreform des 17. und 18. Jahrhunderts', *Medizin, Gesellschaft und Geschichte*, vol. 9, 1990, 7–19.

Giesecke, Michael, *Der Buchdruck in der frühen Neuzeit. Eine historische Fallstudie über die Durchsetzung neuer Information- und Kommunikationstechnologien*, Frankfurt, Suhrkamp, 1991.

Gillispie, Charles Coulston, *Science and Polity in France at the End of the Old Regime*, Princeton, Princeton University Press, 1980.

Ginevra, Donata, 'Mattio Lovat, l'autocrocifisso', *Pensiero spensierato*, [web blog], 8 October 2011, http://www.pensierospensierato.net/2011/10/mattio-lovat-lautocrocifisso/, (accessed 10 September 2017).

Ginnaio, Monica, *La pellagre: Histoire du mal et de la misère en Italie. XIXe siècle – début XXe*, Paris, L'Harmattan, 2014.

Ginzburg, Carlo, 'Ein Plädoyer für den Kasus', in Johannes Süßmann, Susanne Scholz, and Gisela Engel (eds.), *Fallstudien. Theorie – Geschichte – Methode*, Berlin, trafo, 2007, 28–48.

Giormani, Virgilo, 'Contrasti tra l'università di Padova e il collegio dei medici di Venezia nel '700', *Quaderni per la storia dell'università di Padova*, vol. 28, 1995, 23–87.

Giormani, Virgilo, *I collegi dei medici fisici e dei medici chirurghi a Venezia nel settecento*, Pisa and Rome, Fabrizio Serra, 2007.

Giormani, Virgilo, 'I rapporti tra i due collegi veneziani, dei filosofi e medici e dei chirurghi, con l'università di Padova nel settecento', in Gian Paolo Brizzi and Jacques Verger (eds.), *Le università minori in Europa (secoli XV–XIX)*, Soveria Mannelli, Rubbettino, 1998, 169–181.

Goldberg, Ann, *Sex, Religion and The Making of Modern Madness. The Eberbach Asylum and German Society 1815–1849*, Oxford, Oxford University Press, 1999.

Goldmann, Stefan, 'Kasus-Krankengeschichte-Novelle', in S. Dickson, S. Goldman and C. Wingertszahn (eds.), *'Fakta, und kein moralisches Geschwätz'. Zu den Fallgeschichten im 'Magazin für die Erfahrungsseelenkunde' (1783–1793)*, Göttingen, Wallstein, 2011, 33–64.

Goldstein, Jan, *Console and Classify. The French Psychiatric Profession in the Nineteenth Century*, Chicago, University of Chicago Press, 2001.

Goldstein, Jan, 'Enthusiasm or Imagination? Eighteenth-Century Smear Words in Comparative National Context', *Huntington Library Quaterly*, vol. 60, 1997, 29–49.

Goldstein, Jan, *Hysteria Complicated by Ecstasy: The Case of Nanette Leroux*, Princeton, Princeton University Press, 2011.

Gori Bucci, Nina, *Il pittore Teodoro Matteini (1754S–1831)*, Venice, Istituto Veneto di Scienze Lettere ed Arti, 2006.

Gottardi, Michele, *L'Austria a Venezia. Società ed istituzioni nella prima dominazione austriaca, 1798–1806*, F. Angeli Milan, 1993.

Gottardi, Michele (ed.), *Venezia suddita (1798–1866)*, Venice, Marsilio, 1999.

Gregory, James, 'Eccentric Biography and the Victorians', *Biography*, vol. 30, no. 3, 2007, 342–376.

Gregory, James, 'Eccentric Lives: Character, Characters, and Curiosities in Britain, c. 1760–1900', in Waltraud Ernst (ed.), *Histories of the Normal and of the Abnormal. Social and Cultural Histories of Norms and Normativity*, London and New York, Routledge, 2006, 72–100.

Gregory, James, '"Local Characters": Eccentricity and the North-East in the Nineteenth Century', *Northern History*, vol. 42, no. 1, 2005, 163–186.

Greve, Ylva, 'Die Unzurechnungsfähigkeit in der "Criminalpsychologie" des 19. Jahrhunderts', in Michael Niehaus and Hans-Walter Schmidt-Hannisa (eds.), *Unzurechnungsfähigkeiten. Diskursivierungen unfreier Bewusstseinszustände seit dem 18. Jahrhundert*, Frankfurt, Peter Lang, 1998, 107–132.

Grossenbach, Karoline, 'Fromme Quergänger in der Psychiatrie des Vormärz: Religionswahnsinn bei Patienten des großherzoglich-hessischen Hospitals Hofheim', *WerkstattGeschichte*, vol. 33, 2002, 5–21.

Guillemain, Hervé, *Diriger les consciences, guérir les âmes. Une histoire comparée des pratiques thérapeutiques et religieuses, 1830–1939*, Paris, La Découverte, 2006a.

Guillemain, Hervé, 'Médecine Et religion au XIXe aiècle. Le traitement moral de la folie dans les asiles de l'ordre de Saint-Jean de Dieu (1830–1860)', *Le mouvement social*, vol. 215, 2006b, 35–49.

Guthmüller, Marie, 'Der Traum im psychopathologischen Fallbericht des 19. Jahrhunderts: Maurice Macario, Alfred Maury, Sante de Sanctis', in Rudolf Behrens, Nicole Bischoff, and Carsten Zelle (eds.), *Der ärztliche Fallbericht. Epistemische Grundlagen und textuelle Strukturen dargestellter Beobachtung*, Wiesbaden, Harrassowitz, 2012, 171–200.

Hackler, Ruben and Katherina Kinzel (eds.), *Paradigmatische Fälle. Konstruktion, Narration und Verallgemeinerung von Fall-Wissen in den Geistes-und Sozialwissenschaften*, Basel, Schwabe, 2016.

Hagner, Michael, *Der Hauslehrer – Die Geschichte eines Kriminalfalls. Erziehung, Sexualität und Medien um 1900*, Frankfurt, Suhrkamp, 2010.

Hannaway, Caroline and Anne La Berge (eds.), *Constructing Paris Medicine*, Amsterdam, Rodopi, 1998.

Hardtke, Thomas, *Wahn-Glaube-Fiktion. Die Pathologie devianter Religiosität im medizinischen, religiösen und literarischen Diskurs seit 1800*, Freie Universität Berlin, 2016.

Heinz, Daniel, 'MÜNTZER (Münzer)', in Traugott Bautz (ed.), *Biographisch-Bibliographisches Kirchenlexikon*, vol. 6, Herzberg, Traugott Bautz, 1993, 329–345.

Henson, Louise et al., 'Introduction', in Louise Henson et al. (eds.), *Culture and Science in the Nineteenth-Century Media*, Aldershot, Ashgate, 2005, XVII–XXV.

Herrmann, Klaus, Andrea Levèvre, and Raymond Wolff (eds.), *Neuköllner Pitaval. Wahre Kriminalgeschichten aus Berlin*, Hamburg, Rotbuch, 1994.

Hess, Volker, 'Formalisierte Beobachtung. Die Genese der modernen Krankenakte am Beispiel der Berliner und Pariser Medizin (1725–1830)', *Medizinhistorisches Journal*, vol. 45, 2010, 293–340.

Hess, Volker, 'Observatio und Casus: Status und Funktion der medizinischen Fallgeschichte', in Susanne Düwell and Nicolas Pethes (eds.), *Fall – Fallgeschichte – Fallstudie. Theorie und Geschichte einer Wissensform,* Frankfurt, campus, 2014, 34–59.

Hess, V. and J.A. Mendelsohn, 'Case and Series: Medical Knowledge and Paper Technology, 1600-1900', *History of Science*, vol. 48, 2010, 287–314.

Heyd, Michael, *'Be Sober and Reasonable': The Critique of Enthusiasm in the Seventeenth and Early Eighteenth Centuries*, Leiden, Brill, 1995.

Hinks, John, Catherine Armstrong, and Matthew Day (eds.), *Periodicals and Publishers. The Newspaper and Journal Trade 1740–1914*, London, British Library, 2009.

Höcker, Arne, Jeannie Moser, and Philippe Weber (eds.), *Wissen. Erzählen. Narrative der Humanwissenschaften*, Bielefeld, transcript, 2006.

Holländer, Eugen, *Wunder, Wundergeburt und Wundergestalt in Einblattdrucken des 15.-18. Jahrhunderts*, Stuttgart, Enke, 1922.

Huneman, Philippe, 'From a Religious view of Madness to Religious Mania: The Encyclopédie, Pinel, Esquirol', *History of Psychiatry*, vol. 28, no. 2, 2017, 147–165.

Hunt, Lynn, 'Introduction: Obscenity and the Origins of Modernity, 1500–1800', in Lynn Hunt (ed.), *The Invention of Pornography. Obscenity and the Origins of Modernity, 1500–1800*, New York, Zone Books, 1993, 9–45.

Hurwitz, Brian, 'Narrative Constructs in Modern Clinical Case Reporting', *Studies in History and Philosophy of Science* vol. 62, 2017, 65–73.

Infelise, Mario, 'Venezia e la circolazione delle informazioni: tra censura e controllo', *Archivio veneto*, vol. 161, 2003, 231–245.

Jacyna, L. Stephen, 'Pious Pathology. J.L. Alibert's Iconography of Disease', in Caroline Hannaway and Anne Elizabeth Fowler La Berge (eds.), *Constructing Paris Medicine*, Amsterdam and Atlanta, Rodopi, 1998, 185–219.

Jolles, André, *Einfache Formen: Legende, Sage, Mythe, Rätsel, Spruch, Kasus, Memorabile, Märchen, Witz*, Tübingen, Max Niemeyer Verlag, 1968.

Jones, Caroline A. and Peter Galison, 'Introduction. Picturing Science, Producing Art', in Caroline A. Jones and Peter Galison (eds.), *Picturing Science and Producing Art*, New York and London, Routledge, 1998, 1–26.

Jordan, John O., and Robert L Patten. (eds.), *Literature in the Marketplace. Nineteenth-Century British Publishing and Reading Practices*, Cambridge, UK, Cambridge University Press, 1995.

Jouhaud, Christian and Alain Viala (eds.), *De la publication entre renaissance et lumières*, Paris, Fayard, 2002.

Kaufmann, Doris, *Aufklärung, bürgerliche Selbsterfahrung und die 'Erfindung' der Psychiatrie in Deutschland, 1770–1850*, Göttingen, Vandenhoeck & Ruprecht, 1995.

Kaufmann, Doris, 'Wahnsinn und Geschlecht. Eine erfahrungsseelenkundliche Fallgeschichte aus der Entstehungszeit der bürgerlichen Gesellschaft in Deutschland', in Christiane Eifert et al. (eds.), *Was sind Frauen? Was sind Männer? Geschlechterkonstruktionen im historischen Wandel*, Frankfurt, Suhrkamp, 1996, 176–195.

Keel, Othmar, *L'avènement de la médecine clinique moderne en Europe 1750–1815*, Montreal, Presses de l'Université de Montréal, 2001.

Keil, Geert, Lara Keuck, and Rico Hauswald (eds.), *Vagueness in Psychiatry*, Oxford, Oxford University Press, 2017.

Kennaway, James and Jonathan Andrews, '"The Grand Organ of Sympathy": "Fashionable" Stomach Complaints and the Mind in Britain, 1700–1850', *Social History of Medicine*, https://academic.oup.com/shm/article-abstract/doi/10.1093/shm/hkx055/4080244/The-Grand-Organ-of-Sympathy-Fashionable-Stomach?redirectedFrom=fulltext, (accessed 6 October 2017).

Kennedy, Meegan, *Revising the Clinic: Vision and Representation in Victorian Medical Narrative and the Novel*, Columus: Ohio State University Press, 2010.

Kertzer, David I., 'Religion and Society, 1789–1892', in John A. Davis (ed.), *Italy in the Nineteenth Century*, Oxford, Oxford University Press, 2000, 181–205.

King, Andrew and John Plunkett (eds.), *Victorian Print Media. A Reader*, Oxford, Oxford University Press, 2005.

Klein, Lawrence E. and Anthony J La Vopa., 'Introduction', in Lawrence E. Klein and Anthony J. La Vopa (eds.), *Enthusiasm and Enlightenment in Europe, 1650–1850*, San Marino, CA, Huntington Library, 1998, 1–6.

Košenina, Alexander, 'Fallgeschichten. Von der Dokumentation zur Fiktion', *Zeitschrift für Germanistik. Neue Folge*, vol. 19, no. 2, 2009, 283–287.

Košenina, Alexander, *Literarische Anthropologie. Die Neuentdeckung des Menschen*, Berlin, Walter de Gruyter, 2008.

Košenina, Alexander, 'Recht-gefällig. Frühneuzeitliche Verbrechensdarstellung zwischen Dokumentation und Unterhaltung', *Zeitschrift für Germanistik Neue Folge*, vol. 15, no. 1, 2005, 28–47.

Košenina, Alexander, 'Schiller und die Tradition der (kriminal)psychologischen Fallgeschichte bei Goethe, Meißner, Moritz und Spieß', in Alice Stašková (ed.), *Friedrich Schiller und Europa: Ästhetik, Politik, Geschichte*, Heidelberg, Winter, 2007a, 119–139.

Košenina, Alexander, 'Von Bedlam nach Steinhof. Irrenhausbesuche in der Frühen Neuzeit und Moderne', *Zeitschrift Für Germanistik Neue Folge*, vol. 17, 2007b, 322–339.

Krause, Marcus, *Infame Menschen: Zur Epistemologie literarischer Fallgeschichten 1774–1816*, Berlin, Kadmos Kulturverlag, 2017.

Kutzer, Michael, 'Liebeskranke Magd, tobsüchtiger Mönch, schwermütiger Handelsherr: "Psychiatrie" in den Observationes und Curationes des niederländischen "Hippokrates" Pieter van Foreest (1522–1592)', *Medizinhistorisches Journal*, vol. 30, no. 3, 1995, 245–273.

Langewiesche, Dieter, 'Nation', 'Nationalismus', 'Nationalstaat' in der europäischen Geschichte seit dem Mittelalter – Versuch einer Bilanz, http://www.db-thueringen .de/servlets/DerivateServlet/Derivate-1344/langewiesche.pdf, at 68 (accessed 4 June 2018).

Langford, Paul, *Englishness Identified. Manners and Character 1650–1850*, Oxford, Oxford University Press, 2000.

Ledebuhr, Sophie, 'Schreiben und Beschreiben. Zur epistemischen Funktion von psychiatrischen Krankenakten, ihrer Archivierung und deren Übersetzung in Fallgeschichten', *Berichte zur Wissenschaftsgeschichte*, vol. 34, no. 2, 2011, 102–124.

Lepenies, Wolf, *Das Ende der Naturgeschichte. Wandel kultureller Selbstverständlichkeiten in den Wissenschaften des 18. und 19. Jahrhunderts*, Frankfurt, Carl Hanser, 1978.

Lerner, Barron H., *When Illness Goes Public. Celebrity Patients and How We Look at Medicine*, Baltimore, Johns Hopkins University Press, 2008.

Lesky, Erna, 'The Development of Bedside Teaching at the Vienna Medical School from Scholastic Times to Special Clinics', in Charles Donald O'Malley (ed.), *The History of Medical Education: An International Symposium*, Berkeley, University of California Press, 1970, 217–234.

Leventhal, Robert, 'Der Fall des Falls: Neuere Forschung zur Geschichte und Poetik der Fallerzählung im 18. Jahrhundert', *Das Achtzehnte Jahrhundert*, vol. 41, no. 1, 2017, 93–102.

Lind, Vera, *Selbstmord in der frühen Neuzeit. Diskurs, Lebenswelt und kultureller Wandel*, Göttingen, Vandenhoeck & Ruprecht, 1999.

Lorenz, Maren, '"Er ließe doch nicht eher nach biß er was angefangen". Zu den Anfängen gerichtspsychiatrischer Gutachtung im 18. Jahrhundert', in Richard van Dülmen, Erhard Chvojka, and Vera Jung (eds.), *Neue Blicke. Historische Anthropologie in der Praxis*, Cologne, Böhlau, 1997, 200–222.

Lyons, Martyn, *Le triomphe du livre. Une histoire sociologique de la lecture dans la France du XIXe siècle*, Paris, Promodis, 1987.

Lyons, Martyn, *Readers and Society in Nineteenth-Century France. Workers, Women, Peasants*, Basingstoke, Palgrave, 2001.

Lyons, Martyn, *Reading Culture and Writing Practice in Nineteenth-Century France*, Toronto, University of Toronto Press, 2008.

Maccagni, Carlo, 'Francesco Aglietti e il suo tempo', in Istituto Veneto di Scienze Lettere ed Arti (ed.), *Le scienze mediche nel veneto dell'ottocento*, Venice, Istituto Veneto di Scienze Lettere ed Arti, 1990, 155–169.

MacDonald, Michael, 'The Medicalization of Suicide in England: Laymen, Physicians, and Cultural Change, 1500–1870', *The Milbank Quarterly*, vol. 67, Supplement 1, *Framing Disease: The Creation and Negotiation of Explanatory Schemes*, 1989, 69–91.

MacDonald, Michael and Terence R Murphy., *Sleepless Souls: Suicide in Early Modern England*, Oxford and New York, Clarendon, 1990.

Macfarlane, Robert, *Original Copy. Plagiarism and Originality in Nineteenth-Century Literature*, Oxford, Oxford University Press, 2007.

Maclean, Ian, 'The Medical Republic of Letters before the Thirty Years War', *Intellectual History Review*, vol. 18, 2008, 15–30.

Maggiolo, Attilio, *I soci dell'academia pataviana dalla sua fondazione (1599)*, Padua, Accademia Padavina di scienze, lettere, ed arti, 1983.

Maire, Catherine-Laurence, *Les convulsionnaires de Saint-Medard. Miracles, convulsions et propheties à Paris au XVIIIe siècle*, Paris, Gallimard, 1985.

Mandressi, Rafael, 'Le passé, l'enseignement, la science: Félix Vicq d'Azyr et l'histoire de la médecine au XVIIIe siècle', *Medicina nei secoli. Arte e scienza*, vol. 20, no. 1, 2008, 183–212.

Mariani-Costantini, Renato and Aldo Mariani-Costantini, 'An Outline of the History of Pellagra in Italy', *Journal of Anthropological Sciences*, vol. 85, 2007, 163–171.

Markschies, Christoph, *Origenes und sein Erbe. Gesammelte Studien*, Berlin, Walter de Gruyter, 2007.

Marneros, Andreas and Frank Pillmann (eds.), *Das Wort Psychiatrie ... wurde in Halle geboren: von den Anfängen der deutschen Psychiatrie*, Stuttgart, Schattauer, 2005.

Martin, Henri-Jean and Roger Chartier (eds.), *Le temps des éditeurs. Du romantisme à la belle époque*, Paris, Promodis, 1985.

Martschukat, Jürgen, 'Von Seelenkrankheiten und Gewaltverbrechen im frühen 19. Jahrhundert', in Richard van Dülmen, Erhard Chvojka, and Vera Jung (eds.), *Neue Blicke. Historische Anthropologie in der Praxis*, Cologne, Böhlau, 1997, 223–247.

Marx, Julius, *Die Österreichische Zensur im Vormärz*, Vienna, Verlag für Geschichte und Politik, 1959.

Meißner, August Gottlieb, *Ausgewählte Kriminalgeschichten. Mit einem Nachwort von Alexander Košenina*, St. Ingbert, Röhrig, 2003.

Mendelsohn, J. Andrew, 'The World on a Page. Making a General Observation in the Eighteenth Century', in Lorraine Daston and Elizabeth Lunbeck (eds.), *Histories of Scientific Observation*, Chicago, University of Chicago Press, 2001, 396–420.

Minois, Georges, *History of Suicide: Voluntary Death in Western Culture*, trans. L.G. Cochrane, Baltimore, Johns Hopkins University Press, 2001.

Mocek, Reinhard, *Johann Christian Reil (1759–1813). Das Problem des Übergangs von der Spätaufklärung zur Romantik in Biologie und Medizin in Deutschland*, Frankfurt, Peter Lang, 1995.

Morgan, Mary S., 'Introduction. Narrative Science and Narrative Knowing. Introduction to Special Issue on Narrative Science', *Studies in History and Philosophy of Science*, vol. 62, 2017, 1–5.

Moschini, Giannantonio, *Della letteratura veneziana del secolo XVIII fino ai giorni nostri*, vol. 3, Venice, Dalla Stamperia Palese, 1806.

Müchler, Karl Friedrich, *Kriminalgeschichten. Aus gerichtlichen Akten gezogen (1792). Mit einem Nachwort herausgegeben von Alexander Košenina*, Hannover, Wehrhahn, 2011.

Müller, Irmgard et al., 'Protokolle des Unsichtbaren: Visa reperta in der gerichtsmedizinischen Praxis des 18. und 19. Jahrhunderts', in Rudolf Behrens, Nicole Bischoff, and Carsten Zelle (eds.), *Der ärztliche Fallbericht. Epistemische Grundlagen und textuelle Strukturen dargestellter Beobachtung*, Wiesbaden, Harrassowitz, 2012, 36–62.

Murat, Laure, *L'homme qui se prenait pour Napoléon: Pour une histoire politique de la folie*, Paris, Gallimard, 2011.

Muri, Paolo, 'E Mattio sclese di salire sulla croce', *La Repubblica*, 9 June 1992, http://ricerca.repubblica.it/repubblica/archivio/repubblica/1992/06/09/mattio-scelse-di-salire-sulla-croce.html, (accessed 1 August 2017).

Neuhaus, Klaus, *Der Wundenmann: Tradition und Struktur einer Abbildungsart in der medizinischen Literatur,* Münster, Diss. med., 1981.

Nicolas, Serge, 'Les annales médico-psychologiques. Abrégé d'histoire sur la fondation de la première revue française de psychiatrie', *Université Paris Descartes, BIU Santé*, [website], 2006, http://www.biusante.parisdescartes.fr/histoire/medica/annalesmedicopsychologiques.php, (accessed 18 April 2012).

Niehaus, Michael and Hans-Walter Schmidt-Hannisa, 'Einleitung', in Michael Niehaus and Hans-Walter Schmidt-Hannisa (eds.), *Unzurechnungsfähigkeiten. Diskursivierungen unfreier Bewusstseinszustände seit dem 18. Jahrhundert*, Frankfurt, Peter Lang, 1998, 7–13.

Nolte, Karen, 'Vom Verschwinden der Laienperspektive aus der Krankengeschichte: Medizinische Fallberichte im 19. Jahrhundert', in Sibylle Brändli, Barbara Lüthi, and Gregor Spuhler (eds.), *Zum Fall machen, zum Fall werden. Wissensproduktion und Patientenerfahrung in Medizin und Psychiatrie des 19. und 20. Jahrhunderts*, Frankfurt, campus, 2009, 33–61.

Nosenghi, Gianna, *Il grande libro dei misteri di Venezia risolti ed irrisolti*, Rome, Newton Compton Editori, 2010.

Odier, Louis, *Les honoraires médicaux et autres mémoires d'éthique médicale*, Paris, Classiques Garnier, 2011.

Pagel, Julius, 'Schlegel, Julius Heinrich Gottlieb', in Historische Kommission bei der Bayerischen Akademie der Wissenschaften (ed.), *Allgemeine Deutsche Biographie*, vol. 31, Munich, Duncker & Humblot, 1890, 389.

Pantin, Isabelle, 'The Role of Translations in European Scientific Exchanges in the Sixteenth and Seventeenth centuries', in Peter Burke and Ronnie Po-Chia Hsia (eds.),

Cultural Translation in Early Modern Europe, Cambridge, UK, Cambridge University Press, 2007, 163–179.

Passeron, Jean-Claude and Jacques Revel, 'Penser par cas. Raisonner à partir des singularités', in Jean-Claude Passeron and Jacques Revel (eds.), *Penser par cas*, Paris, EHESS, 2005, 9–44.

Pelizza, Andrea, 'Da "alberghi informi di ammalati" a "fortunati nosocomiali ritiri". Gli ospedali maggiori veneziani tra la fine della repubblica veneta e le riforme italiche', *Studi veneziani*, vol. 60, 2010, 415–486.

Pethes, Nicolas, *Literarische Fallgeschichten. Zur Poetik einer epistemischen Schreibweise*, Konstanz, Konstanz University Press, 2016.

Pethes, Nicolas, 'Telling Cases: Writing against Genre in Medicine and Literature', *Literature and Medicine*, vol. 32, no. 1, 2014, 24–45.

Pethes, Nicolas, 'Vom Einzelfall zur Menschheit. Die Fallgeschichte als Medium der Wissenpopularisierung in Recht, Medizin und Literatur', in Gereon Blaseio, Hedwig Pompe, and Jens Ruchatz (eds.), *Popularisierung und Popularität*, Cologne, Dumont, 2005, 63–92.

Pethes, Nicolas, *Zöglinge der Natur. Der literarische Menschenversuch des 18. Jahrhunderts*, Göttingen, Wallstein, 2007.

Pethes, Nicolas and Sandra Richter (eds.), *Medizinische Schreibweisen. Ausdifferenzierung und Transfer zwischen Medizin und Literatur (1600–1900)*. Tübingen, Max Niemeyer Verlag, 2008.

Pocock, John G.A., 'Enthusiasm. The Antiself of Enlightenment', in Lawrence E. Klein and Anthony J. La Vopa (eds.), *Enthusiasm and Enlightenment in Europe, 1650–1850*, San Marino, CA, Huntington Library, 1998, 7–28.

Pohlig, Matthias, 'Individuum und Sattelzeit oder: Napoleon und der Triumph des Willens', in C. Jaser, U. Lotz-Heumann, and M. Pohlig (eds.), *Alteuropa – Vormoderne – Neue Zeit. Epochen und Dynamiken der europäischen Geschichte (1200–1800)*, Berlin, Duncker & Humblot, 2012, 265–282.

Pointon, Marcia, *Hanging the Head: Portraiture and Social Formation in Eighteenth-Century England*, New Haven, Yale University Press, 1993.

Polaschegg, Andrea and Steffen Martus (eds.), *Das Buch der Bücher – gelesen. Lesarten der Bibel in den Wissenschaften und Künsten*, Bern, Lang, 2006.

Polaschegg, Andrea and Daniel Weidner (eds.), *Das Buch in den Büchern. Wechselwirkungen von Bibel und Literatur*, Munich, Wilhelm Fink, 2012.

Pomata, Gianna, 'A Word of the Empirics: The Ancient Concept of Observation and its Recovery in Early Modern Medicine', *Annals of Science*, vol. 68, no. 1, 2011a, 1–25.

Pomata, Gianna, '"Observatio" ovvero "Historia". Note su empirismo e storia in età moderna', *Quaderni storici*, no. 91, 1996, 175–198.

Pomata, Gianna, 'Observation Rising: Birth of an Epistemic Genre, ca. 1500–1650', in Lorraine Daston and Elizabeth Lunbeck (eds.), *Histories of Scientific Observation*, Chicago, University of Chicago Press, 2011b, 45–80.

Pomata, Gianna, '*Praxis Historialis*: The Uses of *Historia* in Early Modern Medicine', Gianna Pomata and Nancy G. Siraisi (eds.), *Empiricism and Erudition in Early Modern Europe*, Cambridge, MA and London, MIT Press, 2005, 105–146.

Pomata, Gianna, 'Sharing Cases: The Observationes in Early Modern Medicine', *Early Science and Medicine*, vol. 15, no. 3, 2010, 193–236.

Pomata, Gianna, 'The Medical Case Narrative: Distant Reading of an Epistemic Genre', *Literature and Medicine*, vol. 32, no. 1, 2014, 1–23.

Pomata, Gianna, 'The Recipe and the Case: Epistemic Genres and the Dynamics of Cognitive Practices', in Kaspar von Greyerz, Silvia Flurbacher, and Philipp Senn (eds.), *Wissenschaftsgeschichte und Geschichte des Wissens im Dialog – Connecting Science and Knowledge*, Göttingen, V&R unipress, 2013, 131–154.

Porter, Roy, 'The Eighteenth Century', in Lawrence I. Conrad et al. (eds.), *The Western Medical Tradition 800 BC to AD 1800*, Cambridge, UK, Cambridge University Press, 1995, 371–476.

Porter, Roy, 'The Rise of Medical Journalism in Britain to 1800', in William F. Bynum, Stephen Lock, and Roy Porter (eds.), *Medical Journals and Medical Knowledge. Historical Essays*, London, Routledge, 1992, 6–28.

Pott, Sandra, *Medizin, Medizinethik und schöne Literatur. Studien zu Säkularisierungsvorgängen vom 17. bis zum frühen 19. Jahrhundert*, Berlin, Walter de Gruyter, 2002.

Priani, E., 'Shrouded in a Dark Fog': Comparison of the Diagnosis of Pellagra in Venice and General Paralysis of the Insane in the United Kingdom, 1840–1900, *History of Psychiatry*, vol. 28, no. 2, 2017, 166–181.

Puttenham, George et al. (eds.), *The Art of English Poesy*, Ithaca, Cornell University Press, 2007.

Raines, Dorit (ed.), *Anatomia di una biblioteca: cinquanta volumi di medicina dalla collezione storica dell'ateneo veneto*, Venice, Ateneo Veneto, 2007.

Raymond, Joad and Noah Moxham, 'New Networks in Early Modern Europe', in Joad Raymond and Noah Moxham (eds.), *News Networks in Early Modern Europe*, Leiden and Boston, Brill, 2016, 1–18.

Retzlaff, Stefanie, *Observieren und Aufschreiben: Zur Poetologie medizinischer Fallgeschichten (1700–1765)*, Munich, Wilhelm Fink, 2018.

Riall, Lucy, 'Martyr Cults in Nineteenth-Century Italy', *Journal of Modern History*, vol. 82, no. 2, 2010, 255–287.

Rieder, Philip Alexander, 'La médecine pratique: Une activité heuristique à la fin du 18e siècle?', *Dix-huitième siècle*, vol. 47, 2015, 135–148.

Rimmele, Marius, 'Geordnete Unordnung. Zur Bedeutungsstiftung im Zusammenhang der Arma Christi', in David Ganz and Felix Pürlemann (eds.), *Das Bild im Plural. Mehrteilige Bildformen zwischen Mittelalter und Gegenwart*, Berlin, Reimer, 2010, 219–242.

Roe, Daphne A., *A Plague of Corn. The Social History of Pellagra*, Ithaca, Cornell University Press, 1973.

Rosada, Bruno, 'Letteratura e vita culturale a Venezia nella prima metà dell'ottocento', in Michele Gottardi (ed.), *Venezia suddita (1798–1866)*, Venice, Marsilio, 1999, 107–126.

Rosenfeld, Hellmut, 'Jolles, André' in *Neue Deutsche Biographie*, vol. 10, 1974, 586 f., https://www.deutsche-biographie.de/pnd122521102.html#ndbcontent (accessed 4 June 2018).

Rousseau, George S., 'Science and the Discovery of the Imagination in Enlightened England', *Eighteenth Century Studies*, vol. 3, no. 1, 1969, 108–135.

Rousseau, George S., '"Stung into Action...": Medicine, Professionalism, and the News', in Joad Raymond (ed.), *News, Newspapers, and Society in Early Modern Britain*, London, Frank Cass and Company, 1999, 176–205.

Ruggiero, Guido, 'Excusable Murder: Insanity and Reason in Early Renaissance Venice', *Journal of Social History*, vol. 16, no. 1, 1982, 109–119.

Rylance, Rick, '"The Disturbing Anarchy of Investigation": Psychological Debate and the Victorian Periodical', in Louise Henson et al. (eds.), *Culture and Science in the Nineteenth-Century Media*, London, British Library, 2009, 239–250.

Rylance, Rick, 'The Theatre and the Granary: Observations on Nineteenth-Century Medical Narratives', *Literature and Medicine*, vol. 25, no. 2, 2006, 255–276.

Saccardo, Rosanna, *La tampa periodica veneziana fino alla caduta della repubblica*, Padua, Tipografia del seminario, 1942.

Saurer, Edith, 'Religiöse Praxis und Sinnesverwirrung. Kommentare zur religiösen Melancholiediskussion', in Richard van Dülmen (ed.), *Dynamik der Tradition. Studien zur historischen Kulturforschung IV*, Frankfurt, Fischer, 1992, 213–239.

Saville, Julia S., 'Eccentricity as Englishness in David Copperfield', *Studies in English Literature 1500–1900*, vol. 42, no. 4, 2002, 781–797.

Savoia, Daniela, 'Dalla parte di Alfredo Comandini. Note per una biografia', in Giuseppina Benassati and Daniela Savoia. (eds.), *L'Italia nei cento anni. Libri e stampe della biblioteca di Alfredo Comandini,* Bologna, grafis, 1998, 1–9.

Scarabello, Giovanni and Veronica Gusso, *Processo al moro. Razzismo, follia, amore e morte*, Rome, Jouvence, 2000.

Schär, Markus, *Seelennöte der Untertanen. Selbstmord, Melancholie und Religion im Alten Zürich, 1500–1800*, Zurich, Chronos, 1985.

Schings, Hans Jürgen, *Melancholie und Aufklärung. Melancholiker und ihre Kritik in Erfahrungsseelenkunde und Literatur des 18. Jahrhunderts*, Stuttgart, Metzler, 1977.

Schipperges, Heinrich, 'Ideler, Karl Wilhelm', in Historische Kommission bei der Bayerischen Akademie der Wissenschaften (ed.), *Neue Deutsche Biographie*, vol. 10, Berlin, Duncker & Humblot, 1974, 116–118.

Schöne, Albrecht, *Säkularisation als sprachbildende Kraft. Studien zur Dichtung deutscher Pfarrersöhne,* Göttingen, Vandenhoeck & Ruprecht, 1958.

Schott, Heinz and Reiner Tölle, *Geschichte der Psychiatrie. Krankheitslehren, Irrwege, Behandlungsformen*, Munich, C.H. Beck, 2006.

Schreiner, Julia, *Jenseits vom Glück. Suizid, Melancholie und Hypochondrie in deutschsprachigen Texten des späten 18. Jahrhunderts*, Munich, R. Oldenbourg, 2003.

Schwarz, Angela, 'Bilden, Überzeugen, Unterhalten: Wissenschaftspopularisierung und Wissenskultur im 19. Jahrhundert', in Carsten Kretschmann (ed.), *Wissenspopularisierung. Konzepte der Wissensverbreitung im Wandel*, Berlin, Akademie Verlag, 2003, 221–234.

Seifert, Arno, *Cognitio Historica: Die Geschichte als Namengeberin der frühneuzeitlichen Empirie*, Berlin, Duncker & Humblot, 1976.

Shepherd, Michael, 'Psychiatric Journals and the Evolution of Psychological Medicine', in William F. Bynum, Stephen Lock, and Roy Porter (eds.), *Medical Journals and Medical Knowledge. Historical Essays*, London and New York, Routledge, 1992, 188–206.

Shinn, Terry and Richard Whitley (eds.), *Expository Science: Forms and Functions of Popularisation*, Dordrecht, Boston, and Lancaster, D. Reidel, 1985.

Siefert, Helmut, 'Emil Kraepelin', in Historische Kommission bei der Bayerischen Akademie der Wissenschaften (ed.), *Neue Deutsche Biographie*, vol. 12, Berlin, Duncker & Humblot, 1980, 639–640.

Signori, Gabriela (ed.), *Trauer, Verzweiflung und Anfechtung. Selbstmord und Selbstmordversuche in mittelalterlichen und frühneuzeitlichen Gesellschaften*, Tübingen, edition diskord, 1994.

Siraisi, Nancy G., *Communities of Learned Experience. Epistolary Medicine in the Renaissance*, Baltimore, Johns Hopkins University Press, 2012.

Siraisi, Nancy G., *History, Medicine and the Traditions of Renaissance Learning*, Ann Arbor, University of Michigan Press, 2007.

Soeur, Laurent, 'La place de la religion catholique dans les asiles d'aliénés au XIXe siècle', *Revue historique*, vol. 289, no. 1, 1993, 141–148.

Stammberger, Birgit, *Monster und Freaks. Eine Wissensgeschichte außergewöhnlicher Körper im 19. Jahrhundert*, Bielefeld, transcript, 2011.

Stefanutti, Ugo, *Documentazioni cronologiche per la storia della medicina, chirurgia e farmacia in Venezia*, Venice, Ongania, 1961.

Steinke, Hubert, *Irritating Experiments. Haller's Concept and the European Controversy on Irritability and Sensibility, 1750–90*, Amsterdam and New York, Rodopi, 2005.

Steinke, Hubert and Martin Stuber, 'Medical Correspondence in Early Modern Europe. An Introduction', *Gesnerus*, vol. 61, 2004, 139–160.

Steinlechner, Gisela, *Fallgeschichten. Krafft-Ebing, Panizza, Freud, Tausk*, Vienna, WUV Universitätsverlag, 1995.

Stengers, Jan and Anne van Neck (eds.), *Storia della masturbazione*, Bologna, Odoya, 2009.

Stockhorst, Stephanie (ed.), *Cultural Transfer through Translation. The Circulation of Enlightened Thought in Enlightened Europe by means of Translation*, Amsterdam and New York, Rodopi, 2010.

Stolberg, Michael, 'Formen und Funktionen medizinischer Fallberichte in der Frühen Neuzeit (1500–1800)', in Johannes Süßmann, Susanne Scholz, and Gisela Engel (eds.), *Fallstudien. Theorie – Geschichte – Methode*, Berlin, trafo, 2007, 81–95.

The New International Version of the Bible, http://www.biblegateway.com/ passage/?search=Matthew%207&version=NIV, (accessed 17 July 2017).

Tromp, Marlene (ed.), *Victorian Freaks. The Social Context of Freakery in Britain*, Columbus, OH, The Ohio State University Press, 2008.

Vanzan Marchini, Nelli-Elena, *Dalla scienza medica alla pratica dei corpi. Fonti e manoscritti per la storia della sanità*, Venice, Neri Pozza, 1993.

Vanzan Marchini, Nelli-Elena, 'Diritto e follia a Venezia nel XVI secolo', *Sanità, scienza e storia*, vol. 1, 1984, 49–76.

Vanzan Marchini, Nelli-Elena, *La follia, una nave, una citta. Storia di pazzi e di pazzie a Venezia nel '700*, Mira, Brenctani editrice, 1981.

Vanzan Marchini, Nelli-Elena, *La memoria della salute. Venezia e il suo ospedale dal XVI al XX secolo*, Venice, Arsenale, 1985.

Vanzan Marchini, Nelli-Elena, 'La politica sanitaria e i medici riformatori', in Nelli-Elena Vanzan Marchini (ed.), *I mali e i rimedi della serenissima*, Venice, Neri Pozza, 1995a, 157–194.

Vanzan Marchini, Nelli-Elena (ed.), *Le leggi di sanità della repubblica di Venezia*, vol. 1, Venice, Neri Pozza, 1995b.

Vanzan, Nelli-Elena, *San Servolo e Venezia. Un' isola e la sua storia*, Venice, Caselle di Sommacampagna, 2004.

Vasset, Sophie, *Medicine and Narration in the Eighteenth Century*, Oxford, Oxford University Press, 2013.

Vasset, Sophie and Alexandre Wenger (eds.), *Raconter la maladie. Dix-huitième siècle n°47*, Paris, La Découverte, 2015.

Vogl, Joseph, 'Einleitung', in Joseph Vogl (ed.), *Poetologien des Wissens um 1800*, Munich, Wilhelm Fink, 1999, 7–16.

Von Krafft-Ebing, Richard, *Lehrbuch der Psychiatrie: auf klinischer Grundlage für praktische Ärzte und Studierende*, Saarbrücken, Verlag Dr. Müller, 2007.

Von Prantl, Carl, 'Hoffbauer, Johann Christoph', Historische Kommission bei der Bayerischen Akademie der Wissenschaften (ed.), *Allgemeine Deutsche Biographie*, vol. 12, Munich, Duncker & Humblot, 1880, 567–568.

Watt, Jeffrey R. (ed.), *From Sin to Insanity: Suicide in Early Modern Europe*, Ithaca, Cornell University Press, 2004.

Weaver, John C., *A Sadly Troubled History: The Meanings of Suicide in the Modern Age*, Montréal and Kingston, McGill-Queen's University Press, 2009.

Weber, Philippe, *Der Trieb zum Erzählen. Sexualpathologie und Homosexualität 1852–1914*, Bielefeld, transcript, 2008.

Weiner, Dora B., *The Citizen-Patient in Revolutionary and Imperial Paris*, Baltimore, Johns Hopkins University Press, 1993.

Weiner, Dora B. and M.J Sauter., 'The City of Paris and the Rise of Clinical Medicine', *Osiris, 2nd Series*, vol. 18, 2003, 23–42.

Wenger, Alexandre, 'From Medical Case to Narrative Fiction: Diderot's *La Religieuse*', *SVEC*, vol. 4, 2013, 17–30.

Werner, Michael, 'Les libraires comme intermédiaires culturels: remarques à propos du rôle des libraires allemands en France au XIXe siècle', in Frédéric Barbier, Sabine Juratic, and Dominique Varry (eds.), *L'Europe et le livre. Réseaux et pratiques du né-goce du librairie XVIe–XIXe siècles*, Paris, Klinksieck, 1996, 527–542.

Werner, Michael and Bénédicte Zimmermann, 'Penser l'histoire croisée: entre empirie et réflexivité', *Annales*, vol. 58, 2003, 7–36.

Werner, Michael and Bénédicte Zimmermann, 'Beyond Comparison. Histoire Croisée and the Challenge of Reflexivity', *History and Theory*, vol. 45, 2006, 30–50.

Wernli, Martina, 'Sammelrezension Fallgeschichten' H-Soz-Kult, 16 February 2017, www.hsozkult.de/publicationreview/id/rezbuecher-26171, (accessed 6 October 2017).

Wernli, Martina, *Schreiben am Rand: Die 'Bernische Kantonale Irrenanstalt Waldau' und ihre Narrative (1895–1936)*, Bielefeld, transcript, 2014.

Wesseling, Klaus-Gunther, 'WESSENBERG[-Ampringen], Ignaz Heinrich Karl Joseph Thaddäus Fidel Dismas Freiherr von, katholischer Aufklärungstheologe und Konstanzer Generalvikar', in Traugott Bautz (ed.), *Biographisch-Bibliographisches Kirchenlexikon*, vol. 13, Herzberg, Traugott Bautz, 1998, 976–988.

Willer, Stefan, 'Fallgeschichte', in Bettina von Jagow and Florian Steger (eds.), *Literatur und Medizin. Ein Lexikon*, Göttingen, Vandenhoeck & Ruprecht, 2005, 231–235.

Williams, Elizabeth A., 'Neuroses of the Stomach: Eating, Gender, and Psychopathology in French Medicine 1800–1870', *Isis*, vol. 98, no. 1, 2007, 54–79.

Wiltenburg, Joy, 'True Crime: The Origins of Modern Sensationalism', *American Historical Review*, vol. 109, 2004, 1377–1404.

Winnicott, Donald W., 'Physical and Emotional Disturbances in an Adolescent Girl', in Clare Winnicott, Ray Shephard, and Madelein Davis (eds.), *Psychoanalytic Explorations*, Cambridge MA, Harvard University Press, 1968, 369–374.

Wöbkemeyer, Rita, *Erzählte Krankheit. Medizinische und literarische Phantasien um 1800*, Stuttgart, Metzler, 1990.

Woloshyn, Tania, 'Le pays du soleil: The Art of Heliotherapy on the Côte d'Azur', *Social History of Medicine*, vol. 26, no. 1, 2013, 74–93.

Wright, David and John C. Weaver, 'Introduction', in John C. Weaver and David Wright (eds.), *Histories of Suicide. International Perspectives on Self-Destruction in the Modern World*, Toronto, University of Toronto Press, 2009, 3–18.

Wübben, Yvonne, *Büchners 'Lenz'. Geschichte eines Falls*, Konstanz, Konstanz University Press, 2016.

Wübben, Yvonne, 'Dementia praecox: Emil Kraepelins Lehrbuchfall', in Carsten Zelle and Ali Zein (eds.), *Casus. Von Hoffmanns Erzählungen bis Freuds Novellen. Eine Anthologie der Fachprosagattung 'Fallerzählung'*. Hannover, Wehrhahn, 2015, 207–213.

Wübben, Yvonne, 'Die kranke Stimme. Erzählinstanz und Figurenrede im Psychiatrie-Lehrbuch des 19. Jahrhunderts', in Rudolf Behrens, Nicole Bischoff, and Carsten Zelle (eds.), *Der ärztliche Fallbericht. Epistemische Grundlagen und textuelle Strukturen dargestellter Beobachtung*, Wiesbaden, Harrassowitz, 2012a, 151–170.

Wübben, Yvonne, 'Einleitung: Aufzeichnen in Pathologie, Psychiatrie und Literatur', in Yvonne Wübben and Carsten Zelle (eds.), *Krankheit schreiben. Aufzeichnungsverfahren in Medizin und Literatur*, Göttingen, Wallstein, 2013a, 13–19.

Wübben, Yvonne, 'Mikrotom der Klinik. Der Aufstieg des Lehrbuches in der Psychiatrie (um 1890)', in Yvonne Wübben and Carsten Zelle (eds.), *Krankheit schreiben. Aufzeichnungsverfahren in Medizin und Literatur*, Göttingen, Wallstein, 2013b, 107–133.

Wübben, Yvonne, 'Ordnen und Erzählen. Emil Kraepelins Beispielgeschichten', *Zeitschrift für Germanistik*, vol. 2, 2009, 381–395.

Wübben, Yvonne, *Verrückte Sprache: Psychiater und Dichter in der Anstalt des 19. Jahrhunderts*, Konstanz, Konstanz University Press, 2012b.

Wübben, Yvonne, 'Writing Cases and Casuistic Reasoning in Karl Philipp Moritz' Journal of Empirical Psychology', in *Early Science and Medicine*, vol. 18, 2013c, 471–486.

Wübben, Yvonne and Carsten Zelle (eds.), *Krankheit schreiben. Aufzeichnungsverfahren in Medizin und Literatur*, Göttingen, Wallstein, 2013.

Zampetti, Pietro, *Guida alle opere d'arte della scuola di S. Fantin*, Venice, Ateneo Veneto, 1973.

Zelle, Carsten, '"Die Geschichte bestehet in einer Erzählung". Poetik der medizinischen Fallerzählung bei Andreas Elias Büchner (1701–1769)', in Rudolf Behrens, Nicole Bischoff, and Carsten Zelle (eds.), *Der ärztliche Fallbericht. Epistemische Grundlagen und textuelle Strukturen dargestellter Beobachtung*, Wiesbaden, Harrassowitz, 2012, 301–316.

Zelle, Carsten, 'Einleitung', in Carsten Zelle and Ali Zein (eds.) *Casus. Von Hoffmanns Erzählungen zu Freuds Novellen. Eine Anthologie der Fachprosagattung "Fallerzählung"*, Hannover, Wehrhahn Verlag, 2015, 7–28.

Zorzi, Alvise, *Napoleone a Venezia*, Milan, Mondadori, 2010.

Zorzi, Alvise, *Österreichs Venedig. Das letzte Kapitel der Fremdherrschaft*, Hamburg, Claassen, 1990.

Zorzi, Alvise, *Venezia scomparsa*, Milan, Mondadori, 1972.

Printed in the United States
By Bookmasters